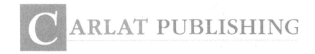

MEDICATION FACT BOOK
FOR PSYCHIATRIC PRACTICE

SIXTH EDITION

Talia Puzantian, PharmD, BCPP

Deputy Editor, *The Carlat Report* newsletters
Co-Author, *The Child Medication Fact Book for Psychiatric Practice*
Professor of Clinical Sciences, Keck Graduate Institute School of Pharmacy and Health Sciences,
Claremont, CA

Daniel J. Carlat, MD

Publisher, *The Carlat Report* newsletters and books
Associate Clinical Professor, Tufts University School of Medicine, Boston, MA

Published by Carlat Publishing, LLC
PO Box 626, Newburyport, MA 01950

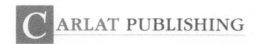
CARLAT PUBLISHING

Medication Fact Book
For Psychiatric Practice
SIXTH EDITION

Published by Carlat Publishing, LLC
PO Box 626, Newburyport, MA 01950

Publisher and Editor-in-Chief: Daniel J. Carlat, MD
Deputy Editor: Talia Puzantian, PharmD, BCPP
Executive Editor: Janice Jutras

This CME/CE activity is intended for psychiatrists, psychiatric nurses, psychologists, and other health care professionals with an interest in mental health. The Carlat CME Institute is accredited by the Accreditation Council for Continuing Medical Education to provide continuing medical education for physicians. Carlat CME Institute maintains responsibility for this program and its content. Carlat CME Institute designates this enduring material educational activity for a maximum of twelve (12) *AMA PRA Category 1 Credits*™. Physicians or psychologists should claim credit commensurate only with the extent of their participation in the activity. The American Board of Psychiatry and Neurology has reviewed the *Medication Fact Book for Psychiatric Practice* and has approved this program as part of a comprehensive Self-Assessment and CME Program, which is mandated by ABMS as a necessary component of maintenance of certification. CME tests must be taken online at www.thecarlatreport.com or http://thecarlatcmeinstitute.com/self-assessment (for ABPN SA course subscribers).

To order, visit www.thecarlatreport.com
or call (866) 348-9279

2 3 4 5 6 7 8 9 10

ISBN #:
Print - 978-1-7329522-8-7
eBook - 978-1-7329522-9-4

PRINTED IN THE UNITED STATES OF AMERICA

Table of Contents

Anxiolytic and Hypnotic Medications

Dementia Medications

LIST OF TABLES

LIST OF TREATMENT ALGORITHMS

Introduction

HOW TO USE THIS BOOK

Medication information is presented in three ways in this book:

- *Fact sheets.* In-depth information for select medications, somatic treatments, and side effects. There are 164 fact sheets in this book. The medication fact sheets don't cover all psychiatric medications, but we have included most of the commonly prescribed and newer medications.
- *Quick-scan medication tables.* These are most often located at the beginning of each therapeutic category and list the very basics: generic and brand names, available strengths, starting doses, and target doses. These tables contain most of the commonly prescribed psychiatric medications.
- *Treatment algorithms.* These quick-reference decision trees can serve as a memory aid and help in clinical decision making. They don't cover every medical nuance but serve as general overviews.

CHANGES AND ADDITIONS TO THE SIXTH EDITION

We've updated the medication fact sheets to reflect availability of newer strengths and formulations, as well as generics. The fact sheets also reflect new clinical data where available. We've expanded our coverage of many categories of medications, including the Side Effect Management chapter; included in this edition are 16 new fact sheets, five new tables, and eight appendices. We've also added a new treatment algorithm to this edition: treatment-resistant depression.

CATEGORIES OF MEDICATIONS

We did our best to categorize medications rationally. However, in some cases a medication can fall into more than one category. In such cases, we categorized the medication with the types of disorders for which it is most often used. If you're having trouble finding a medication in a particular chapter, look in the index to find its page number.

MORE ON THE MEDICATION FACT SHEETS

The goal of these fact sheets is to provide need-to-know information (on a single page) that can be easily and quickly absorbed during a busy day of seeing patients. Please refer to the *PDR (Physicians' Desk Reference)* when you need more in-depth information.

For the most part, each fact sheet contains the following information:

- *Drug names.* Each sheet lists both brand and generic names.
- *Generic availability.* **We include a [G] or (G) if a drug is available as a generic.**
- *Bottom line.* **We begin with a super-condensed summary, including our overall assessment of the drug's value in clinical practice. If you're in a rush, you can get the basics from this alone.**
- *FDA-approved indications.* Psychiatric indications are in bold.
- *Off-label uses.* We list the more common off-label uses, based on both the medical literature and our clinical experience. Just because we list a potential use does not imply that we endorse a medication as being particularly effective for that use. We are simply alerting you to the fact that there is some evidence for efficacy.
- *Dosage forms,* along with available strengths.
- *Dosage guidance.* We provide recommendations on how to dose medications; these are derived from a variety of sources, including package inserts, clinical trials, and common clinical practice. In other words, don't be surprised when our dosing instructions are at odds with what you find in the *PDR*. New to this edition, we have added specific advice on whether to dose certain meds in the morning or at night—a common question from patients.
- *Lab monitoring recommendations.* We include the usual routine monitoring measures for each medication. Of course, you may need to think beyond the "routine" if the clinical picture warrants it.
- *Cost information.* We obtained pricing information for a one-month supply of a common dosing regimen from the website GoodRx (www.goodrx.com), accessed in November 2021. These are the prices patients would have to pay if they had no insurance (GoodRx also offers coupons to purchase certain medications at reduced prices). Because of wide variations in price depending on the pharmacy, we list price categories rather than the price in dollars. The categories are:
  - $: Inexpensive (<$50/month)

- $$: Moderately expensive ($50–$100/month)
- $$$: Expensive ($100–$200/month)
- $$$$: Very expensive ($200–$500/month)
- $$$$$: Extremely expensive ($500/month)

This begs the question, what should you do with knowledge of retail pricing? After all, most patients have some type of insurance and are therefore not going to pay retail price, but rather a co-pay. Since there's no clear source for accurately predicting a co-pay, you can use the retail price as a clue. Meds that are inexpensive will likely require no co-pay, while the most expensive drugs will either require a very expensive co-pay or, more likely, will not be covered at all without an onerous pre-authorization process.

- *Side effects information.* We break down side effects into "most common" vs "rare but serious" side effects. We generally define "most common" side effects as those that occurred in at least 5% of patients in clinical trials, and that were at least double the rate of the placebo group. Such information is usually found in tables in the drugs' package inserts. We also used post-marketing clinical experience as a guide in determining which side effects were common enough to make the list.
- *Mechanism of action.* While the mechanism of action is not well established for most psychiatric drugs, we thought it would be important to report the mechanisms most commonly cited.
- *Pharmacokinetics,* with a focus on drug metabolism and/or half-life.
- *Drug interactions.*
- *Clinical pearls,* which typically comment on advantages or disadvantages of a medication in comparison to others in its therapeutic category, tips for dosing or for avoiding side effects, types of patients who seem to benefit the most, and so forth.
- *Fun facts.*

PREGNANCY AND LACTATION RISK INFORMATION

The risks and benefits of using psychiatric medications during pregnancy and breastfeeding are not as simple or clear as the previously used "ABCDX" letter categories might suggest. The FDA's Pregnancy and Lactation Labeling Rule (PLLR) removed these categories in favor of a more detailed narrative describing available risk data. Rather than putting this information in the fact sheets, we cover the topic separately in Appendix B.

OTHER USEFUL INFORMATION IN THE APPENDICES

- *Drug interactions in psychiatry.* While we do provide some information on drug interactions in the fact sheets, we also have a more extensive discussion of the topic, as well as tables of interactions for commonly prescribed drugs, the most common clinically significant drug interactions in psychiatry, and MAOI dietary and medication considerations, all in Appendix A.
- *Schedules of controlled substances.* Just in case you can't remember which drugs are in which DEA schedule or what each schedule means, we have you covered with a handy table in Appendix C.
- *Lab monitoring for psychiatric medications.* We've included a short easy-reference table listing medications with the recommended labs you should consider ordering, including serum level monitoring, in Appendix D.
- *Urine toxicology screening.* As substance use treatment becomes an ever more important aspect of psychiatric practice, we have a table explaining common urine drug test detection periods, as well as agents that may potentially cause false positives, in Appendix E.
- *Pharmacogenetic testing.* Although we're not big fans of routine pharmacogenetic testing, we provide some basic information on the topic in Appendix F.
- *Anticholinergic agents.* We provide a list of common medications that are highly anticholinergic in Appendix G. These can be particularly problematic in older patients.
- *Dosing of psychotropic medications in patients with hepatic or renal impairment.* Some psychiatric medications require more caution when treating patients with kidney or liver issues. You'll find our recommendations in Appendix H.

FINANCIAL DISCLOSURES

Dr. Puzantian and Dr. Carlat have disclosed that they have no relevant relationships or financial interests in any commercial company pertaining to the information provided in this book.

DISCLAIMER

The medication information in this book was formulated with a reasonable standard of care and in conformity with current professional standards in the field of psychiatry. Medication prescribing decisions are complex, and you should use these fact sheets as only one of many possible sources of medication information. This information is not a substitute for informed medical care. This book is intended for use by licensed professionals only.

If you have any comments or corrections, please let us know by writing to us at info@thecarlatreport.com or *The Carlat Psychiatry Report*, P.O. Box 626, Newburyport, MA 01950.

CONTENT UPDATES AND ADDITIONAL RESOURCES

From time to time we will update content in this book as new research or FDA approvals come out. You can access those updates online at www.thecarlatreport.com/mfb6e, which is also where you'll get access to the 12 CME post-test and the PDF/eBook versions of the book. You will also find additional resources including references and essential reading.

ADHD Medications

GENERAL PRESCRIBING TIPS

Generally, when you have a patient with ADHD symptoms, your first choice will be one of the psychostimulants, because these are usually more effective than the alternatives—atomoxetine, bupropion, clonidine, guanfacine, and viloxazine. Which psychostimulant will you choose? Here are some of the factors that will influence your decision:

1. *Long-acting vs short-acting.* Choosing between long- and short-acting stimulants is more art than science. Trial and error, combined with patient preference, will dictate the final regimen. Adults will often start with a long-acting agent so they can take a single dose in the morning and have it carry through their workday. Kids may do better with short-acting stimulants so that they will have an appetite when the medication wears off at lunch.

2. *Amphetamines vs methylphenidates.* More recent data have suggested that, based on safety and efficacy, methylphenidates are a better choice in kids and adolescents whereas amphetamine-class agents are better in adults. Generally, this is a Coke vs Pepsi decision—some people like one better than the other, and you can't predict their preference ahead of time. We recommend a methylphenidate over an amphetamine because amphetamines may have more side effects and are more likely to be abused or diverted but our algorithm starts with an amphetamine first given the efficacy data.

3. *Stimulants vs non-stimulants.* Stimulants are more effective than non-stimulants, so they will be your first-line choice for most patients. If you have a patient with a substance use disorder, start with atomoxetine. Some special clinical circumstances seem to naturally call for other options. For example, bupropion is helpful for ADHD symptoms, as well as for depression, tobacco use, and being overweight, so it might be a great choice for patients with a combination of these problems. Alpha agonists, such as guanfacine and clonidine, are helpful for both ADHD and insomnia, another potential two-fer, though these meds tend to be used more frequently for children.

4. *Fancy formulations.* Many new formulations of amphetamines and methylphenidates have been introduced over the last few years, including the use of various drug delivery technologies, enantiomers, prodrugs, salts, and dosage forms. While they may have been marketed to increase drug company profits, some of them may have clinical utility. Examples of potentially useful advances include Quillichew ER (a chewable long-acting methylphenidate), Cotempla XR-ODT (an ODT long-acting methylphenidate), Adzenys XR-ODT (an ODT long-acting amphetamine), Dyanavel XR (a long-acting liquid amphetamine), and most intriguingly, Jornay PM (a long-acting methylphenidate you take at night that kicks in the next morning). We cover these formulations in the ADHD Medications table.

5. *Cost.* Most ADHD meds are available generically, but some reasonable choices are still branded and therefore more expensive. The most popular of these is Vyvanse, which is a long-acting amphetamine. Vyvanse appears to have a genuine advantage over many other stimulants, mainly in terms of tolerability and less potential for abuse. However, you'll have a hard time convincing insurance companies to cover the cost of Vyvanse unless you can clearly document intolerance in several other trials of stimulants.

Dose Equivalents and Switching Strategies

Most patients need to try different stimulants, or stimulant formulations, before settling on the one that works best for them. The dose equivalents are, luckily, fairly easy to remember.

1. From one amphetamine to another amphetamine
   - With the exception of Vyvanse, all amphetamines, including both Adderall IR and XR, are roughly equivalent in potency. For example, if a patient is taking Dexedrine 10 mg TID, you can switch this to Adderall 15 mg BID or Adderall XR 30 mg QD. That said, some people believe that Dexedrine, being 100% dextroamphetamine, might be more potent than Adderall, which is 75% d-amphetamine and 25% l-amphetamine (eg, 30 mg/day of Dexedrine may be closer to 40 mg/day of Adderall). In reality, the difference is likely negligible in most people.
   - Vyvanse is composed of both lysine and amphetamine, with amphetamine making up only about 30% of Vyvanse. This means that it's much less potent than straight Dexedrine. So, when switching from another amphetamine to Vyvanse, you have to at least double the dose.

2. From one methylphenidate to another methylphenidate
   - With the exception of Concerta and Focalin, all methylphenidate preparations are roughly equivalent in potency.
   - Concerta, because of its complex delivery system, delivers less methylphenidate than implied by the mg amount you prescribe. The usual conversion percentage used is 83%, meaning that the body sees 83% of Concerta

in methylphenidate equivalents. Thus, Concerta 18 mg is equivalent to methylphenidate 15 mg, 36 mg is equivalent to 30 mg, and so on.

- Focalin is the dextro-isomer of methylphenidate, which is twice as potent as methylphenidate. Thus, use about half the dose when prescribing Focalin.

3. From a methylphenidate to an amphetamine (or vice versa)
   - Methylphenidate is roughly half as potent as amphetamine, so Ritalin 10 mg = Dexedrine 5 mg, etc. Consistent with this equivalency, child psychiatrists often dose methylphenidate at 1 mg/kg, whereas they dose amphetamine at 0.5 mg/kg. Conversely, if you're switching from Dexedrine to Ritalin, you would need to increase the dose by a factor of two.

4. From an oral methylphenidate to the methylphenidate patch (Daytrana)
   - According to a clinical trial of patients switched from various versions of long-acting methylphenidate to the patch, you should dose the patch at about half the dose of the oral medication (Arnold LE et al, *Curr Med Res Opin* 2010;26(1):129–137).

See Table 2 for dose-by-dose breakdowns.

How to Switch

Once you've determined the dose equivalence, the actual switching is easy. You don't have to cross-taper; instead, have your patient take the last dose of stimulant A on day one and start stimulant B on day two. To be prudent, start the new stimulant at a somewhat lower dose than you calculate would be needed based on the equivalent dose rules of thumb. Those equivalencies are based on averages and may not apply to a given individual.

Side Effects and Class Warnings

The following apply to all stimulants:

- *Potential to cause psychosis or aggression.* This is a rare and dose-related effect; it may be more likely in patients with a predisposition for psychosis.

- *Worsening or new-onset Tourette's or tic disorders.* Stimulants may unmask tics. Of stimulants, methylphenidate is favored. The non-stimulant guanfacine is an even better alternative.

- *Seizures.* Stimulants may lower the seizure threshold, although data are contradictory; monitor patients with seizure disorders closely.

- *Growth inhibition or weight loss.* With long-term use, some growth inhibition may occur occasionally in children, but this is generally not a major problem. Monitoring growth and considering "drug holidays" may limit growth suppression.

- *Cardiovascular safety.* The FDA issued a serious class warning in 2006 with regard to cardiovascular safety. However, newer data, both in children and adults, have been reassuring. Cardiac events occurred at virtually the same or lower rates among people who took stimulants compared to those who did not. From a practical perspective, we recommend asking about cardiac problems and consulting the child's pediatrician or cardiologist if a problem exists. Amphetamines should be avoided in patients with known or suspected cardiovascular disease.

- *No refills.* All stimulants are controlled substances (Schedule II), which means they can't be refilled or called in. Patients must be given a new prescription every month. In most states, you are allowed to give patients post-dated prescriptions for convenience.

Adult ADHD Treatment Algorithm

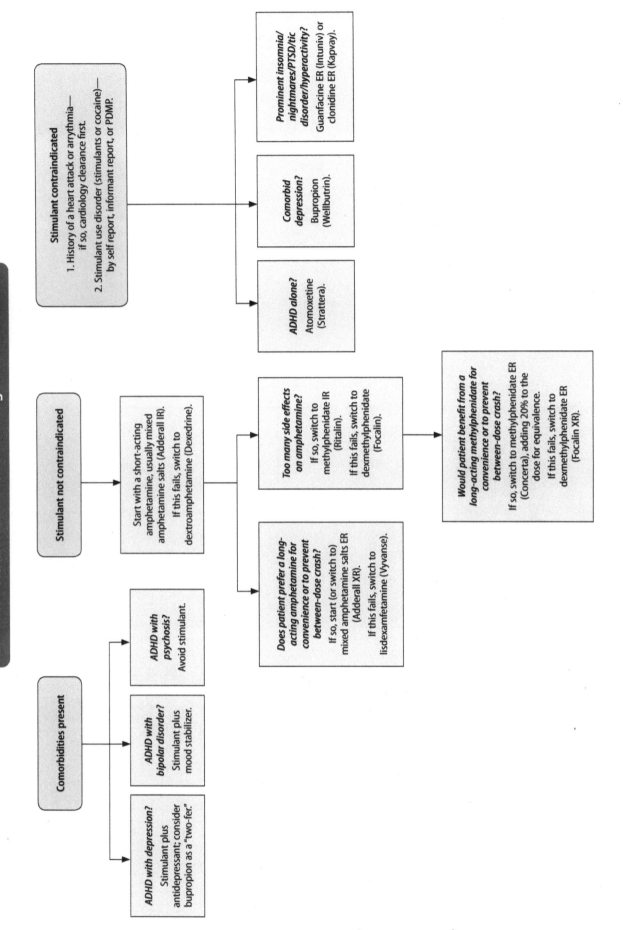

Comorbidities present

ADHD with depression? Stimulant plus antidepressant; consider bupropion as a "two-fer."

ADHD with bipolar disorder? Stimulant plus mood stabilizer.

ADHD with psychosis? Avoid stimulant.

Stimulant not contraindicated

Start with a short-acting amphetamine, usually mixed amphetamine salts (Adderall IR). If this fails, switch to dextroamphetamine (Dexedrine).

Does patient prefer a long-acting amphetamine for convenience or to prevent between-dose crash? If so, start (or switch to) mixed amphetamine salts ER (Adderall XR). If this fails, switch to lisdexamfetamine (Vyvanse).

Too many side effects on amphetamine? If so, switch to methylphenidate IR (Ritalin). If this fails, switch to dexmethylphenidate (Focalin).

Would patient benefit from a long-acting methylphenidate for convenience or to prevent between-dose crash? If so, switch to methylphenidate ER (Concerta), adding 20% to the dose for equivalence. If this fails, switch to dexmethylphenidate ER (Focalin XR).

Stimulant contraindicated
1. History of a heart attack or arrythmia—if so, cardiology clearance first.
2. Stimulant use disorder (stimulants or cocaine)—by self report, informant report, or PDMP.

ADHD alone? Atomoxetine (Strattera).

Comorbid depression? Bupropion (Wellbutrin).

Prominent insomnia/nightmares/PTSD/tic disorder/hyperactivity? Guanfacine ER (Intuniv) or clonidine ER (Kapvay).

Table 1: ADHD Medications

Brand Name (Generic Name, if different than heading) Year FDA Approved [G] denotes generic availability	Available Strengths (mg except where noted)	Usual Dosage Range (starting–max) (mg)	Onset of Action (minutes)	Duration of Action (hours)	Can It Be Split?	Ages Approved for ADHD	Delivery System/Notes (IR = immediate, CR = controlled, DR = delayed, ER = extended release)
Methylphenidates							
Short-Acting							
Focalin [G] (Dexmethylphenidate) 2001	2.5, 5, 10	2.5–10 BID	30–45	3–4	Yes (not scored)	6–17	Tablet; d-enantiomer of Ritalin; 2× more potent than methylphenidate
Methylin CT [G] 2003	2.5, 5, 10	2.5 BID–20 TID	30–45	3–4	Yes	6–17, adults	Chewable, grape-flavored tablet
Methylin oral solution [G] 2002	5 mg/5 mL, 10 mg/5 mL	2.5 BID–20 TID	30–45	3–4	N/A (liquid)	6–17, adults	Clear, grape-flavored liquid
Ritalin [G] 1955	5, 10, 20	2.5 BID–20 TID	30–45	3–4	Yes	6–17, adults	IR tablet
Intermediate-Acting							
Metadate ER [G] 1999 (Branded generic of Ritalin SR)	20	10 QAM–30 BID	60–90	6–8	No	6–17, adults	CR tablet (less predictable because of wax matrix)
Methylin ER [G] 2000 (Branded generic of Ritalin SR)	10, 20	20–60 QAM	60–90	4–8	No	6–17, adults	Hydrophilic polymer tablet; possibly more continuous than others in category
Ritalin SR [G] 1982	10, 20	10–60 QAM	60–90	4–8	No	6–17, adults	CR tablet (less predictable because of wax matrix)
Long-Acting							
Adhansia XR 2019	25, 35, 45, 55, 70, 85	25–85 QAM	45–60	10–16	Can be sprinkled; do not crush or chew	6–17, adults	Capsule of 20% IR beads & 80% DR beads
Aptensio XR 2015	10, 15, 20, 30, 40, 50, 60	10–60 QAM	45–60	8–12	Can be sprinkled; do not crush or chew	6–17, adults	Capsule of 40% IR beads & 60% DR beads
Azstarys (Serdexmethylphenidate/ dexmethylphenidate) 2021	26.1/5.2, 39.2/7.8, 52.3/10.4	39.2/7.8–52.3/10.4 QAM	30–60	8–13	Can be sprinkled or added to water	6–17, adults	Combination of prodrug of dexmethylphenidate (70%) and d-MPH (30%); equivalent to 20, 30, 40 mg dexmethylphenidate (Focalin); twice as potent as methylphenidate
Concerta [G] 2000	18, 27, 36, 54	18–72 QAM	45–60	10–12	No	6–17, adults	CR tablet with 22% IR & 78% DR

¹Strattera dosing: Weight <70 kg, start 0.5 mg/kg, target 1.2 mg/kg, max 1.4 mg/kg; weight >70 kg, 40–100 mg

Brand Name (Generic Name, if different than heading) Year FDA Approved [G] denotes generic availability	Available Strengths (mg except where noted)	Usual Dosage Range (starting–max) (mg)	Onset of Action (minutes)	Duration of Action (hours)	Can It Be Split?	Ages Approved for ADHD	Delivery System/Notes (IR = immediate, CR = controlled, DR = delayed, ER = extended release)
Cotempla XR-ODT 2017	8.6, 17.3, 25.9	17.3–51.8 QAM	45–60	8–12	No (ODT)	6–17	Orally disintegrating; ER with 25% IR & 75% ER
Daytrana patch (Methylphenidate transdermal system) 2006	10, 15, 20, 30	10–30 QAM; remove after 9 hrs	120	8–12	No	6–17	CR patch; duration can be shortened by decreasing wear time; drug effects may persist for 5 hrs after removal
Focalin XR [G] (Dexmethylphenidate XR) 2005	5, 10, 15, 20, 25, 30, 35, 40	6–17 yrs: 5–30 QAM; Adults: 10–40 QAM	30	8–12	Can be sprinkled; do not crush or chew	6–17, adults	Capsule of 50% IR beads & 50% DR beads; mimics BID dosing; twice as potent as methylphenidate
Jornay PM 2018	20, 40, 60, 80, 100	20–100 QPM	8–10 hrs	8–12; after delay in onset	Can be sprinkled; do not crush or chew	6–17, adults	ER capsule of DR beads; taken in evening between 6:30–9:30 p.m.
Metadate CD [G] 2001	10, 20, 30, 40, 50, 60	20–60 QAM	60–90	8–12	Can be sprinkled; do not crush or chew	6–17, adults	Capsule of 30% IR beads & 70% DR beads; mimics BID dosing
Quillichew ER 2015	20, 30, 40	20–60 QAM	45–60	8–12	Yes	6–17, adults	Chewable ER for those who will not swallow pills or take liquids; 30% IR & 70% ER
Quillivant XR 2012	25 mg/5 mL	20–60 QAM	45	8–12	N/A (liquid)	6–17, adults	20% IR & 80% ER in oral solution; shake prior to use
Ritalin LA [G] 2002	10, 20, 30, 40, 60	20–60 QAM	60–90	8–12	Can be sprinkled; do not crush or chew	6–17, adults	Capsule of 50% IR beads & 50% DR beads
Amphetamines							
Short-Acting							
Desoxyn [G] (Methamphetamine) 1943	5	5 QAM–10 BID	30–45	3–5	Yes (scored)	6–17	Tablet
Dexedrine [G] (Dextroamphetamine) 1976	5, 10	3–5 yrs: 2.5 QAM–20 BID; 6–16 yrs: 5 QAM–20 BID	30–45	3–5	Yes	3–16	Scored tablet
Evekeo [G] Evekeo ODT (Amphetamine) 2012, 2019	5, 10 ODT: 2.5, 5, 10, 15, 20	3–5 yrs: 2.5 QAM–20 BID; 6–17 yrs: 5 QAM–20 BID	30–45	3–5	Yes (scored) No (ODT)	3–17	Scored tablet or ODT; 1:1 ratio of l- and d-amphetamine
ProCentra [G] (Dextroamphetamine oral solution) 2008	5 mg/5 mL	5–20 BID	30–45	3–5	N/A (liquid)	3–16	Bubblegum-flavored liquid

[1]Strattera dosing: Weight <70 kg, start 0.5 mg/kg, target 1.2 mg/kg, max 1.4 mg/kg; weight >70 kg, 40–100 mg

Brand Name (Generic Name, if different than heading) Year FDA Approved [G] denotes generic availability	Available Strengths (mg except where noted)	Usual Dosage Range (starting–max) (mg)	Onset of Action (minutes)	Duration of Action (hours)	Can It Be Split?	Ages Approved for ADHD	Delivery System/Notes (IR = immediate, CR = controlled, DR = delayed, ER = extended release)
Zenzedi (Dextroamphetamine) 2013	2.5, 5, 7.5, 10, 15, 20, 30	3–5 yrs: 2.5 QD–20 BID; 6–16 yrs: 5 QAM–20 BID (same as Dexedrine dosing)	30–45	3–5	Yes	3–16	Tablet: 5 mg scored, 10 mg double scored, rest unscored

Intermediate-Acting

Brand Name	Available Strengths	Usual Dosage Range	Onset of Action	Duration of Action	Can It Be Split?	Ages Approved for ADHD	Delivery System/Notes
Adderall [G] (Mixed amphetamine salts) 1960	5, 7.5, 10, 12.5, 15, 20, 30	3–5 yrs: 2.5 QAM–20 BID; 6–17 yrs; Adults: 5 QAM–20 BID	45–60	6–8	Can be crushed	3–17, adults	Tablet; mixed salt of l- and d-amphetamine

Long-Acting

Brand Name	Available Strengths	Usual Dosage Range	Onset of Action	Duration of Action	Can It Be Split?	Ages Approved for ADHD	Delivery System/Notes
Adderall XR [G] (Mixed amphetamine salts) 2001	5, 10, 15, 20, 25, 30	6–12 yrs: 5–30 QAM; 13–17 yrs: 10–40 QAM; Adults: 20–60 QAM	45–60	8–12	Can be sprinkled; do not crush or chew	6–17, adults	Capsule of 50% IR beads & 50% DR beads; mixed salt of l- and d-amphetamine; mimics BID dosing
Adzenys XR-ODT Adzenys ER oral suspension (Amphetamine) 2016, 2017	3.1, 6.3, 9.4, 12.5, 15.7, 18.8 Oral suspension: 1.25 mg/mL	6–12 yrs: 6.3 (5 mL)–18.8 (15 mL) QAM; 13–17 yrs: 6.3 (5 mL)–12.5 (10 mL) QAM; Adults: 12.5 (10 mL) QAM	45–60	8–12	N/A (ODT/liquid)	6–17, adults	50% IR & 50% ER; ER ODT: 3.1 mg is equivalent to 5 mg mixed-salts product; increasing dose preparations are equivalent to 10 mg, 15 mg, 20 mg, 25 mg, and 30 mg respectively. Solution: 1.25 mg is equivalent to 2 mg Adderall XR.
Dexedrine Spansules [G] (Dextroamphetamine) 1976	5, 10, 15	5 QAM–20 BID	30–60	6–8	Can be sprinkled; do not crush or chew	3–16	Capsule of 50% IR & 50% sustained-release beads
Dyanavel XR (Amphetamine) 2015	5, 10, 15, 20 Oral suspension: 2.5 mg/mL	6–17 yrs: 2.5–20 QAM	45–60	8–12	No (oral suspension)	6–17	ER oral suspension allowing once-daily dosing (must shake well); 2.5 mg = 4 mg mixed amphetamine salts
Mydayis (Mixed amphetamine salts) 2017	12.5, 25, 37.5, 50	13–17 yrs: 12.5–25 QAM; Adults: 12.5–50 QAM	45–60	10–16	Can be sprinkled; do not crush or chew	13–17, adults	pH-dependent ER capsule formulation; may have effect up to 16 hrs
Vyvanse (Lisdexamfetamine) 2007	Capsule: 10, 20, 30, 40, 50, 60, 70 Chewable: 10, 20, 30, 40, 50, 60	30–70 QAM	60–90	8–13	Capsules can be dissolved in water	6–17, adults	Lisdexamfetamine is prodrug of dextroamphetamine

'Strattera dosing: Weight <70 kg, start 0.5 mg/kg, target 1.2 mg/kg, max 1.4 mg/kg; weight >70 kg, 40–100 mg

Brand Name (Generic Name, if different than heading) Year FDA Approved [G] denotes generic availability	Available Strengths (mg except where noted)	Usual Dosage Range (starting–max) (mg)	Onset of Action (minutes)	Duration of Action (hours)	Can It Be Split?	Ages Approved for ADHD	Delivery System/Notes (IR = immediate, CR = controlled, DR = delayed, ER = extended release)
Non-Stimulants							
Intuniv [G] (Guanfacine ER) 2009	1, 2, 3, 4	1–4 QD (do not increase faster than 1 mg/wk) (adolescents 7 mg/day max)	N/A	24	No	6–17	ER tablet; do not stop abruptly (rebound hypertension); not a 1:1 conversion from IR; do not give with high-fat meals
Kapvay [G] (Clonidine XR) 2010	0.1, 0.2	0.1 QHS; increase by 0.1 mg/day weekly and give divided BID; max 0.4 QD	N/A	12–16	No	6–17	ER tablet; titrate gradually (orthostatic hypotension); avoid abrupt discontinuation; somnolence
Provigil [G] (Modafinil) 1998	100, 200	100–400 QAM	N/A	18–24	Yes (200 mg tabs are scored)	Not FDA approved for ADHD	Tablet; studies have shown modafinil to be helpful for ADHD, but low incidence of serious rash; minimal data in children
Qelbree (Viloxazine ER) 2021	100, 150, 200	100–400 QAM	N/A	24	Can be sprinkled	6–17, adults	ER capsule; norepinephrine reuptake inhibitor
Strattera [G] (Atomoxetine) 2002	10, 18, 25, 40, 60, 80, 100	Dosage varies; see footnote 1 below	N/A	24	No	6–17, adults	Capsule; norepinephrine reuptake inhibitor
Tenex [G] (Guanfacine IR) 1986	1, 2	1–4 QD (do not increase faster than 1 mg/wk)	N/A	17	Can be crushed	Not FDA approved for kids or ADHD; approved only for adults 18+ for hypertension	Tablet
Wellbutrin [G] (Bupropion) 1985	75, 100	1.4–6 mg/kg/day	N/A	6–9	Yes	Not FDA approved for ADHD	Tablet; bupropion SR & XL versions exist

¹Strattera dosing: Weight <70 kg, start 0.5 mg/kg, target 1.2 mg/kg, max 1.4 mg/kg; weight >70 kg, 40–100 mg

Table 2: **Relative Equivalency and Conversion Guide for Stimulants**[1]

Methylphenidates	
Alternative Formulation	**Regular Methylphenidate Equivalent**
Adhansia XR 25 mg QAM	5 mg IR TID
Adhansia XR 100 mg QAM	20 mg IR TID
Aptensio XR 10 mg QAM	5 mg IR BID or 10 mg ER QAM
Concerta 18, 27, 36, 54 mg tablets	10–15, 15–20, 20–30, 30–45 mg/day, respectively; use 72 mg Concerta for 45–60 mg/day
Cotempla XR-ODT 8.6, 17.3, 25.9 mg tablets	ER 10, 20, 30 mg, respectively
Daytrana patch 10 mg	5 mg IR BID or 10 mg ER QAM
Focalin 5 mg BID	IR 10 mg BID
Focalin XR 10 mg QAM	IR 20 mg QAM
Jornay PM 20 mg QPM	4 mg IR TID
Jornay PM 100 mg QPM	20 mg IR TID
Quillichew ER 20 mg QAM	10 mg IR BID or 20 mg ER QAM
Quillichew ER 30 mg QAM	15 mg IR BID or 30 mg ER QAM
Quillichew ER 40 mg QAM	20 mg IR BID or 40 mg ER QAM
Quillivant XR 10 mg (2 mL) QAM	5 mg IR BID or 10 mg ER QAM
Quillivant XR 20 mg (4 mL) QAM	10 mg IR BID or 20 mg ER QAM
Quillivant XR 30 mg (6 mL) QAM	15 mg IR BID or 30 mg ER QAM
Quillivant XR 40 mg (8 mL) QAM	20 mg IR BID or 40 mg ER QAM
Amphetamines	
Alternative Formulation	**Regular Mixed Amphetamine Salts Equivalent**
Adzenys XR-ODT 3.1 mg QAM	2.5 mg IR BID or 5 mg ER QAM
Adzenys XR-ODT 6.3 mg QAM	5 mg IR BID or 10 mg ER QAM
Adzenys XR-ODT 9.4 mg QAM	7.5 mg IR BID or 15 mg ER QAM
Adzenys XR-ODT 12.5 mg QAM	10 mg IR BID or 20 mg ER QAM
Adzenys XR-ODT 15.7 mg QAM	12.5 mg IR BID or 25 mg ER QAM
Adzenys XR-ODT 18.8 mg QAM	15 mg IR BID or 30 mg ER QAM
Adzenys ER 3.125 mg (2.5 mL) QAM	2.5 mg IR BID or 5 mg ER QAM
Adzenys ER 6.25 mg (5 mL) QAM	5 mg IR BID or 10 mg ER QAM
Adzenys ER 9.375 mg (7.5 mL) QAM	7.5 mg IR BID or 15 mg ER QAM
Adzenys ER 12.5 mg (10 mL) QAM	10 mg IR BID or 20 mg ER QAM
Adzenys ER 15.625 mg (12.5 mL) QAM	12.5 mg IR BID or 25 mg ER QAM
Adzenys ER 18.75 mg (15 mL) QAM	15 mg IR BID or 30 mg ER QAM
Dyanavel XR 6.25 mg (2.5 mL)	5 mg IR BID or 10 mg ER QAM
Dyanavel XR 12.5 mg (5 mL)	10 mg IR BID or 20 mg ER QAM
Dyanavel XR 18.75 mg (7.5 mL)	15 mg IR BID or 30 mg ER QAM
Mydayis 37.5 mg QAM	25 mg ER QAM plus 12.5 mg IR eight hours later
Vyvanse 30 mg QAM	5 mg IR BID or 10 mg ER QAM
Vyvanse 50 mg QAM	10 mg IR BID or 20 mg ER QAM
Vyvanse 70 mg QAM	15 mg IR BID or 30 mg ER QAM

IR = immediate release; ER = extended release

[1] These are approximate equivalencies provided as guidance; taper and titrate each agent based on recommended dosing when switching rather than direct substitution

AMPHETAMINE (Adzenys XR-ODT, Dyanavel XR, Evekeo) Fact Sheet [G]

Bottom Line:

Amphetamine is a 50:50 racemic mixture of dextro- and levo-amphetamine. In clinical practice, the most commonly prescribed amphetamine is Adderall (mixed amphetamine salts; see fact sheet later in this chapter). Based on meta-analyses, amphetamines are clearly the most effective option in both children and adults with ADHD. That doesn't mean they should always be the first choice, though. Methylphenidates are often better tolerated and have relatively less abuse potential. Several newer formulations of amphetamine may be helpful for patients who don't like to swallow pills—but they come with a price tag.

FDA Indications:

ADHD (Adzenys XR-ODT: adults and children ≥6; Dyanavel XR: children ≥6; Evekeo: children ≥3); **narcolepsy** (Evekeo); obesity (Evekeo).

Off-Label Uses:

Treatment-resistant depression.

Dosage Forms:

- **Tablets (Evekeo, [G]):** 5 mg, 10 mg (scored); **(Evekeo ODT):** 2.5 mg, 5 mg, 10 mg, 15 mg, 20 mg.
- **ER tablets (Dyanavel XR):** 5 mg (scored), 10 mg, 15 mg, 20 mg.
- **ER orally disintegrating tablets (Adzenys XR-ODT):** 3.1 mg, 6.3 mg, 9.4 mg, 12.5 mg, 15.7 mg, 18.8 mg.
- **ER oral suspension (Dyanavel XR):** 2.5 mg/mL; **(Adzenys ER):** 1.25 mg/mL.

Dosage Guidance:

- Tablets (Evekeo, [G]):
  - Children 3–5: Start 2.5 mg QAM, increase in 2.5 mg/day increments weekly.
  - Children 6–17: Start 5 mg QAM, increase in 5 mg/day increments weekly to maximum of 40 mg/day in divided doses.
  - Narcolepsy: Start 5 mg QAM (ages 6–12) or 10 mg QAM (ages >12), increase by 5 or 10 mg/day increments weekly, respectively. Maximum 60 mg/day in divided doses.
- ER ODT (Adzenys XR-ODT) or Adzenys ER oral suspension:
  - Start 6.3 mg (5 mL) QAM, increase in 3.1 mg (2.5 mL)–6.3 mg (5 mL) per day increments weekly. Maximum of 18.8 mg (15 mL)/day (ages 6–12) or 12.5 mg (10 mL)/day (ages 13–17 and adults).
- ER oral suspension (Dyanavel XR):
  - Children 6–12: Start 2.5–5 mg QAM, increase in 2.5–10 mg/day increments every four to seven days. Maximum 20 mg/day.

Monitoring: ECG if history of cardiac disease.

Cost: [G]: $$$; others: $$$$

Side Effects:

- Most common: Abdominal pain, decreased appetite, weight loss, insomnia, headache, nervousness.
- Serious but rare: See class warnings in chapter introduction.

Mechanism, Pharmacokinetics, and Drug Interactions:

- Stimulant that inhibits reuptake of dopamine and norepinephrine.
- Metabolized primarily via CYP2D6; t ½: 11 hours.
- Avoid use with MAOIs, antacids.

Clinical Pearls:

- These racemic forms of amphetamine differ from dextroamphetamine in that the l-isomer component is more potent than the d-isomer in peripheral activity (potentially resulting in more cardiovascular effects and tics).
- A racemic mixture may be less appetite suppressing compared to dextroamphetamine.
- Divide IR (Evekeo) doses by intervals of four to six hours.
- Approximate equivalence doses of Adzenys XR-ODT and mixed amphetamine salts XR (Adderall XR) are: 3.1 mg = 5 mg, 6.3 mg = 10 mg, 9.4 mg = 15 mg, 12.5 mg = 20 mg, 15.7 mg = 25 mg, 18.8 mg = 30 mg.
- Dyanavel XR oral suspension: Shake well to get the intended extended-release effect. The approximate equivalence of 2.5 mg/mL is 4 mg of mixed amphetamine salts.

Fun Facts:

The term "amphetamine" is the contracted name of the chemical "alpha-methylphenethylamine." Its first pharmacologic use was in 1934 when pharmaceutical company Smith, Kline and French sold amphetamine under the trade name Benzedrine as a decongestant inhaler.

ATOMOXETINE (Strattera) Fact Sheet [G]

Bottom Line:

Atomoxetine is a non-stimulant ADHD treatment that carries no abuse potential, causes less insomnia and anxiety, and is unlikely to worsen tics. Unfortunately, it is generally less effective than stimulants and takes longer to work (two to four weeks).

FDA Indications:

ADHD (adults and children ≥6 years).

Off-Label Uses:

Treatment-resistant depression.

Dosage Forms:

Capsules (G): 10 mg, 18 mg, 25 mg, 40 mg, 60 mg, 80 mg, 100 mg.

Dosage Guidance:

- Start 40 mg QAM for three days, ↑ to 80 mg QAM, may ↑ to 100 mg/day after two to four weeks if needed (max 100 mg/day); may divide doses >40 mg/day (morning and late afternoon/early evening).
- Special dosing for children <70 kg: Start 0.5 mg/kg QAM for three days, ↑ to 1.2 mg/kg QAM, may ↑ to max 1.4 mg/kg/day or 100 mg/day (whichever is less) after two to four weeks if needed; may divide doses >0.5 mg/kg/day.

Monitoring: Baseline LFTs; follow up if signs of liver disease.

Cost: $

Side Effects:

- Most common: *Children:* Headache, abdominal pain, decreased appetite, fatigue, nausea, vomiting. *Adults:* Nausea, dry mouth, decreased appetite, insomnia, constipation, fatigue, erectile dysfunction, abdominal pain, dizziness, urinary hesitation.
- Serious but rare: Class warning for suicidal ideation in children and teens. Severe hepatic injury including increased hepatic enzymes (up to 40 times normal) and jaundice (bilirubin up to 12 times upper limit of normal). Increased blood pressure (↑ 15–20 mmHg) and heart rate (↑ 20 bpm).

Mechanism, Pharmacokinetics, and Drug Interactions:

- Selective norepinephrine reuptake inhibitor (NRI).
- Metabolized primarily via CYP2D6; t ½: 5 hours.
- Avoid use with MAOIs. Exercise caution with 2D6 inhibitors such as fluoxetine, paroxetine, and quinidine (increased atomoxetine serum levels); use slower titration and do not exceed 80 mg/day in presence of 2D6 inhibitors or in 2D6 poor metabolizers.

Clinical Pearls:

- QAM and BID dosing are equally effective, but BID dosing has better GI tolerability. Can also be dosed at bedtime if it causes fatigue.
- Appears to be more effective in improving attention than in controlling hyperactivity.

Fun Fact:

Atomoxetine was originally known as "tomoxetine"; however, the FDA requested that the name be changed because the similarity to "tamoxifen" could lead to dispensing errors.

CLONIDINE (Catapres, Kapvay) Fact Sheet [G]

Bottom Line:
Clonidine is an alpha-2 agonist that has no abuse potential, does not worsen tics, and does not cause insomnia. However, it's less effective than stimulants and has a delayed onset of effect (two to four weeks); it is often added to a stimulant to prevent insomnia. Clonidine may be used as a second-line option for opioid detoxification if buprenorphine or methadone are not available.

FDA Indications:
Hypertension; **ADHD** (children ages 6–17), as monotherapy or adjunctive therapy to stimulants (not approved for ADHD in adults).

Off-Label Uses:
Conduct disorder; Tourette's and motor tics; pervasive developmental disorders; migraine prophylaxis; opioid withdrawal.

Dosage Forms:
- **IR tablets (Catapres, [G]):** 0.1 mg, 0.2 mg, 0.3 mg.
- **ER tablets (Kapvay, [G]):** 0.1 mg, 0.2 mg.
- **Patch (Catapres-TTS, [G]):** 0.1 mg/day, 0.2 mg/day, 0.3 mg/day.

Dosage Guidance:
- IR: Start 0.1 mg BID, ↑ by 0.1 mg/day at weekly intervals; max 2 mg/day. For opioid withdrawal, may be dosed 0.1–0.2 mg every four to six hours as needed. Daily dosing requirement can be established by tabulating the total amount administered over the first 24 hours and dividing this amount into a TID or QID schedule. Total dose should not exceed 1.2 mg the first 24 hours and 2 mg/day beyond that.
- ER: Start 0.1 mg QHS, ↑ by 0.1 mg/day at weekly intervals; max 0.4 mg/day. May divide doses >0.2 mg/day; divided doses may be unequal with higher dose given at bedtime.

Monitoring: Blood pressure (hold doses for BP <90/60).

Cost: $

Side Effects:
- Most common: Dry mouth, somnolence, dizziness, constipation, fatigue, headache.
- Serious but rare: Hypotension, syncope, orthostasis.

Mechanism, Pharmacokinetics, and Drug Interactions:
- Centrally acting, selective alpha-2 adrenergic agonist.
- Metabolized primarily through CYP2D6; t ½: 6–20 hours.
- Avoid use with MAOIs. Caution with 2D6 inhibitors (eg, paroxetine, fluoxetine, duloxetine).

Clinical Pearls:
- Not a controlled substance.
- Clonidine tends to be more sedating than guanfacine, another alpha agonist.
- When used in detox, clonidine relieves most opioid withdrawal symptoms but is less effective than methadone or buprenorphine. Therefore, adjunctive medications are often used with clonidine to manage insomnia, muscle pain, headache, agitation, and other symptoms. Even so, detox completion rates with clonidine are typically significantly lower than those with buprenorphine or methadone.
- The patch formulation is not typically used (except for hypertension) because clonidine's effects on BP may be prolonged and continue even after patch removal.
- If patient misses two or more consecutive doses, consider repeating titration.
- Minimize side effects, especially somnolence, by administering at bedtime.
- Monitor blood pressure, especially during initial dosing titration.
- Risk of nervousness, anxiety, and possibly rebound hypertension two to four days after abrupt discontinuation. Taper dose in no more than 0.1 mg/day decrements, every three to seven days.

Fun Fact:
The Federal Bureau of Prisons' clinical guidance document, *Detoxification of Chemically Dependent Inmates*, recommends maintaining strict control over medication access to prevent diversion or misuse. It cites the example of inmates eating clonidine patches to obtain a state of euphoria.

DEXMETHYLPHENIDATE (Azstarys, Focalin, Focalin XR) Fact Sheet [G]

Bottom Line:

Dexmethylphenidate (Focalin) is the d-isomer of methylphenidate and is two times more potent than methylphenidate. Azstarys is a newly approved (and expensive) combination of Focalin and a prodrug version of Focalin—the Focalin is absorbed quickly while the prodrug is absorbed more slowly (it's the Vyvanse of methylphenidate). There's no clear advantage of Focalin over Ritalin—the main difference is that Focalin may mean fewer tablets for patients. Focalin XR only recently went generic, so it will likely remain quite expensive for a while. Azstarys may be less abusable than Focalin.

FDA Indications:

ADHD in adults (Azstarys, Focalin XR) and in children ≥6 years (Azstarys, Focalin IR and XR).

Off-Label Uses:

Narcolepsy, obesity, treatment-resistant depression.

Dosage Forms:

- **Dexmethylphenidate tablets (Focalin, [G]):** 2.5 mg, 5 mg, 10 mg.
- **Dexmethylphenidate ER capsules (Focalin XR, [G]):** 5 mg, 10 mg, 15 mg, 20 mg, 25 mg, 30 mg, 35 mg, 40 mg.
- **Serdexmethylphenidate/dexmethylphenidate ER capsules (Azstarys):** 26.1/5.2 mg, 39.2/7.8 mg, 52.3/10.4 mg.

Dosage Guidance:

- d-MPH IR: Start 2.5 mg BID, ↑ by 5–10 mg/day every seven days. Max 20 mg/day; divide IR doses by at least four hours.
- d-MPH ER: Start 10 mg QAM, ↑ by 10 mg/day every seven days. Max 40 mg/day. For children, start 5 mg QAM, ↑ by 5 mg/day every seven days. Max (children) 30 mg/day.
- Serdex-MPH/d-MPH: Start 39.2/7.8 mg QAM, ↑ to max dose of 52.3/10.4 mg after one week if indicated.

Monitoring: ECG if history of cardiac disease.

Cost: IR: $; ER: $$; Azstarys: $$$$

Side Effects:

- Most common: Decreased appetite, insomnia, anxiety, GI distress, irritability, tics, headache, tachycardia, hypertension, dry mouth.
- Serious but rare: See class warnings in chapter introduction.

Mechanism, Pharmacokinetics, and Drug Interactions:

- Stimulant that inhibits reuptake of dopamine and norepinephrine.
- Serdexmethylphenidate (Serdex-MPH) is a prodrug of dexmethylphenidate (d-MPH). d-MPH is metabolized primarily via de-esterification, not CYP450; d-MPH t ½: 2–4.5 hours (2–3 hours in children); d-MPH ER delivers 50% of dose immediately and 50% about five hours later. Azstarys t ½: 6–12 hours; delivers 30% d-MPH immediately and 70% as prodrug.
- Avoid use with MAOIs.

Clinical Pearls:

- d-MPH is the d-isomer of methylphenidate and is two times more potent than methylphenidate, which is why it is prescribed at about half the dose. Serdex-MPH is a prodrug, converted to d-MPH in the lower GI tract.
- Use the same total daily dose of Focalin IR as Focalin XR. The combined dose of Azstarys 26.1/5.2, 39.2/7.8, or 52.3/10.4 mg is equivalent to 20, 30, or 40 mg of Focalin, respectively.
- Focalin XR capsules contain two kinds of beads: Half are IR beads and half are enteric-coated DR beads. A single, once-daily XR capsule provides the same amount of dexmethylphenidate as two IR tablets given four hours apart.
- The ER capsules cannot be split in half. However, they can be opened and the beads sprinkled over food. The patient should then eat all that food—eating half won't work to split the dose accurately because it won't be possible to determine if the eaten portion contains more immediate-release or delayed-release beads.
- Give with food if GI side effects occur.

Fun Fact:

With two stereoactive centers, methylphenidate has four possible stereoisomers. Of the four, dexmethylphenidate is the most active biologically.

DEXTROAMPHETAMINE (Dexedrine, ProCentra, Zenzedi) Fact Sheet [G]

Bottom Line:
Dextroamphetamine is the dextro-isomer of racemic amphetamine. It has a long history of safe use in children, and is available in short- and long-acting formulations as generics.

FDA Indications:
ADHD (children ≥3 years); **narcolepsy** (adults and children ≥6 years).

Off-Label Uses:
Obesity, treatment-resistant depression.

Dosage Forms:
- **Tablets (Dexedrine, [G]):** 5 mg, 10 mg (scored).
- **Tablets (Zenzedi):** 2.5 mg, 5 mg, 7.5 mg, 10 mg, 15 mg, 20 mg, 30 mg (5 mg scored, 10 mg double scored; rest unscored).
- **ER capsules (Dexedrine Spansules, [G]):** 5 mg, 10 mg, 15 mg.
- **Liquid (ProCentra, [G]):** 5 mg/5 mL.

Dosage Guidance:
- ADHD (IR and ER):
  - Adults and children ≥6 years: Start 5 mg QAM, ↑ by 5 mg/day at weekly intervals to max 60 mg/day, though doses ≥40 mg/day are rarely more effective. Divide IR dose QD–TID.
  - Children 3–5 years: Start 2.5 mg QAM, ↑ by 2.5 mg/day weekly to max 60 mg/day, though doses >40 mg/day are rarely more effective. Divide IR dose QD–TID.
- Narcolepsy (IR and ER):
  - Start 10 mg QAM, ↑ by 10 mg/day weekly to max 60 mg/day. Divide IR dose QD–TID.

Monitoring: ECG if history of cardiac disease.

Cost: IR/ER: $ (Zenzedi and ProCentra: $$$$)

Side Effects:
- Most common: Abdominal pain, anorexia, nausea, tics, insomnia, tachycardia, headache.
- Serious but rare: See class warnings in chapter introduction.

Mechanism, Pharmacokinetics, and Drug Interactions:
- Stimulant that inhibits reuptake of dopamine and norepinephrine.
- Metabolized primarily through CYP450 2D6 (minor) and glucuronidation; t ½: 12 hours.
- Avoid use with MAOIs, antacids.

Clinical Pearls:
- Dextroamphetamine is the more potent d-isomer of amphetamine; it has potentially less peripheral effects (eg, motor tics) than a racemic mix (eg, mixed amphetamine salts like Adderall, amphetamine, or methamphetamine).
- IR tablets and oral solution: Doses can be given at intervals of four to six hours.
- Dextroamphetamine is the only stimulant, other than Adderall IR, approved for children <6 years (approved for children ≥3 years).
- The newer Zenzedi brand offers more dosing flexibility options, but it is more expensive than generic IR tablets.
- Also available as D,L racemic mixture of amphetamine as Evekeo tablets, Adzenys XR-ODT, and Dyanavel XR oral suspension (see amphetamine fact sheet).

Fun Fact:
Dexys Midnight Runners, the British band famous for its song "Come On Eileen" (1982), derived their name from Dexedrine—"Dexys" after the drug's name and "Midnight Runners" in reference to the energy it provides.

GUANFACINE (Intuniv, Tenex) Fact Sheet [G]

Bottom Line:

Guanfacine is an alpha-2 agonist that has no abuse potential, does not worsen tics, and does not cause insomnia. However, it is less effective than stimulants and has a delayed onset of effect (two to four weeks). Guanfacine ER is now available in generic and is easier to use than IR.

FDA Indications:

ADHD (children ages 6–17), as monotherapy or adjunctive therapy to stimulants (not approved for ADHD in adults).

Off-Label Uses:

Conduct disorder; Tourette's and motor tics; pervasive developmental disorders; migraine prophylaxis; opioid withdrawal.

Dosage Forms:

• **IR tablets (Tenex, [G]):** 1 mg, 2 mg.
• **ER tablets (Intuniv, [G]):** 1 mg, 2 mg, 3 mg, 4 mg.

Dosage Guidance:

• IR dosing depends on weight:
  – 27–40.5 kg (55–90 lbs): Start 0.5 mg QHS, ↑ by 0.5 mg/day at weekly intervals up to 1.5 mg/day, may ↑ to 2 mg/day after two weeks; max 2 mg/day in two to four divided doses.
  – 40.5–45 kg (90–99 lbs): Start 0.5 mg QHS, ↑ by 0.5 mg/day at weekly intervals; max 1 mg per dose, 3 mg/day.
  – >45 kg (>99 lbs): Start 1 mg QHS, ↑ by 1 mg/day at weekly intervals up to 3 mg/day, may ↑ to 4 mg/day after 2 weeks; max 1 mg per dose, 4 mg/day.
• ER: Start 1 mg QHS, ↑ by 1 mg/day at weekly intervals; max 4 mg/day. Alternative: 0.05–0.12 mg/kg QD or QHS; max 4 mg/day. Doses up to 7 mg/day ER studied as monotherapy in adolescents.

Monitoring: Blood pressure.

Cost: $

Side Effects:

• Most common: Dry mouth, somnolence, dizziness, constipation, fatigue, headache.
• Serious but rare: Hypotension, syncope, orthostasis.

Mechanism, Pharmacokinetics, and Drug Interactions:

• Centrally acting, selective alpha-2 adrenergic agonist.
• Metabolized primarily through CYP3A4; t ½: 13–14 hours in children (16–18 hours in adults).
• Avoid use with MAOIs. Caution with 3A4 inhibitors (eg, clarithromycin, fluvoxamine) and inducers (eg, St. John's wort, carbamazepine).

Clinical Pearls:

• Not a controlled substance.
• Guanfacine IR and ER are not interchangeable on a mg:mg basis. When switching from one formulation to the other, taper and re-titrate.
• Guanfacine tends to be less sedating than clonidine, another alpha agonist.
• If patient misses two or more consecutive doses, consider repeating titration.
• ER tablets should not be taken with a high-fat meal due to increased medication exposure.
• Minimize side effects, especially somnolence, by administering at bedtime.
• Monitor blood pressure, especially during initial dosing titration.
• Risk of nervousness, anxiety, and possibly rebound hypertension two to four days after abrupt discontinuation. Taper dose in 1 mg/day decrements, every three to seven days.

Fun Fact:

Some prescribers have taken advantage of guanfacine's sympatholytic properties for the treatment of nightmares and dissociative symptoms in PTSD.

LISDEXAMFETAMINE (Vyvanse) Fact Sheet

Bottom Line:

Vyvanse may have a gentler, "smoother" side effect profile than other amphetamines, and it probably has a lower risk of diversion or abuse. However, its high cost means insurance companies don't like to pay for it without prior authorization.

FDA Indications:

ADHD (adults and children ≥6 years); **binge eating disorder** (BED).

Off-Label Uses:

Narcolepsy; obesity; treatment-resistant depression.

Dosage Forms:

- **Capsules:** 10 mg, 20 mg, 30 mg, 40 mg, 50 mg, 60 mg, 70 mg.
- **Chewtabs:** 10 mg, 20 mg, 30 mg, 40 mg, 50 mg, 60 mg.

Dosage Guidance:

- ADHD (adults and children ≥6 years): Start 30 mg QAM, ↑ by 10–20 mg/day at weekly intervals. Target lowest effective dose; max 70 mg/day.
- BED: Start 30 mg QAM, ↑ by 20 mg/day at weekly intervals to target 50 mg/day; max 70 mg/day.

Monitoring: ECG if history of cardiac disease.

Cost: $$$$

Side Effects:

- Most common: Headache, insomnia, anorexia, abdominal pain, irritability, agitation, tics, decreased appetite, increased heart rate, jitteriness, anxiety.
- Serious but rare: See class warnings in chapter introduction.

Mechanism, Pharmacokinetics, and Drug Interactions:

- Stimulant that inhibits reuptake of dopamine and norepinephrine.
- Metabolized primarily through non-CYP-mediated hepatic and/or intestinal metabolism; t ½: lisdexamfetamine (inactive prodrug) <1 hour; dextroamphetamine (active metabolite) 12 hours. Dextroamphetamine metabolized by CYP2D6.
- Avoid use with MAOIs and antacids. Caution with antihypertensives (decreased efficacy of antihypertensive). Caution with 2D6 inhibitors, which may increase stimulant effects.

Clinical Pearls:

- Lisdexamfetamine is dextroamphetamine with the chemical lysine bound to it, which renders it inactive. It remains inactive until GI enzymes cleave off lysine and convert it to active dextroamphetamine. This means that drug abusers can't get high by snorting or injecting it.
- Anecdotally, Vyvanse has a more gradual onset and offset than other stimulants, and it may cause fewer side effects than other amphetamines.
- Taking with food decreases the effect slightly and delays peak levels by an hour. If patients feel it's not "kicking in" fast enough, have them take it earlier or on an empty stomach.
- Lisdexamfetamine 70 mg is equivalent to 30 mg of mixed amphetamine salts (Adderall).
- While indicated for BED, it is not approved for use as a weight loss or anti-obesity agent.

Fun Fact:

The manufacturer of Vyvanse pursued an indication as an add-on medication for depression, but disappointing results in clinical trials put an end to this effort.

METHAMPHETAMINE (Desoxyn) Fact Sheet [G]

Bottom Line:

Methamphetamine is highly addictive when used in its crystal form ("crystal meth"), because it causes an immediate and intense high when snorted or smoked. Its use is generally not recommended. Watch the television show "Breaking Bad" if you're not convinced!

FDA Indications:

ADHD (children ≥6 years); obesity (adults and adolescents ≥12 years).

Dosage Forms:

Tablets (G): 5 mg.

Dosage Guidance:

ADHD (adults and children ≥6 years): Start 5 mg QAM–BID, ↑ by 5 mg/day at weekly intervals to max 20 mg/day, divided BID.

Monitoring: ECG if history of cardiac disease.

Cost: $$$$

Side Effects:

- Most common: Anorexia, tachycardia, dizziness, insomnia, tremor, tics, restlessness, headache, constipation (decreased GI motility). Dental complications, such as poor dental hygiene, diffuse cavities, bruxism, and tooth wear, may develop with abuse.
- Serious but rare: See class warnings in chapter introduction.

Mechanism, Pharmacokinetics, and Drug Interactions:

- Stimulant that inhibits reuptake of dopamine and norepinephrine.
- Metabolized primarily through CYP2D6 to active metabolite (amphetamine); t ½: 4–5 hours.
- Avoid use with MAOIs and antacids. Caution with 2D6 inhibitors, which may increase stimulant effects.

Clinical Pearls:

- High risk of abuse.
- Not widely used (DEA reports that there were only 16,000 prescriptions written in 2012). When prescribed for obesity, the recommendation is for short-term use only (ie, a few weeks) and as an adjunct to caloric restriction due to its high addiction and diversion potential.
- Methamphetamine's CNS-stimulating effect is approximately equal to or greater than that of amphetamine but less than that of dextroamphetamine; less blood pressure elevation than with amphetamine.

Fun Facts:

Desoxyn is the same as the abused street drug methamphetamine, just pharmaceutical grade. Although methamphetamine and amphetamine were long thought to be available only via laboratories, methamphetamine has been reported to occur naturally in certain acacia trees that grow in West Texas.

METHYLPHENIDATE IR (Methylin, Ritalin) Fact Sheet [G]

Bottom Line:
Methylphenidate has a better side effect profile and somewhat lower abuse potential than amphetamines. However, patients often prefer the "kick" they get from Adderall.

FDA Indications:
ADHD (adults and children ≥6 years); **narcolepsy**.

Off-Label Uses:
Obesity; treatment-resistant depression.

Dosage Forms:
- **Tablets (Ritalin, [G]):** 5 mg, 10 mg, 20 mg.
- **Chewable tablets (Methylin CT, [G]):** 2.5 mg, 5 mg, 10 mg.
- **Oral solution (Methylin, [G]):** 5 mg/5 mL, 10 mg/5 mL.

Dosage Guidance:
- ADHD:
  - Adults: Start 5–10 mg BID, ↑ by 10 mg/day at weekly intervals to max 60 mg/day.
  - Children ≥6 years: Start 0.3 mg/kg BID or 2.5–5 mg BID before breakfast and lunch, increase by 0.1 mg/kg/dose or 5–10 mg/day at weekly intervals to a max of 2 mg/kg/day or 60 mg/day.
- Narcolepsy: Same dosing as ADHD.

Monitoring: ECG if history of cardiac disease.

Cost: $; chewable tabs: $$$

Side Effects:
- Most common: Insomnia, headache, nervousness, abdominal pain, nausea, vomiting, anorexia, weight loss, affect lability, tics.
- Serious but rare: See class warnings in chapter introduction.

Mechanism, Pharmacokinetics, and Drug Interactions:
- Stimulant that inhibits reuptake of dopamine and norepinephrine.
- Hepatic metabolism via carboxylesterase CES1A1, not CYP450 isoenzymes; t ½: 2–4 hours.
- Avoid use with MAOIs, antacids.

Clinical Pearls:
- Methylphenidate generally causes fewer side effects than amphetamine preparations—patients are less likely to report feeling "wired."
- While all stimulants may cause tics, a Cochrane review of eight randomized trials showed that methylphenidate did not worsen tics in children with ADHD and a tic disorder; in some cases it even improved tics.
- Methylin chewable tablets: Administer with at least eight ounces of water or other fluid.

Fun Fact:
Methylphenidate was synthesized by Ciba (now Novartis) chemist Leandro Panizzon. His wife, Marguerite, had low blood pressure and would take the stimulant before playing tennis. He named the substance "Ritaline" (yes, with the "e" on the end) after his wife's nickname, Rita.

METHYLPHENIDATE ER (Concerta, Ritalin SR and LA, others) Fact Sheet [G]

Bottom Line:
There are many longer-acting methylphenidate preparations. Two good options are Concerta and Ritalin LA, both of which are now available generically.

FDA Indications:
ADHD (adults and children ≥6 years); **narcolepsy**.

Off-Label Uses:
Obesity; treatment-resistant depression.

Dosage Forms (more commonly used):
• **Tablets**
 – **Ritalin SR, Metadate ER, Methylin ER, [G]:** 10 mg, 20 mg.
 – **Concerta, [G]:** 18 mg, 27 mg, 36 mg, 54 mg (22% IR/78% ER).
• **Capsules**
 – **Ritalin LA, [G]:** 10 mg, 20 mg, 30 mg, 40 mg, 60 mg (50% IR/50% ER).
 – **Metadate CD, [G]:** 10 mg, 20 mg, 30 mg, 40 mg, 50 mg, 60 mg (30% IR/70% ER).
 – **Aptensio XR:** 10 mg, 15 mg, 20 mg, 30 mg, 40 mg, 50 mg, 60 mg (40% IR/60% ER).
 – **Adhansia XR:** 25 mg, 35 mg, 45 mg, 55 mg, 70 mg, 85 mg (20% IR/80% ER).
 – **Jornay PM:** 20 mg, 40 mg, 60 mg, 80 mg, 100 mg (onset delayed 10 hours).
• **Oral solution (Quillivant XR):** 25 mg/5 mL (20% IR/80% ER).
• **Chewable tablets (Quillichew ER):** 20 mg, 30 mg (scored), 40 mg (scored) (30% IR/70% ER).
• **Orally disintegrating tablets (Cotempla XR-ODT):** 8.6 mg, 17.3 mg, 25.9 mg (25% IR/75% ER).

Dosage Guidance:
• Intermediate-acting (Ritalin SR, Metadate ER, Methylin ER):
 – Titrate to effective daily dose with IR, then switch to equivalent eight-hour SR or ER dose QAM–BID.
• Long-acting (Aptensio XR, Metadate CD, Ritalin LA, Quillivant XR, Quillichew ER):
 – Start 10–20 mg QAM, ↑ by 10–20 mg/day at weekly intervals; max 60 mg/day.
• Long-acting (Adhansia XR):
 – Start 25 mg QAM, ↑ by 10–15 mg/day at weekly intervals; max 70 mg/day (children) and 85 mg/day (adults).
• Long-acting (Cotempla XR-ODT):
 – Start 17.3 mg QAM, ↑ by 8.6–17.3 mg/day at weekly intervals; max 51.8 mg/day.
 – 8.6 mg, 17.3 mg, 25.9 mg equivalent to 10 mg, 20 mg, 30 mg of other methylphenidate formulations, respectively.
• Long-acting (Concerta):
 – Start 18–36 mg QAM, ↑ by 18 mg/day at weekly intervals; max 72 mg/day.
 – Children ≥6 years: Start 18 mg QAM, ↑ by 18 mg/day in weekly intervals to max 54 mg/day (ages 6–12) or 72 mg/day (age 13+).
• Jornay PM:
 – Start 20 mg daily in the evening and increase by 20 mg/day up to maximum of 100 mg/day. Adjust timing between 6:30 and 9:30 p.m.
• Narcolepsy: Start 10–20 mg ER QAM, ↑ by 10 mg/day at weekly intervals; max 60 mg/day.

Monitoring: ECG if history of cardiac disease.

Cost: $$; Concerta: $$$; Aptensio XR, Cotempla XR-ODT, Jornay PM, Quillivant XR, Quillichew ER: $$$$

Side Effects and Mechanism, Pharmacokinetics, and Drug Interactions:
See methylphenidate IR fact sheet.

Clinical Pearls:
• **ER capsules** contain a mixture of 30% IR and 70% ER beads. **Aptensio XR** contains a mixture of 40% IR and 60% ER beads, whereas Adhansia XR contains 20% IR and 80% ER. **Ritalin LA** and its generic ER capsules are a combination of 50% IR and 50% DR beads. These products mimic BID dosing of IR. **Cotempla XR-ODT** delivers a mixture of 25% IR and 75% ER in an orally disintegrating extended-release formulation. **Jornay PM** is dosed in the evening; if early-morning awakening occurs, dose earlier in evening.
• **Concerta** is based on the OROS osmotic delivery system (also used for Invega). 22% of the dose is immediate (with effects in one to two hours) and 78% is delayed.

METHYLPHENIDATE TRANSDERMAL (Daytrana) Fact Sheet

Bottom Line:
Daytrana is helpful for kids who, for whatever reason, cannot use any of the wide variety of oral stimulant preparations. Otherwise, we don't recommend it due to high cost, lag time for onset of effect, and the side effect of rash, which is pretty common and unpleasant.

FDA Indications:
ADHD (children ≥6 years).

Dosage Forms:
Transdermal patch: 10 mg, 15 mg, 20 mg, 30 mg/9 hour.

Dosage Guidance:
Start 10 mg/9 hour patch QAM (for initial therapy or for patients switching from other methylphenidate preparations, regardless of dose). Apply to hip two hours before an effect is needed and remove nine hours after application (drug effects may persist for five hours after removal). Increase dose at weekly intervals by using next higher dose system. May be removed sooner if shorter duration is desired or if late-day side effects occur. Rotate application sites. Max 30 mg QD.

Monitoring: ECG if history of cardiac disease.

Cost: $$$$

Side Effects:
- Most common: Headache, insomnia, irritability, decreased appetite, anorexia, nausea, tics, application site reaction (10%–40% incidence in children).
- Serious but rare: Allergic contact dermatitis/sensitization, characterized by intense local reactions (eg, edema, papules) that may spread beyond patch site; sensitization may subsequently manifest systemically with other routes of methylphenidate administration.

Mechanism, Pharmacokinetics, and Drug Interactions:
- Stimulant that inhibits reuptake of dopamine and norepinephrine.
- Hepatic metabolism via carboxylesterase CES1A1, not CYP450 isoenzymes; t ½: 3–4 hours.
- Avoid use with MAOIs, antacids.

Clinical Pearls:
- Apply patch to clean, dry area of the hip; don't apply to waistline or to areas under tight clothes, as it may rub off. Alternate sites daily (eg, opposite hip). Absorption not affected by perspiration. Remove after nine hours. If dislodged, replace with a new patch but remove within the nine-hour total wear time.
- Clinical effect usually seen in two hours and lasts approximately 12 hours.
- Exposure of application site to a heat source (eg, hair dryer, heating pad, electric blanket) may increase the amount of drug absorbed.
- For localized skin reactions (redness at site), use cortisone cream (1%–2%). For more severe or systemic reactions, discontinue patch.
- In June 2015, the FDA added a warning that Daytrana could cause chemical leukoderma, a permanent loss of skin color. These reactions are irreversible and not harmful but can be disfiguring. Instruct patients to contact their physician if they notice skin color changes or lightening of skin areas; in such cases an alternative medication should be considered.

Fun Fact:
Since 2006, Shire Pharmaceuticals has issued at least 10 recalls of Daytrana patches because users have had difficulty removing the protective cover from the patch. Recall costs have reached into the millions.

MIXED AMPHETAMINE SALTS (Adderall, Adderall XR, Mydayis) Fact Sheet [G]

Bottom Line:

Adderall contains 75% dextroamphetamine and 25% levoamphetamine. This ratio of amphetamine isomers is effective but is probably the most abused and diverted of all prescription stimulants.

FDA Indications:

ADHD (adults and children ≥3 years for IR, ≥6 years for XR, ≥13 years for Mydayis); **narcolepsy** (adults and children ≥6 years).

Off-Label Uses:

Obesity; treatment-resistant depression.

Dosage Forms:

- **Tablets (G):** 5 mg, 7.5 mg, 10 mg, 12.5 mg, 15 mg, 20 mg, 30 mg.
- **ER capsules (G):** 5 mg, 10 mg, 15 mg, 20 mg, 25 mg, 30 mg.
- **ER capsules (Mydayis):** 12.5 mg, 25 mg, 37.5 mg, 50 mg.

Dosage Guidance:

- ADHD:
  - Rule of thumb for both preparations: Initial dose should be 0.5 mg/kg, but shoot for a target dose of 1.0–1.2 mg/kg.
  - Adults:
    - IR: Start 5 QAM–BID, max 40 mg/day divided BID.
    - ER: Start 20 mg QAM, increase to max 60 mg/day QAM. For Mydayis, start 12.5 mg QAM, increase in increments of 12.5 mg/day weekly, to max 50 mg/day.
  - Children and adolescents:
    - IR: Start 2.5–5 mg BID, max 40 mg/day divided BID.
    - ER: Start 5–10 mg QAM, increase gradually to max 30 mg/day, or 40 mg/day QAM in adolescents. For Mydayis (adolescents ≥13 years), start 12.5 mg QAM, increase in increments of 12.5 mg/day weekly, to max 25 mg/day.
- Narcolepsy: Start 10 mg QAM, increase by 10 mg/day at weekly increments; max 60 mg/day.

Monitoring: ECG if history of cardiac disease.

Cost: IR/ER: $; Mydayis: $$$$

Side Effects:

- Most common: Insomnia, headache, decreased appetite, abdominal pain, weight loss, agitation.
- Serious but rare: See class warnings in chapter introduction.

Mechanism, Pharmacokinetics, and Drug Interactions:

- Stimulant that inhibits reuptake of dopamine and norepinephrine.
- Metabolized primarily through CYP2D6; t ½: 9–14 hours. Duration of action: 6–8 hours (IR), 8–12 hours (XR).
- Avoid use with MAOIs, antacids. Caution with 2D6 inhibitors, which may increase stimulant effects.

Clinical Pearls:

- Each dose contains a mixture of amphetamine salts, resulting in a 75:25 ratio of dextro- and levo-isomers of amphetamine.
- When converting from IR to ER, use the same total daily dose, given QAM.
- Adderall may provide more of a "kick" than methylphenidate preparations. Roughly twice as potent (per mg) as methylphenidate.
- Mydayis is formulated with pH-dependent drug-releasing beads, with IR and DR beads that release drug at pH 5.5 and 7.0. Duration of effect may be up to 16 hours.
- Dextroamphetamine and mixed amphetamine salts are the only stimulants approved for children <6 years (approved for children ≥3 years), with the exception of Mydayis, which causes very high rates of side effects (insomnia, reduced appetite) in children <13 years and should only be used in children ≥13 years.

Fun Fact:

Was briefly pulled from the market in Canada in 2005 because of cardiac concerns.

VILOXAZINE XR (Qelbree) Fact Sheet

Bottom Line:
Like the first norepinephrine reuptake inhibitor for ADHD, atomoxetine, viloxazine has no abuse potential and is less likely than stimulants to cause insomnia, anxiety, or tics. However, it is generally less effective than stimulants and takes longer to work. It's unclear if it has any advantage, and unlike atomoxetine, there's no option for a cheaper generic.

FDA Indications:
ADHD (adults, children ≥6 years).

Off-Label Uses:
Treatment-resistant depression.

Dosage Forms:
ER capsules: 100 mg, 150 mg, 200 mg.

Dosage Guidance:
- Children 6–11: Start 100 mg QD, ↑ by 100 mg/day at weekly intervals to max 400 mg QD.
- Children 12–17: Start 200 mg QD, ↑ by 200 mg after one week to max 400 mg QD.

Monitoring: Baseline renal function.

Cost: $$$$

Side Effects:
- Most common: Somnolence, decreased appetite, fatigue, nausea, vomiting, insomnia, irritability.
- Serious but rare: Class warning for suicidal ideation in children and teens. Mania reported. May increase pulse and BP.

Mechanism, Pharmacokinetics, and Drug Interactions:
- Selective norepinephrine reuptake inhibitor (NRI).
- Metabolized primarily via CYP2D6, UGT1A9, UGTB15; t ½: 7 hours.
- Avoid use with MAOIs. Strong 1A2 inhibitor; exercise caution with 1A2 substrates with narrow therapeutic index (eg, clozapine, duloxetine, ramelteon, tasimelteon, tizanidine, theophylline) as combination may increase side effects of substrate.

Clinical Pearls:
- ER capsules, so do not cut, crush, or chew; can open and sprinkle contents in applesauce.
- Adjust dose in severe renal impairment (eGFR <30 mL/min); max 200 mg/day.
- Data from one of four studies suggest viloxazine may work a bit faster than atomoxetine (week one vs week three), but this finding is not based on head-to-head data and it's hard to know whether it is clinically significant.

Fun Fact:
Viloxazine has been studied for various indications since the 1970s and originally received an FDA orphan drug designation for narcolepsy.

Antidepressants

GENERAL PRESCRIBING TIPS

It's particularly hard to suggest a first-line antidepressant prescription because antidepressants are effective for so many other conditions. Nonetheless, it's helpful to review the most common clinical scenarios.

Medication-Naïve Patients With "Just" Depression

For these patients (admittedly unusual in a psychiatric practice), you want something effective and with minimal side effects. This means either an SSRI or bupropion. While most of us start with an SSRI, we recommend considering bupropion as your go-to first-line agent. With bupropion, you get an effective antidepressant with essentially no sexual side effects, no weight gain, no sedation, and a boost in attention. While it has not been approved for any anxiety disorders, bupropion is just as effective as SSRIs for the nonspecific anxiety that usually accompanies depression. On the downside, you have potential insomnia, and, at doses above 300 mg/day, a small risk of seizure.

If you start with an SSRI, go with escitalopram or sertraline. Both have minimal side effects and minimal drug-drug interactions.

Patients Who Have Comorbid Conditions

Patients with depression plus another psychiatric disorder can be tried on "two-fer" meds—that is, antidepressants that have clear efficacy for two conditions. Here are some of the common secondary conditions and meds that are effective for them: anxiety disorders (TCAs, SSRIs), bulimia (fluoxetine), smoking cessation (bupropion), ADHD (bupropion), fibromyalgia (duloxetine), diabetic neuropathic pain (duloxetine), and premenstrual dysphoric disorder (SSRIs). Finally, mirtazapine—an antidepressant sometimes shunned because it causes weight gain—is an excellent choice for patients with depression who are underweight and have insomnia, and it has the benefit of no sexual side effects.

Patients Who Have Been on Other Antidepressants

"Treatment-resistant depression" is usually defined as the failure of at least two prior trials of antidepressants at adequate doses and for adequate lengths of time. There are unfortunately no convincing data on what your next step should be. The STAR*D trial tried to tease out strategies such as switching vs augmenting, but it could not find statistical differences between the techniques. That means we're left with a combination of the few clinical trials that have been published, leavened with a great deal of personal preference. Here's a reasonable approach:

- First, try switching to an antidepressant in a different class (though some clinicians believe that the best next step is to augment; see the bullet below). Assuming the treatment failures were on SSRIs, the usual sequence of subsequent trials would be: 1) bupropion or mirtazapine; 2) an SNRI (venlafaxine, duloxetine, levomilnacipran); 3) an MAOI or a tricyclic.

- Second, try a combination. A suggested order of combinations is: 1) SSRI/SNRI + bupropion; 2) SSRI/SNRI + second-generation antipsychotic; 3) SSRI/SNRI + lithium or thyroid supplementation (we've included a thyroid fact sheet in this chapter). There are many more combination possibilities, but these are probably the highest-yield options with which to begin.

- Third, consider the neurostimulation devices, such as ECT, TMS, and others. You'll find more details on these options in our chapter on somatic treatments.

Class Warnings

There are some side effects or warnings that apply to **all** antidepressants. They are listed here in order to minimize repetition in the fact sheets that follow:

- *Suicide risk.* In 2004, the FDA added a black box warning to the labeling of all antidepressants regarding an increased risk of suicidal ideation in children and adolescents. The warning was based on retrospective reports that showed a very slight increase in suicidal ideation in patients on nine different antidepressants. The warning was revised in 2007 to include adolescents and young adults, up to age 24. Since then, more prospective data have emerged that do not support an association, and this warning has been called into question. For now, however, the warning remains and is applied to the labeling of all medications approved for the treatment of depression. Thus, you should monitor all patients closely—especially early in therapy or after medication discontinuation—for clinical worsening, changes in behavior, or suicidality.

- *Mania switch.* Activation of mania or hypomania may occur with the use of any antidepressant in individuals who are at risk. Antidepressants should be used with caution in patients with a history of mania or hypomania, or in those with a family history of bipolar disorder.

- *Serotonin syndrome.* A rare but potentially life-threatening condition called serotonin syndrome (agitation, hallucinations, other mental status changes, hyperthermia, tachycardia, labile BP, myoclonus, hyperreflexia, incoordination, nausea, vomiting, diarrhea) has been reported when serotonergic antidepressants are used with other serotonergic agents (including SSRIs, SNRIs, buspirone, lithium, and MAOIs). See our new fact sheet on serotonin syndrome in the Side Effect Management chapter.

- *Discontinuation syndrome.* Abrupt discontinuation of antidepressants, particularly SSRIs and SNRIs, may result in a discontinuation syndrome. These symptoms usually begin within a few days of stopping the antidepressant. While not medically dangerous and generally self-limiting, the syndrome may be uncomfortable for patients. Symptoms include dizziness, nausea, headache, irritability, insomnia, diarrhea, agitation, sensory disturbances (eg, electric shock sensations), lethargy, and abnormal dreams. In general, symptoms are more severe with higher-dose and longer-term antidepressant use. Agents that are particularly short-acting may have a higher likelihood of causing a discontinuation syndrome (eg, paroxetine, venlafaxine) compared to longer-acting agents (eg, fluoxetine). In cases of planned discontinuation, antidepressant dose should be gradually reduced; a rule of thumb is to taper by 25% each week for a four-week taper, but if there are discontinuation symptoms, you may have to slow this down to a several-month taper.

Table 3: Risk of Discontinuation Syndrome With Various Antidepressants and Recommendations for Management

Antidepressant	Possibility of Discontinuation Syndrome	Recommendations
Paroxetine, fluvoxamine, venlafaxine	Highest risk	Very gradual taper (4–12 weeks); consider switching to fluoxetine, then taper
Citalopram, duloxetine, escitalopram, MAOIs, sertraline, TCAs, vilazodone, vortioxetine	Moderate risk	Gradual taper (1–4 weeks)
Bupropion, mirtazapine	Low risk	Rapid taper (2–7 days)
Fluoxetine	Lowest risk	Can be stopped abruptly

Strategies for minimizing discontinuation symptoms:

- Switch to fluoxetine for one to two weeks. Fluoxetine can then typically be stopped abruptly without discontinuation symptoms because it self-tapers due to a long half-life and active metabolite with even longer half-life.
- Benzodiazepines can be helpful in mitigating discontinuation symptoms such as anxiety and insomnia.

- *Bleeding risk.* Increased bleeding episodes (eg, GI bleed, bruising, nosebleed) have been reported with serotonergic antidepressants, particularly when they are used concomitantly with aspirin, NSAIDs, anticoagulants, or antiplatelet agents. Occasionally, surgeons will request that patients stop SSRIs before surgery in order to decrease the bleeding risk. While this practice does not reflect the standard of care, it might be reasonable in situations where the risk of bleeding is especially high.

- *Hyponatremia.* Antidepressants can cause hyponatremia particularly in elderly patients; the risk seems to be greater with SSRIs and SNRIs. In rare severe cases, this can lead to delirium, seizures, or death. Use caution in the elderly, especially if there is a comorbid risk for hyponatremia (eg, diuretic use, congestive heart failure, renal impairment, dehydration) and check the sodium level if a patient presents with confusion, weakness, or lethargy.

Switching Antidepressants

When switching from one antidepressant to another, you have two main choices: an immediate switch or a cross-taper. The immediate switch is usually associated with switching between two meds with the same mechanism of action. For example, consider a patient who is switched from 50 mg of sertraline to 20 mg of citalopram. On the morning she starts citalopram, there will still be some sertraline in her serum, but there's no significant drug interaction between them, and both drugs block serotonin reuptake. On the other hand, when switching from paroxetine to vortioxetine, you may need more caution. Any paroxetine in the serum could slow down vortioxetine's metabolism, potentially causing doubling of vortioxetine levels and increasing risk of nausea. In this case, you would taper down the dose of paroxetine before starting vortioxetine—at a lower dose than normal.

In the table below, we list a variety of switching situations along with recommendations on how the switching should be accomplished.

Table 4: Recommended Strategies for Switching Antidepressants

Switch From...	Switch To...	Recommended Strategy
SSRI	Other SSRI, SNRI, bupropion, mirtazapine, vortioxetine, vilazodone	Immediate switch (stop SSRI, start new antidepressant the next day); exception is paroxetine, which should be tapered gradually
SSRI	TCA	Immediate switch if switching from citalopram, escitalopram, or sertraline; cross-taper if switching from fluoxetine or paroxetine (due to inhibition of TCA metabolism)
SNRI	SNRI	Immediate switch (stop SNRI, start new SNRI the next day)
Bupropion	All antidepressants	Switching to or from bupropion can be immediate, with the exception of switching from fluoxetine or paroxetine, both of which can increase blood levels and potentially incur the risk of seizure
MAOIs	All antidepressants	At least 1 week washout of SSRI (6 weeks if fluoxetine) and other antidepressants before starting MAOI; 2 weeks washout if switching from MAOI to other agents due to irreversible inhibition of monoamine oxidase enzymes and the 2 weeks it takes to regenerate enzymes

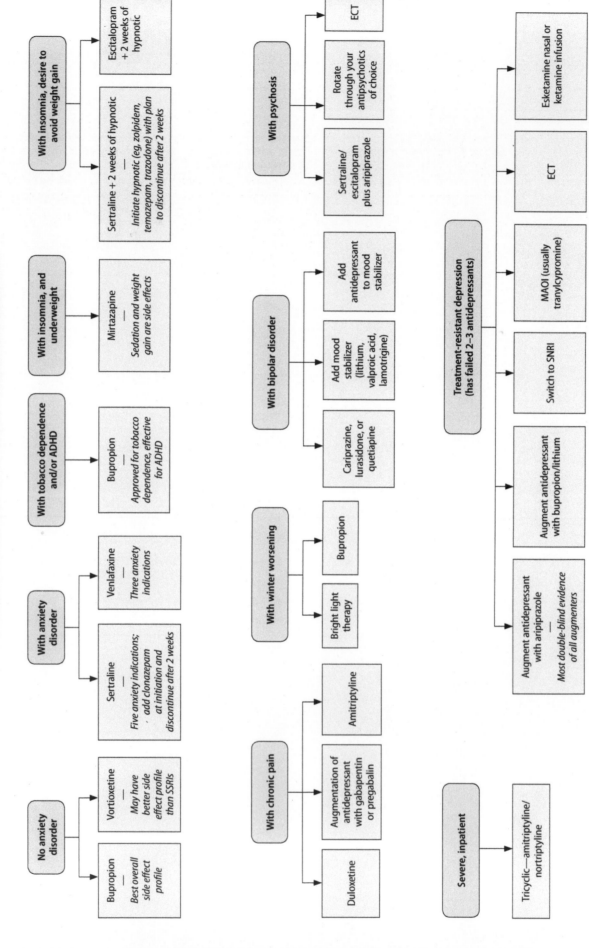

Depression Treatment Algorithm

No anxiety disorder
- Bupropion — Best overall side effect profile
- Vortioxetine — May have better side effect profile than SSRIs

With anxiety disorder
- Sertraline — Five anxiety indications; add clonazepam at initiation and discontinue after 2 weeks
- Venlafaxine — Three anxiety indications

With tobacco dependence and/or ADHD
- Bupropion — Approved for tobacco dependence, effective for ADHD

With insomnia, and underweight
- Mirtazapine — Sedation and weight gain are side effects

With insomnia, desire to avoid weight gain
- Sertraline + 2 weeks of hypnotic — Initiate hypnotic (eg, zolpidem, temazepam, trazodone) with plan to discontinue after 2 weeks
- Escitalopram + 2 weeks of hypnotic

With chronic pain
- Duloxetine
- Augmentation of antidepressant with gabapentin or pregabalin
- Amitriptyline

With winter worsening
- Bright light therapy
- Bupropion

With bipolar disorder
- Cariprazine, lurasidone, or quetiapine
- Add mood stabilizer (lithium, valproic acid, lamotrigine)
- Add antidepressant to mood stabilizer

With psychosis
- Sertraline/ escitalopram plus aripiprazole
- Rotate through your antipsychotics of choice
- ECT

Severe, inpatient
- Tricyclic—amitriptyline/ nortriptyline

Treatment-resistant depression (has failed 2–3 antidepressants)
- Augment antidepressant with aripiprazole — Most double-blind evidence of all augmenters
- Augment antidepressant with bupropion/lithium
- Switch to SNRI
- MAOI (usually tranylcypromine)
- ECT
- Esketamine nasal or ketamine infusion

Treatment-Resistant Depression Treatment Algorithm

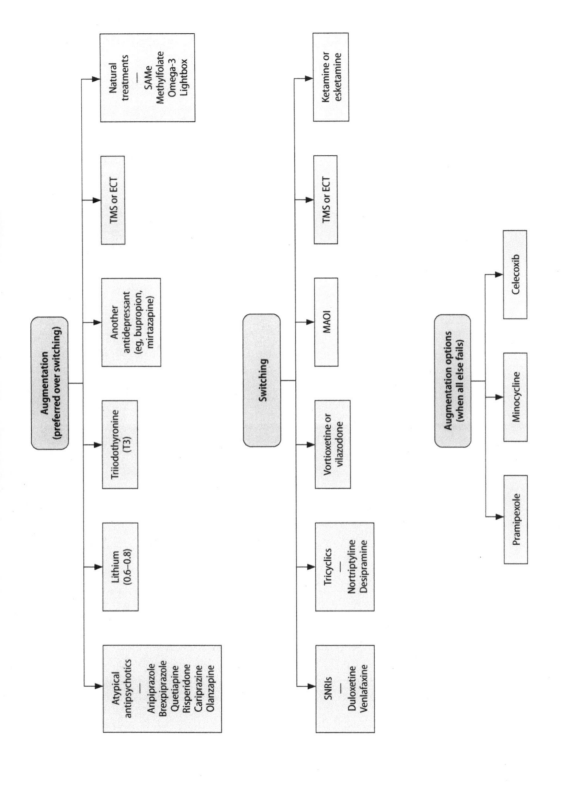

Augmentation (preferred over switching)

- Atypical antipsychotics
  —
  Aripiprazole
  Brexpiprazole
  Quetiapine
  Risperidone
  Cariprazine
  Olanzapine
- Lithium (0.6–0.8)
- Triiodothyronine (T3)
- Another antidepressant (eg, bupropion, mirtazapine)
- TMS or ECT
- Natural treatments
  —
  SAMe
  Methylfolate
  Omega-3
  Lightbox

Switching

- SNRIs
  —
  Duloxetine
  Venlafaxine
- Tricyclics
  —
  Nortriptyline
  Desipramine
- Vortioxetine or vilazodone
- MAOI
- TMS or ECT
- Ketamine or esketamine

Augmentation options (when all else fails)

- Pramipexole
- Minocycline
- Celecoxib

Table 5: Antidepressants

Generic Name (Brand Name) Year FDA Approved [G] denotes generic availability	Relevant FDA Indication(s)	Available Strengths (mg)	Usual Adult Dosage Range (starting–max) (mg)
Selective Serotonin Reuptake Inhibitors (SSRIs)			
Citalopram [G] (Celexa) 1998	MDD	10, 20, 40, 10/5 mL	20–40
Escitalopram [G] (Lexapro) 2002	MDD (12+ yrs), GAD	5, 10, 20, 5/5 mL	10–20
Fluoxetine [G] (Prozac) 1987	MDD (8+ yrs), OCD (7+ yrs), panic disorder, bulimia, PMDD	10, 20, 40, 60, 20/5 mL	20–80
Fluoxetine DR [G] (Prozac Weekly) 2001	MDD maintenance	90 DR	90 Qweek
Fluvoxamine [G] Luvox brand discontinued; generic only 1994	OCD (8+ yrs)	25, 50, 100	50–300
Fluvoxamine ER [G] (Luvox CR) 2008	OCD	100, 150 ER	100–300
Paroxetine [G] (Paxil) 1992 (Pexeva) 2003 (Brisdelle) 2013	MDD, OCD, panic disorder, social anxiety, GAD, PTSD, PMDD, menopausal hot flashes (as Brisdelle)	7.5 (Brisdelle), 10, 20, 30, 40, 10/5 mL	20–60
Paroxetine CR [G] (Paxil CR) 1999	MDD, panic disorder, social anxiety, PMDD	12.5, 25, 37.5 ER	25–62.5
Sertraline [G] (Zoloft) 1991	MDD, OCD (6+ yrs), panic disorder, PTSD, PMDD, social anxiety	25, 50, 100, 150, 200, 20/mL	50–200
Serotonin Norepinephrine Reuptake Inhibitors (SNRIs)			
Desvenlafaxine [G] (Pristiq) 2008	MDD	25, 50, 100 ER	50–100
Duloxetine [G] (Cymbalta) 2004 (Drizalma Sprinkle) 2019	MDD, GAD (7+ yrs) (also diabetic peripheral neuropathy, fibromyalgia, chronic musculoskeletal pain)	20, 30, 40, 60 DR	40–120
Levomilnacipran (Fetzima) 2013	MDD	20, 40, 80, 120 ER	20–120
Venlafaxine [G] 1993 Effexor brand discontinued; generic only	MDD	25, 37.5, 50, 75, 100	75–375
Venlafaxine ER [G] (Effexor XR) 1997	MDD, GAD, social anxiety disorder, panic disorder	37.5, 75, 150, 225 ER	75–225
Tricyclic Antidepressants (TCAs)			
Amitriptyline [G] Elavil brand discontinued; generic only 1961	MDD	10, 25, 50, 75, 100, 150	50–300
Clomipramine [G] (Anafranil) 1989	OCD (10+ yrs)	25, 50, 75	25–250
Desipramine [G] (Norpramin) 1964	MDD	10, 25, 50, 75, 100, 150	50–300

Generic Name (Brand Name) Year FDA Approved [G] denotes generic availability	Relevant FDA Indication(s)	Available Strengths (mg)	Usual Adult Dosage Range (starting–max) (mg)
Imipramine [G] Tofranil brand discontinued; generic only 1984	MDD	10, 25, 50, 75, 100, 125, 150	25–300
Nortriptyline [G] (Pamelor) 1977	MDD	10, 25, 50, 75, 10/5 mL	25–150
Monoamine Oxidase Inhibitors (MAOIs)			
Isocarboxazid (Marplan) 1959	MDD	10	20–60
Phenelzine [G] (Nardil) 1961	MDD	15	45–90
Selegiline transdermal (Emsam) 2006	MDD	6, 9, 12/24 hr patch	6–12/24 hr
Tranylcypromine [G] (Parnate) 1961	MDD	10	30–60
Other Antidepressants			
Brexanolone (Zulresso) 2019	Postpartum depression	100 mg/20 mL vial for injection	30–90 mcg/kg/hr continuous intravenous infusion over 60 hours
Bupropion [G] (Wellbutrin) 1985	MDD	75, 100	200–450
Bupropion SR [G] (Wellbutrin SR) 1996	MDD, smoking cessation	100, 150, 200	150–400
Bupropion XL [G] (Forfivo XL, Wellbutrin XL) 2003	MDD, seasonal affective disorder	150, 300 (Wellbutrin XL), 450 (Forfivo XL)	150–450
Esketamine (Spravato) 2019	Treatment-resistant depression, MDD with suicidality; used in conjunction with oral antidepressant	28 mg per nasal spray device	56–84 twice weekly to every 2 weeks
Ketamine [G] (Ketalar) 1970	Not indicated but used for severe or suicidal depression	10, 50, 100 mg/mL vial for injection	0.5 mg/kg intravenous infusion over 40 minutes
Mirtazapine [G] (Remeron) 1996	MDD	7.5, 15, 30, 45	15–45
Mirtazapine ODT [G] (Remeron SolTab) 2001	MDD	15, 30, 45	15–45
Nefazodone [G] Serzone brand discontinued; generic only 1994	MDD	50, 100, 150, 200, 250	200–600
Trazodone [G] Desyrel brand discontinued; generic only 1981	MDD	50, 100, 150, 300	50–600
Vilazodone (Viibryd) 2011	MDD	10, 20, 40	10–40
Vortioxetine (Trintellix) 2013	MDD	5, 10, 20	10–20

Antidepressants

Table 5A: Selective Serotonin Reuptake Inhibitors (SSRIs)

Generic Name (Brand Name) [G] denotes generic availability	Uses (FDA-indicated uses in bold)	Usual Dosage Range (starting–max) (mg)	Metabolized by (major pathways in bold)	Inhibits (potent inhibition in bold)	Elimination Half-Life	Cost (for generic, unless otherwise specified)
Citalopram [G] (Celexa)	**MDD**, OCD, PTSD, social anxiety, GAD, panic disorder, PMDD	20–40 QD Increase by 20 mg/day in 7 days	**2C19, 3A4**	2D6 (weak)	35 hrs	$
Escitalopram [G] (Lexapro)	**MDD (12+ yrs), GAD,** OCD, PTSD, social anxiety, panic disorder, PMDD	10–20 QD Increase by 10 mg/day in 7 days	**2C19, 3A4**	2D6 (weak)	27–32 hrs	$ Liquid: $$
Fluoxetine [G] (Prozac, Prozac Weekly)	**MDD (8+ yrs), OCD (7+ yrs),** panic disorder, bulimia, **PMDD,** PTSD, social anxiety	20–80 QAM Increase by 10 mg/day after several weeks (Starting dose DR: 90 Qweek)	**2D6**	**2C9/19, 2D6,** 3A4	4–6 days fluoxetine; 9 days norfluoxetine (metabolite)	$ Weekly: $$$ Sarafem: $$$$$
Fluvoxamine [G] (Luvox, Luvox CR)	**MDD, OCD (8+ yrs), panic disorder, GAD,** PTSD	50–300 QHS Increase by 50 mg/day Qweek (Starting dose CR: 100 QHS)	**1A2, 2D6**	**1A2, 2C9, 2C19, 3A4**	16 hrs	$ ER: $$$
Paroxetine [G] (Brisdelle, Paxil, Paxil CR, Pexeva)	**MDD, OCD, panic disorder, social anxiety, GAD, PTSD, PMDD, menopausal hot flashes (as Brisdelle),** premature ejaculation	20–60 QHS CR: 25–62.5 QD Increase by 10 mg/day Qweek; CR: 12.5 mg/day Qweek	**2D6**	**2D6**	21 hrs	$ ER: $$ Brisdelle: $$$ Liquid, Pexeva: $$$$
Sertraline [G] (Zoloft)	**MDD, OCD (6+ yrs), panic disorder, PTSD, PMDD, social anxiety,** GAD	50–200 QD Increase by 50 mg/day Qweek	**2C19,** 2D6, 3A4	2D6 (weak; moderate at high dose), 3A4 (weak)	26 hrs	$

Table 6: Relative Side Effects of Antidepressants

Drug	Nausea/Diarrhea	Insomnia/Agitation	Sedation/Drowsiness	Sexual Dysfunction	Weight Gain	Anticholinergic	Orthostatic Hypotension	Increased BP, P, Sweating	QT Prolongation
Selective Serotonin Reuptake Inhibitors (SSRIs)									
Citalopram [G] (Celexa)	+	+	-	+++	+	-	-	-	+++
Escitalopram [G] (Lexapro)	+	+	-	+++	+	-	-	-	++
Fluoxetine [G] (Prozac)	+	+++	-	+++	-	-	-	-	+
Fluvoxamine [G] (Luvox, Luvox CR)	+	+	++	+++	+	-	-	-	+
Paroxetine [G] (Paxil, Paxil CR)	+	+	++	++++	++	+	+	-	+
Sertraline [G] (Zoloft)	++	+	-	+++	+	-	-	-	+
Serotonin Norepinephrine Reuptake Inhibitors (SNRIs)									
Desvenlafaxine [G] (Pristiq)	++	+	+	++	+	-	-	+	-
Duloxetine [G] (Cymbalta, Drizalma)	++	+	-	++	+	-	-	+	-
Levomilnacipran (Fetzima)	++	+	-	++	+	-	-	++	-
Venlafaxine [G] (Effexor, Effexor XR)	++	+	+	++	+	-	-	+	+
Tricyclic Antidepressants (TCAs)									
Amitriptyline [G] (Elavil)	-	-	++++	+++	+++	++++	+++	-	+++
Clomipramine [G] (Anafranil)	-	+	++++	+++	+++	++++	+++	-	+++
Desipramine [G] (Norpramin)	-	+	++	+++	+++	++	++	-	++
Imipramine [G] (Tofranil)	-	-	++++	+++	+++	++++	+++	-	+++
Nortriptyline [G] (Pamelor)	-	-	++	+++	+++	++	++	-	++
Monoamine Oxidase Inhibitors (MAOIs)									
Isocarboxazid (Marplan)	-	++	+	+++	++	+	++	-	-

Drug	Nausea/ Diarrhea	Insomnia/ Agitation	Sedation/ Drowsiness	Sexual Dysfunction	Weight Gain	Anticholinergic	Orthostatic Hypotension	Increased BP, P, Sweating	QT Prolongation
Phenelzine [G] (Nardil)	-	+	++	+++	++	+	++	-	-
Selegiline transdermal (Emsam)	-	+	-	-	-	+	+	-	-
Tranylcypromine [G] (Parnate)	-	++	+	+++	+	+	++	-	-
Other Antidepressants									
Bupropion [G] (Wellbutrin SR, XL, Forfivo)	+	+++	-	-	-	-	-	-	-
Mirtazapine [G] (Remeron)	-	-	+++	-	+++	-	-	-	-
Nefazodone [G] (Serzone)	++	-	+++	-	-	-	++	-	-
Trazodone [G] (Desyrel)	+	-	++++	+	-	-	++	-	+
Vilazodone (Viibryd)	++++	++	-	++	-	-	-	-	-
Vortioxetine (Trintellix)	++++	-	-	++	-	-	-	-	-

BREXANOLONE (Zulresso) Fact Sheet

Bottom Line:

Brexanolone is a novel, fast-acting option that is given intravenously for women with severe postpartum depression. However, its utility is limited by the lengthy infusion (60 hours) in a health care setting, potential for severe reactions and associated need for close monitoring, high cost ($34,000 for the drug alone, plus costs associated with providers and health care facilities), and lack of follow-up data beyond 30 days.

FDA Indications:

Postpartum depression.

Dosage Forms:

Vial for injection: 100 mg/20 mL.

Dosage Guidance:

Dosing is gradually titrated up and then tapered off over a 60-hour administration period. Start 30 mcg/kg/hour for hours 0–4, 60 mcg/kg/hour for hours 4–24, 90 mcg/kg/hour for hours 24–52 (can use 60 mcg/kg/hour for those who don't tolerate 90 mcg/kg/hour), 60 mcg/kg/hour for hours 52–56, and 30 mcg/kg/hour for hours 56–60.

Monitoring: Pulse oximetry.

Cost: $$$$$

Side Effects:

- Most common: Sedation, somnolence, dry mouth, loss of consciousness, flushing.
- Serious but rare: Excessive sedation or loss of consciousness, hypoxia.

Mechanism, Pharmacokinetics, and Drug Interactions:

- Gamma-aminobutyric acid A (GABA$_A$) modulator.
- Metabolized by non-CYP450 pathways; t ½: 9 hours.
- Use caution or avoid use with CNS depressants such as benzodiazepines, which may have additive effects.

Clinical Pearls:

- Brexanolone is a neurosteroid that is chemically identical to endogenous allopregnanolone, a hormone whose levels rise during pregnancy and then fall abruptly after childbirth.
- Approval was based on positive results in two trials of pregnant women with moderate to severe postpartum depression; a statistically significant higher percentage of brexanolone patients remitted compared to placebo (51% vs 16% with 60 mcg/kg/hour and 61% vs 38% with 90 mcg/kg/hour infusion). In the higher-dose patients, 94% maintained response at 30 days.
- Zulresso's use is restricted to patients and health care facilities enrolled in the Zulresso REMS program (www. zulressorems.com). Monitoring for sedation, sudden loss of consciousness, and hypoxia using continuous pulse oximetry with an alarm is required for the duration of the 60-hour infusion.
- If patient experiences excessive sedation during non-sleep periods, the infusion should be stopped and can be resumed at the same or lower dose as clinically appropriate once symptoms resolve.
- For women wishing to breastfeed, sparse data involving 12 women indicate that brexanolone transfer to breast milk is minimal with a relative infant dose of 1%–2% of maternal weight-adjusted dosage. While the risks of adverse effects are not known, the concentrations of the drug in breast milk are low.
- The DEA has designated brexanolone as a Schedule IV controlled substance.
- Zuranolone, a two-week, once-daily oral medication with similar mechanism of action, is in development for postpartum depression.

Fun Fact:

Many psychiatric medications owe their discovery to chance or serendipity. Not so with brexanolone, which was developed by design starting with a series of basic and translational neuroscience studies dating back to the 1980s.

BUPROPION (Wellbutrin, others) Fact Sheet [G]

Bottom Line:
May be particularly useful for individuals whose depression is associated with fatigue and poor concentration. Absence of sexual side effects and weight gain make this an appealing option for many depressed patients. Although not effective for anxiety disorders, it is effective for the anxiety that often accompanies depression. The seizure risk is not a concern for most patients when dosed appropriately.

FDA Indications:
Major depression; seasonal affective disorder; smoking cessation (as Zyban).

Off-Label Uses:
ADHD; sexual dysfunction; bipolar depression.

Dosage Forms:
- **Tablets (G):** 75 mg, 100 mg.
- **SR tablets (G):** 100 mg, 150 mg, 200 mg.
- **ER tablets (G):** 150 mg, 300 mg; **Forfivo XL:** 450 mg.
- **ER tablets, hydrobromide salt formulation (Aplenzin):** 174 mg, 348 mg, 522 mg (equivalent to 150 mg, 300 mg, 450 mg, respectively).

Dosage Guidance:
- General comment: Timing of the dose can be tricky, because taking too much at once increases seizure risk (the risk increases from 300 mg on up). But splitting the dose BID can cause insomnia. For this reason, some clinicians choose to start all patients on the ER formulation, which is released slowly and minimizes peak serum levels—single doses of up to 450 mg are safe.
  - IR: Start 100 mg BID, ↑ to 100 mg TID after >3 days; max dose 450 mg/day, 150 mg/dose; separate doses by at least six hours to minimize seizure risk.
  - SR: Start 150 mg QAM, ↑ to 150 mg BID (usual target dose) as early as fourth day; max dose 400 mg/day, 200 mg/dose; separate doses by at least eight hours to minimize seizure risk.
  - ER: Start 150 mg QAM, ↑ to 300 mg QAM as early as fourth day; max dose 450 mg QAM.
- Seasonal affective disorder: Start 150 mg XR QAM, ↑ to 300 mg XR QAM after seven days (fall through spring). Taper to 150 mg XR QAM for two weeks to discontinue.
- Smoking cessation: Start 150 mg SR QAM for three days, ↑ to 150 mg BID for seven to 12 weeks. Stop smoking after five to seven days of treatment.

Monitoring: No routine monitoring recommended unless clinical picture warrants.

Cost: IR/SR/ER: $; Forfivo: $$$; Aplenzin: $$$$$

Side Effects:
- Most common: Agitation, insomnia, headache, nausea, vomiting, tremor, tachycardia, dry mouth, weight loss.
- Serious but rare: Seizures; risk higher with rapid and large dose increases and in patients at risk for seizures, including those with a seizure history and patients with eating disorders (mainly those with purging-type bulimia). Risk of seizure depends on dose and formulation: IR: 300–450 mg/day (0.4%) vs 450–600 mg/day (4%). SR/ER: 100–300 mg/day (0.1%) vs 400 mg/day (0.4%). Do not chew, divide, or crush SR or ER tablets as risk of seizures may be increased.

Mechanism, Pharmacokinetics, and Drug Interactions:
- Dopamine and norepinephrine receptor uptake inhibitor.
- Metabolized primarily through CYP2B6; inhibits CYP2D6; t ½: 21 hours.
- Avoid use with MAOIs.

Clinical Pearls:
- Before prescribing bupropion, ask patients if they've ever had a seizure or if they've had bulimia—both of which are relative contraindications.
- Forfivo XL offers ease of use (one pill a day) for patients taking 450 mg/day, but it is more expensive.
- Aplenzin brand could also be a one-pill-a-day solution (the 522 mg is equivalent to 450 mg Wellbutrin) but otherwise doesn't offer any real clinical advantage as a different salt (hydrobromide) formulation.
- Give ER dose as early in the morning as possible to minimize insomnia.
- Bupropion can cause false-positive urine test results for amphetamines.

Not-So-Fun Fact:
There have been case reports of teenagers, prisoners, and others snorting crushed tablets of bupropion (believing it to be a stimulant), with subsequent seizures.

CITALOPRAM (Celexa) Fact Sheet [G]

Bottom Line:

Citalopram has a favorable profile in that it's not particularly sedating or activating and has a low risk for drug interactions. However, it has fewer FDA indications than other SSRIs, and its higher risk for QT prolongation makes us favor escitalopram.

FDA Indications:

Major depression.

Off-Label Uses:

OCD; PTSD; social anxiety; generalized anxiety disorder; panic disorder; PMDD.

Dosage Forms:

- **Tablets (G):** 10 mg, 20 mg (scored), 40 mg (scored).
- **Oral solution (G):** 10 mg/5 mL.

Dosage Guidance:

- Start 10–20 mg QD; may ↑ by increments of 10–20 mg/day weekly to max 40 mg QD.
- Most patients take it in the morning, but bedtime dosing is OK if there is no insomnia.
- Max dose is 20 mg/day in patients >60 years of age or in those taking CYP2C19 inhibitors, or who are CYP2C19 poor metabolizers.

Monitoring: Sodium in patients at risk; ECG in patients on doses >40 mg/day, CYP2C19 poor metabolizers, or if cardiac disease.

Cost: $

Side Effects:

- Most common: Nausea, somnolence, sexual side effects, headache.
- Serious but rare: Hyponatremia, mainly in the elderly; gastrointestinal bleeding, especially when combined with NSAIDs such as ibuprofen.

Mechanism, Pharmacokinetics, and Drug Interactions:

- Serotonin reuptake inhibitor.
- Metabolized primarily through CYP2C19 and 3A4; t ½: 35 hours.
- Avoid use with MAOIs (two-week washout period); avoid other serotonergic agents (serotonin syndrome).
- Use caution in patients taking CYP2C19 inhibitors including cimetidine, omeprazole (will increase citalopram levels and potential for QT prolongation).

Clinical Pearl:

The FDA reduced citalopram's maximum daily dose from 60 mg/day to 40 mg/day in August 2011 due to data suggesting increased QTc interval prolongation at doses >40 mg/day. Mean QTc interval prolongation at 60 mg/day was 18.5 msec (vs ziprasidone, which has been shown to increase this interval by 20.6 msec). As of this writing, no comparable warning has been issued for escitalopram.

Fun Fact:

Citalopram given as an intravenous infusion in treatment-resistant OCD and depression has been studied over the last 20 years and is available for use throughout Europe.

CLOMIPRAMINE (Anafranil) Fact Sheet [G]

Bottom Line:
Clomipramine, which has more side effects than SSRIs, is usually considered a second-line medication for OCD.

FDA Indications:
OCD.

Off-Label Uses:
Cataplexy in narcolepsy; sleep terrors; sleepwalking; major depression; panic disorder; pain.

Dosage Forms:
Capsules (Anafranil, [G]): 25 mg, 50 mg, 75 mg.

Dosage Guidance:
- Start 25 mg QHS and ↑ by 25 mg/day every four to seven days to target dose 150–250 mg/day; max 250 mg/day.
- Using divided doses (BID to TID) may help with tolerability during initiation and titration, but can convert to QHS dosing to minimize daytime sedation.

Monitoring: Check clomipramine/norclomipramine levels (trough levels, 12 hours after last dose) in patients on higher doses (150 mg or higher) or in those with significant side effects. Optimal ranges: clomipramine + norclomipramine 220–500 ng/mL. Check ECG if history of cardiac disease.

Cost: $$

Side Effects:
- Most common: Sedation, dry mouth, constipation, weight gain, sexual side effects, urinary hesitation, blurred vision.
- Serious but rare: Seizure (especially at doses greater than 250 mg/day), cardiac effects including orthostasis, arrhythmias, QT prolongation, AV block.

Mechanism, Pharmacokinetics, and Drug Interactions:
- As a tricyclic antidepressant, causes both serotonin and norepinephrine reuptake inhibition (more selective for serotonin).
- Metabolized by CYP1A2, 2C19, 2D6, 3A4; t ½: 32 hours (69 hours for active metabolite).
- Avoid MAOIs and other serotonergic agents. Caution with other anticholinergic agents or potent CYP inhibitors.

Clinical Pearls:
- Clomipramine is the only tricyclic antidepressant that is FDA approved for OCD. Efficacy is likely due to greater selectivity for serotonin reuptake inhibition.
- Used to be considered more effective than SSRIs for OCD, but recent studies show equivalent efficacy.
- Overdose toxicity with potentially serious cardiac effects or fatality with as little as 10-day supply.
- Pharmacokinetics are nonlinear, meaning higher-than-expected levels, longer t ½, and drug accumulation in the higher end of dosing range. Full effects of dosage increase in the higher range may not be seen for two weeks or longer.
- Like other serotonergic agents, discontinuation syndrome may occur with abrupt discontinuation; slow taper recommended.

Fun Fact:
Clomipramine is on the World Health Organization's Model List of Essential Medicines. This list includes the medications considered to be most effective and safe to meet the most important needs in a health system and is frequently used by countries to help determine local essential medicines.

DESVENLAFAXINE (Pristiq) Fact Sheet [G]

Bottom Line:

Desvenlafaxine is the active metabolite of venlafaxine, and it has some minor advantages in terms of drug interactions, ease of dosing, and longer half-life. One disadvantage is lack of FDA approval for anxiety disorders. At least for depression, since desvenlafaxine is now available in a low-cost generic version, some clinicians prefer it over venlafaxine XR.

FDA Indications:

Major depression.

Off-Label Uses:

Fibromyalgia; vasomotor symptoms of menopause; generalized anxiety disorder (GAD); social anxiety disorder; panic disorder; PTSD; PMDD.

Dosage Forms:

ER tablets (G): 25 mg, 50 mg, 100 mg.

Dosage Guidance:

Start 50 mg QD, usually best in the morning due to risk of insomnia. Some patients require increase to 100 mg QD, but dosing above this is not recommended as it only increases side effects without being more efficacious.

Monitoring: Periodic blood pressure.

Cost: $

Side Effects:

- Most common: Nausea, dizziness, insomnia, excessive sweating, constipation, dry mouth, somnolence, decreased appetite, anxiety, sexual side effects.
- Serious but rare: Dose-related increases in systolic and diastolic blood pressure (as likely with desvenlafaxine as venlafaxine). Monitor BP regularly, and if increases are sustained, consider reducing dose or discontinuing.

Mechanism, Pharmacokinetics, and Drug Interactions:

- Serotonin and norepinephrine reuptake inhibitor.
- Active metabolite of venlafaxine, metabolized primarily through conjugation and oxidation via CYP3A4 (minor). Minimally inhibits CYP2D6; t ½: 11 hours.
- Avoid use with MAOIs, other serotonergic medications. Not likely to cause other clinically significant interactions.

Clinical Pearls:

- Potential advantages vs venlafaxine: not significantly metabolized by 2D6, so less concern about drug interactions; less dosage titration needed (starting dose is usually effective, occasionally need to increase to 100 mg daily); longer half-life (11 vs six hours), so potentially less severe discontinuation syndrome.
- Potential disadvantages vs venlafaxine: FDA approval limited to major depression (vs major depression plus GAD, panic disorder, and social anxiety disorder for venlafaxine); flat dose-response curve.
- Desvenlafaxine has not been shown to be any more effective than venlafaxine.
- Recent low-cost generic versions of desvenlafaxine make it about as cheap as venlafaxine.
- Desvenlafaxine is available in two forms: a succinate salt (Pristiq) and a base (Khedezla). Aside from small differences in half-life, there is no difference between these products—all efficacy studies were based on the original Pristiq studies.

Fun Fact:

Desvenlafaxine's manufacturer withdrew its application for approval in the European Union, where regulatory bodies had said that desvenlafaxine was likely less effective than venlafaxine with no advantages in terms of safety and tolerability.

DULOXETINE (Cymbalta, Drizalma Sprinkle) Fact Sheet [G]

Bottom Line:
Duloxetine is the main SNRI alternative to venlafaxine/desvenlafaxine. It has a niche for depressed patients with various comorbid pain syndromes. However, you should balance this advantage against its potentially serious (though rare) hepatic side effects.

FDA Indications:
Major depression; generalized anxiety disorder (GAD) (children ages 7+ and adults); diabetic peripheral neuropathic pain; fibromyalgia; chronic musculoskeletal pain (including osteoarthritis and chronic low back pain).

Off-Label Uses:
Other neuropathic or chronic pain disorders; other anxiety disorders; stress urinary incontinence.

Dosage Forms:
Delayed-release capsules (Drizalma Sprinkle, [G]): 20 mg, 30 mg, 40 mg, 60 mg.

Dosage Guidance:
- Depression and GAD: Start 40–60 mg/day; may be divided (20 or 30 mg BID) or given as a single daily dose; target dose 60 mg QD; for doses >60 mg/day, titrate in increments of 30 mg/day over one week to max 120 mg/day, although doses >60 mg/day not shown to be more effective.
- Fibromyalgia and chronic pain: Start 30 mg QD, increase to target 60 mg QD; max dose 60 mg/day.
- Diabetic neuropathy: Start, target, and maximum dose of 60 mg QD.
- Dose timing: Depends on patient preference, since it causes drowsiness in some but insomnia in others. Let patients experiment until they get it right.

Monitoring: LFTs if suspect liver disease; periodic blood pressure.

Cost: $; Drizalma Sprinkle: $$$

Side Effects:
- Most common: Nausea, dry mouth, constipation, diarrhea, decreased appetite, vomiting, fatigue, insomnia, dizziness, agitation, sweating, headache, urinary hesitation, and sexual side effects.
- Serious but rare: Rare cases of hepatic failure (including fatalities) have been reported (too rare to require routine LFTs in all patients). Hepatitis with abdominal pain, hepatomegaly, elevated transaminases >20 times normal, with and without jaundice observed. May cause orthostatic hypotension or syncope, especially in first week of therapy and after dose increases. Urinary retention reported; hospitalization and/or catheterization were necessary in some cases.

Mechanism, Pharmacokinetics, and Drug Interactions:
- Serotonin and norepinephrine reuptake inhibitor.
- Metabolized primarily through CYP1A2 and 2D6; inhibitor of CYP2D6; t ½: 12 hours.
- Avoid use with MAOIs, other serotonergic medications. Caution with drugs metabolized by CYP2D6 (eg, paroxetine, fluoxetine, aripiprazole, iloperidone, risperidone, atomoxetine, beta blockers) as their levels may be increased. Potent inhibitors of CYP2D6 (eg, paroxetine, fluoxetine, quinidine) and CYP1A2 (eg, fluvoxamine, ciprofloxacin) may increase duloxetine levels.

Clinical Pearls:
- Duloxetine advantages vs venlafaxine: milder discontinuation symptoms; less hypertension; less toxic in overdose; FDA indications for pain syndromes. Duloxetine disadvantages vs venlafaxine: potential hepatic toxicity; greater potential for drug interactions.
- Since capsules are delayed release, they should be swallowed whole; do not chew or crush. Although the manufacturer does not recommend opening the capsules, their contents may be sprinkled on applesauce or in apple juice and swallowed immediately.
- Avoid in patients with a history of heavy alcohol use or chronic hepatic disease because of the possibility that duloxetine and alcohol may interact, causing hepatic injury, or the possibility that duloxetine may aggravate preexisting hepatic disease.
- Drizalma Sprinkle is a new formulation for use in patients with swallowing difficulty, either by sprinkling over applesauce or administering via nasogastric tube.

Fun Fact:
Duloxetine is approved in Europe for stress urinary incontinence, but the FDA refused this indication in the US because of concerns regarding liver toxicity and potential suicidal ideation.

ESCITALOPRAM (Lexapro) Fact Sheet [G]

Bottom Line:
Escitalopram is a good first-line SSRI option. It has the tolerability and minimal drug interaction potential of citalopram with less QTc prolongation risk.

FDA Indications:
Major depression (12+ years); generalized anxiety disorder.

Off-Label Uses:
OCD; PTSD; social anxiety disorder; panic disorder; PMDD.

Dosage Forms:
- **Tablets (G):** 5 mg, 10 mg (scored), 20 mg (scored).
- **Oral solution (G):** 5 mg/5 mL.

Dosage Guidance:
- Adults: Start 5–10 mg QD; may ↑ by increments of 5–10 mg/day weekly to target dose of 10 mg QD or max 20 mg QD.
- Ages 6–9 (off-label): Start 2.5 mg QD, increase by 5 mg/day increments weekly; max 20 mg/day.
- Ages 12–17: Start 5 mg QD, increase by 5–10 mg/day increments weekly; max 20 mg/day.
- Dose timing: Usually well tolerated in the morning.

Monitoring: Sodium in patients at risk.

Cost: $

Side Effects:
- Most common: Nausea, sweating, insomnia, somnolence, sexual side effects, headache.
- Serious but rare: Hyponatremia, mainly in the elderly; gastrointestinal bleeding, especially when combined with NSAIDs such as ibuprofen.

Mechanism, Pharmacokinetics, and Drug Interactions:
- Serotonin reuptake inhibitor.
- Metabolized primarily through CYP2C19 and 3A4; t ½: 27–32 hours.
- Avoid use with MAOIs (two-week washout); avoid other serotonergic agents (serotonin syndrome).

Clinical Pearls:
- Escitalopram (which is purified from the racemic mixture, citalopram) is considered the "purest" SSRI and has few, if any, drug-drug interactions.
- Similar to citalopram, escitalopram demonstrates dose-related QTc prolongation, but to a lesser extent (6.6 msec with 20 mg escitalopram vs 12.6 msec with equivalent 40 mg citalopram). Generally, this amount of prolongation is not clinically significant in patients who don't have additional risk factors.

Fun Fact:
A systematic review and network meta-analysis compared the safety and efficacy of nearly two dozen antidepressants and found escitalopram and sertraline were the most effective (Cipriani A et al, *Lancet* 2018; 391(10128):1357–1366).

ESKETAMINE (Spravato) Fact Sheet

Note: See separate fact sheet for information on off-label ketamine treatment.

Bottom Line:
Esketamine is the s-enantiomer of ketamine, given as a nasal spray. It is only modestly effective for treatment-resistant depression and suicidality; its main advantage is its speed of onset, which is typically 24 hours. FDA requirements mandate that it be given in a health care facility and that patients be monitored for two hours after each treatment. Most clinicians consider it less effective than the unapproved intravenous use of ketamine.

FDA Indications:
Treatment-resistant major depression (TRD) or major depression with acute suicidal ideation or behavior (MDSI), to be used in conjunction with an oral antidepressant.

Off-Label Uses:
Pain, migraine headache.

Dosage Forms:
Nasal spray device: 28 mg per device, to be given in two sprays (one 14 mg spray in each nostril).

Dosage Guidance:
• TRD:
  – Induction phase (weeks one to four): 56 mg on day one, then 56 mg or 84 mg twice a week.
  – Maintenance phase (subsequent weeks): 56 or 84 mg weekly or every two weeks, depending on response.
• MDSI:
  – Start and continue 84 mg twice weekly for four weeks.
• Use two devices (each 28 mg) for a 56 mg dose and three devices for an 84 mg dose, with a five-minute rest period after using each device to allow medication to absorb.
• Patients must be observed by a health care provider when they take the medication and for at least two hours after administration, and they will require transportation after treatment.
• Patients cannot take the nasal spray device home; they must come into the office for all doses.
• Patients should avoid food for two hours before administration and liquids 30 minutes prior, because of the risk of nausea and vomiting.
• Check patients' blood pressure (for possible hypertension) both before dose and 40 minutes after dose.

Monitoring: BP (see Spravato REMS, mentioned in clinical pearls).

Cost: $$$$

Side Effects:
• Most common: Sedation, dissociation (including depersonalization and derealization), increased blood pressure (transient, lasts about four hours), cognitive impairment, impaired ability to drive.
• Serious but rare: Hypertensive crisis. Contraindicated in aneurysmal vascular disease and history of intracerebral hemorrhage. Treatment-emergent suicidality may be more common than with standard antidepressants.

Mechanism, Pharmacokinetics, and Drug Interactions:
• N-methyl-D-aspartate (NMDA) receptor antagonist.
• Time to maximum concentration: 20–40 minutes.
• Metabolized primarily by CYP2B6 and CYP3A4; t ½: 7–12 hours.
• Avoid use with CNS depressants (eg, benzodiazepines, opioids, alcohol), MAOIs, and psychostimulants.

Clinical Pearls:
• Esketamine is the s-isomer of ketamine (which is a mixture of both s-ketamine and r-ketamine). One rationale for the development of esketamine is that the s-isomer is a more potent NMDA antagonist than the r-isomer of ketamine.
• Efficacy: In three four-week trials, patients with TRD were randomly assigned to an oral antidepressant plus either esketamine or placebo nasal spray. Esketamine outperformed placebo in one of these trials. In a longer-term maintenance trial, patients were less likely to relapse when continuing on esketamine than placebo.
• Efficacy may be seen as early as 24 hours after first dose. Appropriate duration of treatment remains unknown.
• Only available through a restricted distribution system, under a Risk Evaluation and Mitigation Strategy (REMS) program. In order to provide esketamine to patients, your clinic must become a "certified Spravato treatment center" (online certification: www.spravatorems.com).
• Controlled substance (Schedule III) due to potential for misuse.

Fun Fact:
Esketamine was granted "breakthrough status" by the FDA. This designation is given to agents intended to treat a serious disease if preliminary evidence suggests they provide substantial improvement over existing treatments.

FLUOXETINE (Prozac, Prozac Weekly) Fact Sheet [G]

Bottom Line:

Fluoxetine's wide spectrum of indications and its long track record make it a go-to SSRI, and it is often favored in patients who could use some activation. Its main disadvantage is its high potential for drug interactions.

FDA Indications:

Major depression (8+ years); OCD (7+ years); panic disorder; bulimia; PMDD (as Sarafem).

Off-Label Uses:

PTSD; social anxiety disorder.

Dosage Forms:

- **Capsules (G):** 10 mg, 20 mg, 40 mg.
- **Tablets (G):** 10 mg, 20 mg, 60 mg.
- **Oral solution (G):** 20 mg/5 mL.
- **Delayed-release capsules (G):** 90 mg.

Dosage Guidance:

- Start 10–20 mg QAM; may ↑ by 10–20 mg/day increments after several weeks; max dose 50 mg/day (depression), 60 mg/day (bulimia, panic disorder). Target and max dose in OCD: 80 mg/day.
- Start 5–10 mg QAM in panic disorder to minimize increased anxiety and panic.
- DR capsules (Prozac Weekly): Start 90 mg Qweek seven days after last dose of 20 mg QAM.
- PMDD (Sarafem): 20 mg QAM continuously or only on cycle days 15–28 (14 days prior to anticipated onset of menstruation).
- In children ages 6–7 (off-label): Start 5 mg QD, increase by 5 mg/day increments weekly; max 30 mg/day. Ages 8–17: Start 10 mg QD, increase by 10 mg/day increments weekly; max 60 mg/day. Many children and adolescents will show good treatment response at 10 mg/day.
- Dose timing: Most respond best to morning dosing given its activating effects.

Monitoring: Sodium in patients at risk.

Cost: $; DR: $$

Side Effects:

- Most common: Nausea, diarrhea, nervousness, insomnia, abnormal dreams, anorexia, sweating, tremor, sexual side effects, headache, rash.
- Serious but rare: Hyponatremia, mainly in the elderly; gastrointestinal bleeding, especially when combined with NSAIDs such as ibuprofen.

Mechanism, Pharmacokinetics, and Drug Interactions:

- Serotonin reuptake inhibitor.
- Metabolized primarily through CYP2D6; potent inhibitor of CYP2C9/2C19 and 2D6; t ½: 4–6 days (fluoxetine), 9 days (norfluoxetine metabolite).
- Avoid use with MAOIs (five-week washout if switching to MAOI); avoid other serotonergic agents (serotonin syndrome). Caution with substrates of 2C9/19 and 2D6.

Clinical Pearls:

- Generally less favored in patients with bipolar disorder, as they may switch to mania due to fluoxetine's long half-life (compared to other antidepressants that can be washed out more quickly).
- Also due to long half-life, effects of dose changes will not be fully reflected for several weeks.
- The benefit of the long half-life is that patients are much less likely to experience serotonin discontinuation symptoms after a missed dose or when discontinuing treatment.
- Of the SSRIs, fluoxetine is most likely to cause rash.
- Fluoxetine/olanzapine combination (Symbyax) is approved for acute depression in bipolar disorder and treatment-resistant depression. See olanzapine fact sheet in Antipsychotics chapter.
- Often considered a first-line agent for kids with depression and anxiety disorders.

Fun Fact:

Eli Lilly was criticized for reformulating fluoxetine in a pink color and calling it "Sarafem" for PMDD. The drug's aggressive marketing campaign included a commercial featuring a harried woman asking herself whether she has PMDD while grocery shopping.

FLUVOXAMINE (Luvox, Luvox CR) Fact Sheet [G]

Bottom Line:
Fluvoxamine is used less often due to twice-daily dosing, sedation, risk for drug interactions, and fewer data for uses other than OCD, even though it's likely just as effective as other SSRIs.

FDA Indications:
OCD (8+ years).

Off-Label Uses:
Major depression; panic disorder; generalized anxiety disorder; PTSD.

Dosage Forms:
- **Tablets (G):** 25 mg, 50 mg (scored), 100 mg (scored).
- **ER capsules (G):** 100 mg, 150 mg.

Dosage Guidance:
- Start 50 mg QHS; may ↑ by 50 mg/day increments every four to seven days as tolerated; max dose 300 mg/day. Daily doses over 100 mg should be divided BID.
- ER: Start 100 mg QHS; may ↑ by 50 mg/day increments weekly; max dose 300 mg/day.
- Children and adolescents (8–17 years): Start 25 mg QHS, ↑ by 25 mg/day increments every four to seven days; max 200 mg/day (8–11 years) or 300 mg/day (12–17 years). Daily doses over 50 mg should be divided BID. Due to limited dose availability, ER not appropriate for children.

Monitoring: Sodium in patients at risk.

Cost: $; ER: $$

Side Effects:
- Most common: Nausea, vomiting, somnolence, insomnia, nervousness, sexual side effects, sweating, tremor, headache.
- Serious but rare: Hyponatremia, mainly in the elderly; gastrointestinal bleeding, especially when combined with NSAIDs such as ibuprofen.

Mechanism, Pharmacokinetics, and Drug Interactions:
- Serotonin reuptake inhibitor.
- Metabolized primarily through CYP1A2 and 2D6; potent inhibitor of CYP1A2 and 2C19; moderate inhibitor of CYP2C9 and 3A4; t ½: 16 hours.
- Avoid use with MAOIs (two-week washout if switching to MAOI); avoid other serotonergic agents (serotonin syndrome). Caution with substrates of CYP1A2 and 2C19.

Clinical Pearls:
- Discontinuation symptoms tend to be worse with fluvoxamine compared to other SSRIs.
- Consider using ER in patients who experience daytime sedation or for whom twice-daily dosing is a challenge.
- Always ask patients about other medications, as fluvoxamine can interact with many of them.
- Fluvoxamine is effective and approved for use in other countries for treating depression.
- Low-dose fluvoxamine (25–50 mg/day) has been used to inhibit the metabolism of clozapine to norclozapine (metabolite associated with adverse effects) in order to achieve an optimal 1.5:2 ratio of clozapine to norclozapine.

Fun Fact:
Preliminary data showed fluvoxamine use resulted in less clinical deterioration in patients with symptomatic COVID-19 compared to placebo. Investigators are looking into whether its binding and activation of sigma-1 receptors and subsequent reduced cytokine production may help mitigate the severe inflammatory process associated with COVID-19 infection.

KETAMINE (Ketalar) Fact Sheet [G]

Note: See separate fact sheet for information on FDA-approved esketamine.

Bottom Line:
Ketamine is an intravenous agent that appears uniquely effective for patients who need an ultra-rapid antidepressant, such as patients who are acutely suicidal. Its disadvantages are that it is not FDA approved for depression, and that it requires close medical monitoring during administration.

FDA Indications:
Anesthesia.

Off-Label Uses:
Major depression, chronic pain, severe agitation (eg, in the ICU).

Dosage Forms:
Vials for injection (G): 10 mg/mL, 50 mg/mL, 100 mg/mL.

Dosage Guidance:
- Most commonly used dose in depression trials: 0.5 mg/kg given intravenously (IV) over 40 minutes, which is lower than the typical anesthetic dose (2 mg/kg).
- Administration may be repeated periodically, though there is no clear guidance regarding how often it should be given, nor how many total infusions should be given. Currently available data and clinical practice suggest dosing two to three times weekly over two to four weeks.

Monitoring: ECG, blood pressure, and oxygen blood saturation are typically monitored during infusion because of concerns regarding spikes in blood pressure and heart rate.

Cost: $$$$

Side Effects:
- Most common: Confusion, blurred vision, poor coordination, feeling weird or spaced out, cardiac issues (30% of patients in three clinical trials experienced a spike in blood pressure over 180/100 mmHg and heart rates over 110 beats per minute, but vital signs normalize quickly).
- Serious but rare: Serious reactions (dream-like states, delirium, respiratory depression) are typically associated with higher (anesthetic) doses.

Mechanism, Pharmacokinetics, and Drug Interactions:
- N-methyl-D-aspartate (NMDA) receptor antagonist.
- In one recent study, co-administration of ketamine with naltrexone (an opiate blocker) prevented its antidepressant effect, implying that ketamine may work in part via opioid receptors (Williams NR et al, *Am J Psych* 2018;175(12):1205–1215. Epub 2018 Aug 29).
- Non-CYP450 metabolism; t ½: 2.5 hours.

Clinical Pearls:
- Efficacy: Meta-analyses of placebo-controlled trials have reported that IV ketamine has an ultra-rapid antidepressant response (at 40 minutes) but that the response attenuates over the course of about one week (Kishimoto T et al, *Psychol Med* 2016;46(7):1459–1472. Epub 2016 Feb 12). Relapse rates are up to 90% four weeks following the ketamine treatment.
- Continuation therapy appears to be effective, with one study showing robust improvement over placebo after 15 days when ketamine was administered two or three times per week.
- The most common patient experience seems to be a sense of dissociation or disconnection from their bodies, lives, and problems. The therapeutic effect may relate to being able to more objectively examine the sources of their psychic pain.
- "Ketamine: A Tale of Overcoming Treatment Resistance" is a brief documentary about ketamine for depression (www.youtube.com/watch?v=fTRCXr4dVF8).
- Can be prescribed in an intranasal formulation available from compounding pharmacies (but we recommend using esketamine product formulated for nasal administration).
- Schedule III controlled substance due to potential for misuse.

Fun Fact:
Ketamine was developed in the 1960s and gained a reputation as an unusually safe anesthetic, because it did not slow down breathing or lower blood pressure. For that reason, it was implemented as a "buddy drug" in the Vietnam War, when each soldier carried a vial of ketamine for use in case another soldier required it while awaiting transport to a field hospital.

LEVOMILNACIPRAN (Fetzima) Fact Sheet

Bottom Line:

Levomilnacipran is an enantiomer of milnacipran (Savella), which is an SNRI approved in the US for fibromyalgia and in other countries for depression. Levomilnacipran is effective for depression, but its higher cost, tendency to cause nausea, need for titration, and urinary effects make it a second-line SNRI after venlafaxine or duloxetine. It is the most adrenergic of all the SNRIs, which may explain its high side effect potential.

FDA Indications:

Major depression.

Off-Label Uses:

Fibromyalgia; anxiety disorders; vasomotor symptoms of menopause; diabetic peripheral neuropathy; chronic musculoskeletal pain.

Dosage Forms:

ER capsules: 20 mg, 40 mg, 80 mg, 120 mg.

Dosage Guidance:

Start 20 mg QD; increase to 40 mg QD after two days, then by increments of 40 mg/day every two or more days to max 120 mg QD.

Monitoring: Periodic blood pressure and pulse.

Cost: $$$$

Side Effects:

- Most common: Nausea, vomiting, constipation, sweating, increased heart rate (7–9 beats/minute), erectile dysfunction, and urinary hesitation.
- Serious but rare: Urinary retention; increased blood pressure and tachycardia possible.

Mechanism, Pharmacokinetics, and Drug Interactions:

- Serotonin and norepinephrine reuptake inhibitor.
- Metabolized primarily through CYP3A4; t ½: 12 hours.
- Avoid use with MAOIs, other serotonergic medications. Use lower doses (no more than 80 mg/day) in presence of potent 3A4 inhibitors (eg, ketoconazole).

Clinical Pearls:

- Three eight-week studies showed greater efficacy than placebo at doses of 40 mg/day and greater. No head-to-head studies versus other antidepressants are available to date.
- According to the manufacturer, levomilnacipran has greater potency for norepinephrine reuptake inhibition than for serotonin reuptake inhibition.
- Noradrenergic effects may contribute to urinary hesitation or retention in 4%–6% of patients and is dose related.
- Nausea may be severe for many patients, especially early in treatment. Start 20 mg/day and titrate slowly to minimize, as patients may develop tolerance.
- Do not cut, crush, chew, or dissolve; swallow extended-release tablets whole with fluid.

Fun Facts:

Milnacipran is the parent compound of levomilnacipran and is a 50-50 racemic mix of levo- and dextro-milnacipran. Due to placebo-controlled studies showing efficacy, it has been approved for depression in 45 countries worldwide. However, since it was reaching the end of its patent life, the manufacturer did not submit it for FDA approval in the US, opting instead to isolate the l-isomer for testing and ultimate FDA approval. Fetzima enjoys market exclusivity until 2023.

MIRTAZAPINE (Remeron) Fact Sheet [G]

Bottom Line:
Mirtazapine tends to cause weight gain and sedation, but no sexual dysfunction or GI side effects, and thus is particularly useful in depressed patients with anxiety or insomnia, those who have had sexual side effects with other antidepressants, and those who may benefit from appetite stimulation (eg, elderly, cancer patients).

FDA Indications:
Major depression.

Off-Label Uses:
Panic disorder; PTSD; generalized anxiety disorder; insomnia; nausea; appetite stimulant; methamphetamine use disorder.

Dosage Forms:
- **Tablets (G):** 7.5 mg, 15 mg, 30 mg, 45 mg.
- **Orally disintegrating tablets (Remeron SolTab, [G]):** 15 mg, 30 mg, 45 mg.

Dosage Guidance:
Start 15 mg QHS, ↑ by 7.5 or 15 mg/day every one to two weeks. Max 45 mg/day. Best given at bedtime.

Monitoring: Weight.

Cost: $

Side Effects:
- Most common: Somnolence, increased appetite, weight gain.
- Serious but rare: Agranulocytosis or severe neutropenia (with or without infection) reported very rarely.

Mechanism, Pharmacokinetics, and Drug Interactions:
- Noradrenergic (via central presynaptic alpha-2 adrenergic receptor antagonist activity) and specific serotonergic (via postsynaptic 5-HT2 and 5-HT3 antagonist effects) antidepressant.
- Metabolized primarily through CYP1A2, 2D6, and 3A4; t ½: 20–40 hours.
- Avoid use with MAOIs. Caution with inducers of 1A2 or 3A4 (eg, carbamazepine), which could reduce efficacy of mirtazapine.

Clinical Pearls:
- One large meta-analysis reported that mirtazapine has a faster onset of action than other antidepressants.
- Rumor has it that higher doses of mirtazapine may be paradoxically less sedating than lower doses. However, there is no empirical support for this theory, which is based on the fact that mirtazapine has increased noradrenergic effect relative to antihistaminergic effect at higher doses.
- The strategy of adding mirtazapine to venlafaxine (sometimes called "California Rocket Fuel" and a combination used in the STAR*D trial) was a promising one but has failed to show benefit in a handful of newer larger studies.
- Two small studies in men with methamphetamine use disorder have shown promising effects of mirtazapine 30 mg nightly in reducing methamphetamine use.

Fun Fact:
Esmirtazapine, the s-enantiomer, was under development for the treatment of insomnia and hot flashes associated with menopause, but the company pulled the plug in 2010.

MONOAMINE OXIDASE INHIBITORS (MAOIs) Fact Sheet [G]

Bottom Line:
MAOIs are not commonly used due to side effects, dietary restrictions, and drug interactions; however, they should be considered for appropriate patients who do not tolerate or respond to other antidepressants.

FDA Indications:
Major depression.

Off-Label Uses:
Treatment-resistant depression; panic disorder; social anxiety disorder.

Dosage Forms:
- **Isocarboxazid, tablets (Marplan):** 10 mg (scored).
- **Phenelzine, tablets (Nardil, [G]):** 15 mg.
- **Tranylcypromine, tablets (Parnate, [G]):** 10 mg.

Dosage Guidance:
- Isocarboxazid: Start 10 mg BID, ↑ by 10 mg/day every two to four days, to 40 mg/day by end of the first week (divided BID–QID). After first week, may ↑ by up to 20 mg weekly to max 60 mg/day. Use caution in patients on >40 mg/day.
- Phenelzine: Start 15 mg BID, ↑ by 15 mg/day every two to four days, up to 60–90 mg/day divided BID.
- Tranylcypromine: Start 10 mg BID, ↑ by 10 mg/day every two to three weeks to maximum of 60 mg/day divided BID.
- Dose timing: Tranylcypromine is the best tolerated of the MAOIs, but it can be activating, so prescribe it in the morning initially. Since larger doses may cause orthostasis if taken at once, you may need to split up the dose as you titrate up, but the PM dose should be taken no later than noon.

Monitoring: No routine monitoring recommended unless clinical picture warrants.

Cost: Isocarboxazid: $$$$$; phenelzine: $; tranylcypromine: $$$

Side Effects:
- Most common: Dizziness, headache, orthostatic hypotension, dry mouth, constipation, drowsiness, tremor, sweating, peripheral edema, sexual side effects, weight gain.
- Serious but rare: Hypertensive crisis (see drug interactions).
- Tranylcypromine is the best tolerated for most patients.

Mechanism, Pharmacokinetics, and Drug Interactions:
- Non-selective monoamine oxidase inhibitors.
- Metabolized primarily through liver, limited data though likely through oxidative CYP450; t ½ irrelevant as irreversible inhibition effects continue for two weeks after discontinuation.
- Avoid with other antidepressants, serotonergic agents, stimulants, sympathomimetics, dextromethorphan, disulfiram, and meperidine. Do not use within five weeks of fluoxetine discontinuation or two weeks of other antidepressant discontinuation. Discontinue at least 10 days prior to elective surgery. Antihypertensives may exaggerate hypotensive effects.
- Avoid use with foods or supplements high in tyramine, tryptophan, phenylalanine, or tyrosine. Examples include aged cheese, air-dried or cured meats (eg, salami), fava or broad bean pods, tap/draft beers, Marmite concentrate, sauerkraut, soy sauce, or spoiled foods.
- See Table A3 in Appendix A for more information on diet and drug interactions with MAOIs.

Clinical Pearls:
- Studies in the 1970s and 1980s showed that MAOIs were more effective than TCAs for atypical depression, characterized by overeating, oversleeping, rejection sensitivity, and mood reactivity.
- Rough dose equivalents: 20 mg of tranylcypromine = 40 mg of isocarboxazid = 45 mg phenelzine.
- When switching from an MAOI to another antidepressant, wait two weeks after MAOI discontinuation. This is because monoamine enzymes are irreversibly inhibited by MAOIs, and regeneration of enzymes takes two to three weeks after discontinuation.

Fun Fact:
MAOIs were the first antidepressants developed, after tuberculosis patients given the antibacterial agent isoniazid (INH) were found to have an elevated mood. Isoniazid was found to be an MAOI and was developed as the first antidepressant in the late 1950s.

NEFAZODONE (Serzone) Fact Sheet [G]

Bottom Line:
Nefazodone was once popular due to the lack of sexual side effects, but is now rarely used due to rare hepatic effects.

FDA Indications:
Major depression.

Off-Label Uses:
Anxiety; insomnia.

Dosage Forms:
Tablets (G): 50 mg, 100 mg, 150 mg, 200 mg, 250 mg.

Dosage Guidance:
Start 50–100 mg BID, increase in 50–100 mg/day increments weekly. Usual dose 300–500 mg/day; maximum 600 mg/day divided BID.

Monitoring: LFTs, BP.

Cost: $$

Side Effects:
- Most common: Nausea, somnolence, dry mouth, dizziness, lightheadedness, constipation, blurred vision, confusion; less orthostasis than trazodone.
- Serious but rare: Black box warning for hepatic toxicity; 1/200,000 to 1/300,000 risk (three to four times general incidence); cases of severe hepatotoxicity resulting in death or need for transplant have been reported; seems to occur early in treatment; not necessarily associated with increased LFTs.

Mechanism, Pharmacokinetics, and Drug Interactions:
- Norepinephrine and serotonin reuptake inhibitor and 5-HT2 antagonist.
- Metabolized by CYP3A4; potent inhibitor of CYP3A4; t ½: 2–4 hours.
- Caution with CYP3A4 inhibitors, inducers, and substrates. Avoid MAOIs and other serotonergic agents.

Clinical Pearls:
- Similar to trazodone in chemical structure, but less sedating.
- Minimal sexual side effects.
- If patient tolerates, may be used QHS rather than BID to minimize daytime sedation and improve nighttime sleep.
- Avoid in patients with active liver disease or elevated LFTs; monitor all patients for symptoms of hepatic impairment (jaundice, anorexia, GI complaints, lethargy). If patient is symptomatic or LFTs increase to three or more times upper limit of normal, discontinue and monitor patient; do not re-treat.

Fun Fact:
After the drug was removed from the market in Canada and Europe, the nonprofit organization Public Citizen sued the FDA for failing to remove it from the US market. The suit was later withdrawn, but the manufacturer of the branded product Serzone stopped production due to weak sales; generic sales continue.

PAROXETINE (Brisdelle, Paxil, Paxil CR, Pexeva) Fact Sheet [G]

Bottom Line:

Paroxetine is the least favored SSRI due to its side effect profile (greatest sexual side effects, weight gain, sedation, constipation), drug interaction profile, and risk for discontinuation syndrome. However, its wide range of FDA anxiety indications leads some clinicians to favor it for patients with significant anxiety.

FDA Indications:

Major depression; OCD; panic disorder; social anxiety disorder; generalized anxiety disorder (GAD); PTSD; PMDD; vasomotor symptoms associated with menopause (Brisdelle).

Off-Label Uses:

Premature ejaculation.

Dosage Forms:

- **Tablets (Paxil, Pexeva, [G]):** 10 mg, 20 mg, 30 mg, 40 mg.
- **Capsules (Brisdelle, [G]):** 7.5 mg.
- **Oral suspension (Paxil, [G]):** 10 mg/5 mL.
- **ER tablets (Paxil CR, [G]):** 12.5 mg, 25 mg, 37.5 mg.

Dosage Guidance:

- Start 10–20 mg QD in evening or bedtime; may ↑ by 10 mg/day increments weekly.
- ER: Start 12.5–25 mg QD; may ↑ by 12.5 mg/day increments weekly.
- Max dose: 50 mg/day (depression, GAD, PTSD); 60 mg/day (OCD, panic disorder, social anxiety disorder); 75 mg/day (ER). Max dose in elderly: 40 mg/day (IR); 50 mg/day (ER).
- PMDD: Start 12.5 mg ER QD; may ↑ to max 25 mg/day after one week. Or, 12.5–25 mg ER QD on cycle days 15–28 (14 days prior to anticipated onset of menstruation).
- Vasomotor menopausal symptoms: 7.5 mg QHS.
- Dose timing: Usually best given at bedtime due to sedation.

Monitoring: Sodium in patients at risk; ECG in patients on citalopram >40 mg/day or if cardiac disease.

Cost: $; capsule: $$; oral suspension: $$$$

Side Effects:

- Most common: Nausea, constipation, dry mouth, somnolence, sedation, sexual side effects, weight gain, sweating, tremor, headache.
- Serious but rare: Hyponatremia, mainly in the elderly; gastrointestinal bleeding, especially when combined with NSAIDs such as ibuprofen.

Mechanism, Pharmacokinetics, and Drug Interactions:

- Serotonin reuptake inhibitor.
- Metabolized primarily through 2D6; potent inhibitor of 2D6; t ½: 21 hours.
- Avoid use with MAOIs (two-week washout if switching to MAOI); avoid other serotonergic agents (serotonin syndrome). Caution with substrates of 2D6.

Clinical Pearls:

- Paroxetine has the widest range of FDA-approved indications; however, it is not approved for any use in children or adolescents.
- Ideal medication for thin patients with insomnia and significant anxiety who are not very sexually active.
- Caution with medications that require CYP2D6 to convert into active drug or active metabolite (eg, tamoxifen, tramadol, hydrocodone, codeine) as therapeutic effects will be lowered by paroxetine's potent inhibition of CYP2D6. This is the opposite effect of the majority of 2D6 substrates, which will have their levels increased when combined with paroxetine.
- Paroxetine seems to pose the greatest risk to a fetus in terms of cardiovascular malformation. Unless the benefits of paroxetine outweigh discontinuation or alternative antidepressants, a switch to another antidepressant should be considered.

Fun Fact:

In 2012, paroxetine manufacturer GlaxoSmithKline was fined $3 billion by the U.S. Department of Justice for unlawfully promoting its use in kids based on misleading data from its infamous Study 329. *New Scientist* wrote in 2015: "You may never have heard of it, but Study 329 changed medicine."

SELEGILINE TRANSDERMAL (Emsam) Fact Sheet

Bottom Line:
Emsam is an MAOI patch with less likelihood of dietary interactions at 6 mg, and possibly at higher doses too. Probably fewer side effects than other MAOIs, such as weight gain and sexual side effects, and other potential advantages, including better compliance among patients who do not like swallowing pills and less suicide risk (it's harder to overdose on a patch than with pills). When MAOIs are indicated, this may be the least risky option to try.

FDA Indications:
Major depression.

Off-Label Uses:
Treatment-resistant depression; panic disorder; treatment-resistant anxiety disorders.

Dosage Forms:
Transdermal patch: 6 mg, 9 mg, 12 mg/24 hour patch.

Dosage Guidance:
- Start 6 mg/24 hours QD; may ↑ in increments of 3 mg/24 hours every two weeks or more, up to max 12 mg/24 hours.
- Apply to clean, dry, intact skin to upper torso (below neck and above waist), upper thigh, or outer surface of upper arm; apply at the same time each day and rotate application sites; wash hands with soap and water after handling; avoid touching sticky side of patch.

Monitoring: No routine monitoring recommended unless clinical picture warrants.

Cost: $$$$$

Side Effects:
- Most common: Headache, insomnia, application site reaction, hypotension, diarrhea, dry mouth.
- Serious but rare: Orthostatic hypotension; caution in patients at risk (elderly, cerebrovascular disease, cardiovascular disease, hypovolemia).

Mechanism, Pharmacokinetics, and Drug Interactions:
- Non-selective MAOI.
- Metabolized primarily through CYP2B6 (also 2C9, 3A4/5) to active (N-desmethylselegiline, amphetamine, methamphetamine) and inactive metabolites; t ½: 18–25 hours.
- Interactions with food: When using the 6 mg/day patch, no special diet is required. When using higher doses, a tyramine-restricted diet should be followed. See Table A3 in Appendix A for more information.
- Interactions with other meds are identical to oral MAOIs, so avoid with other antidepressants, serotonergic agents, stimulants, sympathomimetics, dextromethorphan, disulfiram, meperidine, and carbamazepine. Do not use within five weeks of fluoxetine discontinuation or two weeks of other antidepressant discontinuation. Discontinue at least 10 days prior to elective surgery. Antihypertensives may exaggerate hypotensive effects. For doses higher than 6 mg, avoid use with foods or supplements high in tyramine, tryptophan, phenylalanine, or tyrosine.
- Wait two weeks after discontinuing transdermal selegiline before initiating therapy with serotonergic or any other contraindicated drug.

Clinical Pearls:
- Oral selegiline (Eldepryl) used in Parkinson's disease (≤10 mg/day) is a selective inhibitor of MAO-B, which metabolizes dopamine. When used transdermally as Emsam, selegiline achieves higher blood levels and non-selectively inhibits both MAO-A and MAO-B. Its antidepressant effect is thought to be due to its MAO-A inhibition, which blocks the breakdown of other centrally active neurotransmitters (norepinephrine, serotonin).
- Patch may contain conducting metal (eg, aluminum); avoid exposure of application site to external heat source, which may increase the amount of drug absorbed.

Fun Fact:
Named "Emsam" after Emily and Samuel, the children of the CEO of Somerset Pharmaceuticals (original manufacturer).

Antidepressants

SERTRALINE (Zoloft) Fact Sheet [G]

Bottom Line:

Sertraline is a good first-line SSRI option for many patients due to its range of indications, flexible dosing, low drug interaction potential, and relative tolerability.

FDA Indications:

Major depression; OCD (6+ years); panic disorder; PTSD; PMDD; social anxiety disorder.

Off-Label Uses:

Generalized anxiety disorder.

Dosage Forms:

- **Tablets (G):** 25 mg (scored), 50 mg (scored), 100 mg (scored).
- **Capsules (G):** 150 mg, 200 mg.
- **Oral solution concentrate (G):** 20 mg/mL (must be diluted prior to administration).

Dosage Guidance:

- Start 25–50 mg QD; may ↑ by 25–50 mg/day increments weekly; max 200 mg/day.
- Ages 6–12: Start 12.5–25 mg QD, increase by 25–50 mg/day increments weekly; max 200 mg/day.
- Ages 13–17: Start 25–50 mg QD, increase by 25–50 mg/day increments weekly; max dose: 200 mg/day.
- PMDD: Start 50 mg QD; may ↑ by 25–50 mg/day increments weekly; max 150 mg/day. Or, intermittent dosing 50 mg QD during luteal phase only (days 15–28); max 100 mg/day.
- Dose timing: Can be taken in the morning or night, depending on patient preference.

Monitoring: Sodium in patients at risk.

Cost: $; capsule: $$$

Side Effects:

- Most common: Nausea, diarrhea, tremor, decreased appetite, sexual side effects, headache.
- Serious but rare: Hyponatremia, mainly in the elderly; gastrointestinal bleeding, especially when combined with NSAIDs such as ibuprofen.

Mechanism, Pharmacokinetics, and Drug Interactions:

- Serotonin reuptake inhibitor.
- Metabolized primarily through CYP2C19 and to a lesser extent 2D6 and 3A4; moderate inhibitor of CYP2D6 at high doses (>150 mg/day); t ½: 26 hours.
- Avoid use with MAOIs (two-week washout if switching to MAOI); avoid other serotonergic agents (serotonin syndrome).

Clinical Pearls:

- A meta-analysis of 12 newer antidepressants showed that sertraline and escitalopram have best efficacy and tolerability in acute depression (Cipriani A et al, *Lancet* 2018;391(10128):1357–1366).
- Considered one of the safest antidepressants to use during breastfeeding due to low levels of exposure to the fetus.
- If using oral concentrate, use calibrated dropper (has 25 mg and 50 mg graduation marks only) and mix with 4 ounces (½ cup) of water, ginger ale, lemon/lime soda, lemonade, or orange juice ONLY. After mixing, a slight haze may appear, which is normal.
- Oral concentrate is formulated in 12% alcohol. Avoid use with disulfiram.

Fun Fact:

During the COVID-19 pandemic in 2020, there was increased demand for sertraline. The active pharmaceutical ingredients were in short supply, and the medication was backordered off and on for several months.

THYROID (Cytomel, Synthroid, others) Fact Sheet [G]

Bottom Line:

Thyroid augmentation is often chosen for patients with depression-associated lethargy and fatigue. The usual formulation used is T3 (Cytomel). Response rates in clinical trials are mixed and only modest, but thyroid augmentation is inexpensive and well tolerated and may be worth a try, especially for patients on tricyclics (the evidence is less impressive for SSRI augmentation).

FDA Indications:

Treatment of hypothyroidism.

Off-Label Uses:

Augmentation and acceleration of antidepressant response.

Dosage Forms:

- T3: Triiodothyronine (preferred for psychiatric uses):
  Liothyronine tablets (Cytomel, [G]): 5 mcg, 25 mcg, 50 mcg.
- T4: Thyroxine (preferred for hypothyroidism):
  Levothyroxine tablets (Synthroid, Levoxyl, Levothroid, [G]): 25 mcg, 50 mcg, 75 mcg, 88 mcg, 100 mcg, 112 mcg, 125 mcg, 137 mcg, 150 mcg, 175 mcg, 200 mcg, 300 mcg.
- Note: T4 is converted to T3 in the body.
- Thyroid product equivalencies: 100 mcg levothyroxine = 25 mcg liothyronine.

Dosage Guidance:

T3: 25 mcg daily for one to two weeks, increase to 50 mcg if no response (in elderly, start at 12.5 mg and increase gradually up to 50 mcg). Give in the morning.

Monitoring: Check TSH (thyroid stimulating hormone) level before treatment. Repeat every six to 12 months.

Cost: $

Side Effects:

- Most common: At doses used in augmentation, there are rarely any side effects.
- Serious but rare: Reduced bone density; hyperthyroidism, which might theoretically occur (watch for these symptoms: tremor, palpitations, heat intolerance, sweating, anxiety, increased frequency of bowel movements, shortness of breath, and exacerbation of cardiac arrhythmia).
- Contraindications: Recent MI, adrenal insufficiency.

Mechanism, Pharmacokinetics, and Drug Interactions:

- Mechanism for depression not well understood; it may work by generally stimulating metabolism and energy.
- Metabolized by CYP450; t ½: 1 day.
- Caution in patients with warfarin as blood thinning effects may be increased.

Clinical Pearls:

- Efficacy: Mixed evidence.
- After two failed courses of antidepressants, augmentation with T3 or lithium was compared in the STAR*D trial. Remission rates were modest and numerically, but not statistically, higher with T3: 25% with T3 vs 16% with lithium, and lithium patients had more side effects.
- Majority of T3 augmentation studies were in patients taking TCAs, though there are some data with SSRIs and other antidepressants.
- Efficacy for augmentation in partial or non-responders is independent of baseline TSH. Goal TSH is at or below lower limit of normal range, but caution to avoid hyperthyroid symptoms.

Fun Fact:

You may have patients ask you about taking "natural" thyroid. They may be referring to dessicated thyroid, which is derived from extracts of bovine or porcine thyroid glands and contains T3 and T4 in a 1:4 ratio (60 mg contains about 38 mcg of T4 and 9 mcg of T3).

Antidepressants

TRAZODONE (Desyrel) Fact Sheet [G]

Bottom Line:
Trazodone is most commonly used as a hypnotic at low doses (25–50 mg), but at higher doses it is effective for depression, and has the advantage of fewer sexual side effects and less weight gain compared to other serotonergic antidepressants.

FDA Indications:
Major depression.

Off-Label Uses:
Insomnia; anxiety.

Dosage Forms:
Tablets (G): 50 mg, 100 mg, 150 mg, 300 mg (scored).

Dosage Guidance:
* Depression: Start 50 mg TID; ↑ by 50 mg/day every three to four days until response (usually 300–400 mg/day); max 600 mg/day.
* Insomnia (off-label): Start 25–50 mg QHS; may ↑ by 50 mg increments up to 200 mg QHS.
* Dose timing: Generally best given at bedtime, though some patients find the medication stimulating and need to take it in the morning.

Monitoring: No routine monitoring recommended unless clinical picture warrants.

Cost: $

Side Effects:
* Most common: Drowsiness, dry mouth, dizziness or lightheadedness, orthostatic hypotension, headache, blurred vision, nausea, or vomiting.
* Serious but rare: Reports of priapism (painful erection lasting longer than six hours); may require surgical or pharmacologic (eg, epinephrine) intervention and may result in impotence or permanent impairment of erectile function. Orthostatic hypotension and syncope reported (less at hypnotic doses).

Mechanism, Pharmacokinetics, and Drug Interactions:
* Serotonin reuptake inhibitor, alpha-1 adrenergic receptor antagonist, and serotonin 5-HT2A and 5-HT2C receptor antagonist.
* Metabolized primarily through CYP3A4 to active metabolite (mCPP), which in turn is metabolized by 2D6; induces P-glycoprotein; t ½: 7–10 hours.
* Avoid use with MAOIs.

Clinical Pearls:
* Food delays absorption of trazodone for one to two hours, so it's best taken on an empty stomach when used for insomnia. Trazodone's hypnotic effects are not due to anticholinergic or antihistaminergic effects.
* Rarely used as antidepressant due to risk for over-sedation and orthostasis at therapeutic doses; majority of use currently is for insomnia.

Fun Fact:
As a consequence of the production of mCPP as a metabolite, patients taking trazodone may test positive on urine tests for the presence of MDMA (ecstasy).

TRICYCLIC ANTIDEPRESSANTS (TCAs) Fact Sheet [G]

Bottom Line:

Not commonly used due to side effects and overdose toxicity risk; however, TCAs should be considered for appropriate patients who do not respond to other antidepressants.

FDA Indications:

Major depression.

Off-Label Uses:

Headache; migraine; neuropathic pain; fibromyalgia; anxiety disorders; insomnia; nocturnal enuresis; urinary incontinence.

Note: There are nine TCAs approved by the FDA for depression (amitriptyline, amoxapine, desipramine, doxepin, imipramine, maprotiline, nortriptyline, protriptyline, trimipramine) and one approved for OCD (clomipramine). We've selected six TCAs to cover in this book. Doxepin is in the Anxiolytic and Hypnotic Medications chapter, clomipramine is in this chapter, and in this sheet we include four of the more commonly prescribed TCAs.

Dosage Forms:
- Tertiary TCAs (more sedating):
  - **Amitriptyline tablets (G):** 10 mg, 25 mg, 50 mg, 75 mg, 100 mg, 150 mg.
  - **Imipramine tablets and capsules (G):** 10 mg, 25 mg, 50 mg, 75 mg, 100 mg, 125 mg, 150 mg.
- Secondary TCAs (less sedating):
  - **Desipramine tablets (Norpramin, [G]):** 10 mg, 25 mg, 50 mg, 75 mg, 100 mg, 150 mg.
  - **Nortriptyline capsules (Pamelor, [G]):** 10 mg, 25 mg, 50 mg, 75 mg, and 10 mg/5 mL oral solution.

Dosage Guidance:
- Amitriptyline or imipramine: Start 25–50 mg QHS and ↑ by 25–50 mg/day intervals every two to three days to target dose 150–200 mg/day; max 300 mg/day.
- Desipramine: Start 25–50 mg QHS and ↑ by 25–50 mg/day intervals every two to three days to target dose 150–200 mg/day; max 300 mg/day.
- Nortriptyline: Start 25–50 mg QHS and ↑ by 25–50 mg/day intervals every two to three days to target dose 50–150 mg/day; max 150 mg/day.
  - Once you reach a dose of 100 mg/day, check nortriptyline serum level to maintain in optimal therapeutic range of 50–150 ng/mL (check trough level and wait for steady state after a given dose, about five days).

Monitoring: ECG if history of cardiac disease. Nortriptyline level as described above.

Cost: $

Side Effects:
- Most common: Sedation, dry mouth, constipation, weight gain, sexual side effects, urinary hesitation, blurred vision.
- Serious but rare: Seizure; cardiac effects including orthostasis, arrhythmias, QT prolongation, AV block.

Mechanism, Pharmacokinetics, and Drug Interactions:
- Serotonin and norepinephrine reuptake inhibitors.
- Metabolized primarily through liver (limited data, though likely through oxidative CYP2D6 primarily); t ½: 18–44 hours.
- Avoid use with other serotonergic antidepressants or agents with hypotensive or anticholinergic effects.

Clinical Pearls:
- Using divided doses (BID to TID) may help with tolerability during initiation and titration; but can convert to QHS dosing to minimize daytime sedation.
- Tertiary amines amitriptyline and imipramine are metabolized to secondary amines nortriptyline and desipramine, respectively. Secondary amines are generally better tolerated.
- Value of serum level monitoring most clearly established for nortriptyline; utility of monitoring for other TCAs is controversial.
- Overdose toxicity with potentially serious cardiac effects or fatality with as little as 10-day supply.

Fun Fact:

Imipramine was the first antidepressant approved in the US, developed by tweaking the molecular structure of the antipsychotic Thorazine. It didn't work for psychosis, but was the first "wonder drug" for depression and anxiety.

VENLAFAXINE (Effexor, Effexor XR) Fact Sheet [G]

Bottom Line:

Venlafaxine is probably somewhat more effective than SSRIs for depression, but its side effect disadvantages, such as blood pressure elevation and discontinuation symptoms, relegate it to second-line use. Venlafaxine's active metabolite, desvenlafaxine, may be preferred by some over the parent compound—see our desvenlafaxine fact sheet in this chapter.

FDA Indications:

Major depression; social anxiety disorder; generalized anxiety disorder; panic disorder.

Off-Label Uses:

PTSD; PMDD; vasomotor symptoms of menopause; diabetic peripheral neuropathy.

Dosage Forms:

- **Tablets (G):** 25 mg, 37.5 mg, 50 mg, 75 mg, 100 mg (scored).
- **ER tablets (G):** 37.5 mg, 75 mg, 150 mg, 225 mg.

Dosage Guidance:

- Depression:

  Start 75 mg/day in two or three divided doses or as XR once daily; ↑ dose by 75 mg/day at intervals of four or more days; max 375 mg/day (divided TID) or 225 mg/day XR given once daily. IR may be switched to nearest equivalent daily dose of XR QD.

- Anxiety:

  XR: Start 75 mg QD, ↑ by 75 mg/day at weekly intervals; max 225 mg/day; for panic disorder, to minimize exacerbation of panic, start 37.5 mg QD, ↑ to 75 mg QD after one week then by 75 mg/day at weekly intervals; max 225 mg/day.

Monitoring: Periodic blood pressure.

Cost: $

Side Effects:

- Most common: Anorexia, constipation, dizziness, dry mouth, nausea, nervousness, somnolence, sweating, sexual side effects, headache, insomnia.
- Serious but rare: Sustained, dose-related hypertension reported. May cause hyponatremia or SIADH; use with caution in patients who are volume depleted, elderly, or taking diuretics.

Mechanism, Pharmacokinetics, and Drug Interactions:

- Serotonin and norepinephrine reuptake inhibitor.
- Metabolized primarily through CYP2D6 to O-desmethylvenlafaxine (ODV), major active metabolite (an SNRI, marketed as Pristiq), and also by CYP3A4; t ½: 5 hours (11 hours for ODV).
- Avoid use with MAOIs, other serotonergic agents. Caution with CYP2D6 or 3A4 inhibitors, which may increase venlafaxine levels. Inhibits CYP2D6.

Clinical Pearls:

- For patients with nausea, start at lower dose, titrate more slowly, and give with food.
- May cause false-positive PCP in urine drug screen.
- Increase in blood pressure much more likely in doses >225 mg/day.
- Significant discontinuation syndrome, even with XR formulation.
- Theoretically functions as an SSRI in low doses (75 mg/day) and as an SNRI in moderate doses (150–225 mg/day), and affects all monoamines in high doses (>225 mg/day).
- No additional benefit seen with doses >225 mg/day in moderately depressed outpatients, but patients with more severe depression may respond to higher doses (350 mg/day).

Fun Fact:

Venlafaxine is structurally related to the atypical opioid analgesic tramadol (Ultram, itself a serotonergic agent), but not to any other antidepressant drugs.

VILAZODONE (Viibryd) Fact Sheet

Bottom Line:
Vilazodone is essentially an SSRI with the addition of some buspirone-type effects. Early claims of sexual side effect advantages over other SSRIs are unproven. Disadvantages include the slow titration schedule, the need to take it with food in order to achieve a therapeutic blood level, and the many drug interactions. Until further notice, vilazodone should remain a second-line antidepressant.

FDA Indications:
Major depression.

Off-Label Uses:
OCD; other anxiety disorders.

Dosage Forms:
Tablets: 10 mg, 20 mg, 40 mg.

Dosage Guidance:
* Start 10 mg QD for seven days; ↑ to 20 mg QD for seven days, then to recommended dose of 20–40 mg QD (with food). Purpose of dose titration is to minimize GI effects.
* Must take with food, otherwise serum levels are reduced by up to 50%.
* Dose timing: Best taken in the morning due to activating effects.

Monitoring: No routine monitoring recommended unless clinical picture warrants.

Cost: $$$$

Side Effects:
* Most common: Diarrhea, nausea, vomiting, dry mouth, insomnia, dizziness.
* Serious but rare: Possible hyponatremia or SIADH; use with caution in patients who are volume depleted, elderly, or taking diuretics.

Mechanism, Pharmacokinetics, and Drug Interactions:
* SSRI plus 5-HT1A partial agonist (buspirone is also 5-HT1A partial agonist).
* Metabolized primarily through CYP3A4; t ½: 25 hours.
* Avoid use with MAOIs, other serotonergic agents. More P450 drug interactions possible with vilazodone than some other SSRIs. Use with 3A4 inhibitors or inducers may require dose adjustment.

Clinical Pearls:
* Sometimes marketed as having no or few sexual side effects, but FDA officials wrote an article for the *Journal of Clinical Psychiatry* clarifying that studies do not support this claim.
* Although the buspirone-like 5-HT1A effect suggests vilazodone may be especially effective in anxious depression, some patients report feeling a wired or somewhat stimulated effect like fluoxetine.
* Patients who experience nausea or activation, both dose-related effects, may not be able to reach a daily dose of 40 mg due to tolerability but may respond to 20–30 mg per day.

Fun Guess:
The brand name "Viibryd" likely has two origins. First, it rhymes with "hybrid," and the mechanism of action is a hybrid of SSRI and 5-HT1A partial agonism. Second, the word calls to mind "virile," which could be a subliminal suggestion that it does not worsen sexual functioning.

VORTIOXETINE (Trintellix) Fact Sheet

Bottom Line:

Vortioxetine is a newer "multimodal" antidepressant with diverse effects on neurotransmitters. Recent data suggest that vortioxetine may have pro-cognitive effects and may be less likely to cause sexual side effects than SSRIs. It is reasonable to try the drug in patients who have complained of SSRI-induced sexual dysfunction. A high prevalence of nausea and the high brand-name price tag are negative factors to consider.

FDA Indications:

Major depression.

Off-Label Uses:

Generalized anxiety disorder; other anxiety disorders.

Dosage Forms:

Tablets: 5 mg, 10 mg, 15 mg, 20 mg.

Dosage Guidance:

Start 10 mg QD; ↑ to 20 mg QD as tolerated. Consider 5 mg/day for those unable to tolerate higher doses (eg, due to nausea). May be taken in the morning or night.

Monitoring: No routine monitoring recommended unless clinical picture warrants.

Cost: $$$$

Side Effects:

- Most common: Nausea, constipation, vomiting, sexual side effects, dry mouth, headache.
- Serious but rare: Serotonergic antidepressants have been rarely associated with bruising or bleeding.

Mechanism, Pharmacokinetics, and Drug Interactions:

- Multimodal antidepressant.
- Metabolized primarily through CYP2D6 and, to a lesser extent, via 3A4/5, 2C9/19, 2A6, 2C8, and 2B6; t ½: 66 hours.
- Avoid use with MAOIs, other serotonergic medications. Use lower doses in presence of potent 2D6 inhibitors.

Clinical Pearls:

- Vortioxetine is a "multimodal" antidepressant or a "serotonin modulator and stimulator." This means it has effects on several receptor sites. Like SSRIs, it is a serotonin reuptake inhibitor, but it also is an agonist at 5-HT1A receptors, a partial agonist at 5-HT1B receptors, and an antagonist at 5-HT3A, 5-HT1D, and 5-HT7 receptors.
- The Trintellix labeling was updated twice in 2018. First, data from studies examining cognitive functioning in patients treated for depression were included to note improved processing speed with vortioxetine. The second update was made to include head-to-head data showing greater improvement in treatment-emergent sexual side effects when patients were switched from SSRI to vortioxetine over escitalopram.
- The degree of cognitive improvement seen with vortioxetine has been compared to that of caffeine from a shot of espresso. Whether or how much that results in functional improvement remains to be seen.
- Negative findings in some studies were attributed to dose being too low (5–10 mg/day). Higher-dose studies showed vortioxetine to be as effective as both duloxetine and agomelatine, an antidepressant approved in Europe.
- Compared to SSRIs, vortioxetine has more GI side effects, including nausea, vomiting, diarrhea, and constipation. This may mean that some patients won't be able to get beyond 5 or 10 mg per day.
- Two studies looked at vortioxetine for cognitive symptoms in perimenopausal depression. One found benefits and the other did not, but both were small observational studies, not randomized and with no placebo group.

Fun Fact:

The original brand name of vortioxetine, Brintellix, was apparently crafted to subliminally suggest that the drug helps cognition ("**br**ing **intelli**gence"). It was changed to Trintellix in 2016 because of reports of dispensing errors between Brintellix and Brilinta, the antiplatelet medication ticagrelor.

Antipsychotics

GENERAL PRESCRIBING TIPS

Which antipsychotic should you choose? There are dozens of options and approved indications. Here are some of the factors you should weigh as you decide which antipsychotic to prescribe for a given patient:

- Efficacy
- Side effects
- Cost

Efficacy

While there's some debate about this, most experts consider clozapine to be the only antipsychotic that is clearly more effective than the others. Unfortunately, clozapine also happens to have one of the worst side effect profiles in psychiatry. Weight gain is the most prominent: You can expect half of all patients who take clozapine to have a 20% or more weight gain over time (Umbricht DS et al, *J Clin Psychiatry* 1994;55(suppl B):157–160). When you consider its other major side effects, like sedation, drooling, and life-threatening neutropenia, not to mention the necessity of monthly blood draws, it's no wonder that clozapine is used relatively rarely. Nonetheless, it's incredibly helpful for certain treatment-resistant patients.

Next on the list of drugs that might be more effective than others is olanzapine, another side effect overachiever. It doesn't cause as much weight gain as clozapine, but it's close. In the CATIE trial, 30% of patients gained at least 7% of their initial weight.

Beyond this, there's no consensus that any of the other second-generation antipsychotics (SGAs) differ in efficacy, at least for core symptoms of psychosis. It's possible that SGAs have a broader spectrum of efficacy, given that many are approved for various mood syndromes as well as psychosis. Some people believe that SGAs are more effective than first-generation antipsychotics (FGAs) for negative symptoms. This probably stems from the fact that FGAs are more likely to cause side effects, like extrapyramidal symptoms (EPS), which can mimic negative symptoms. It is becoming more reasonable to choose SGAs over FGAs for most patients as more of the former go generic.

Side Effects

Below are some of the key antipsychotic side effects along with our best estimates of the liabilities of specific agents. You'll find a more detailed comparison of relative side effects in Table 10.

- *Weight gain/hyperlipidemia/diabetes:*
  - Most weight gain: Clozapine, olanzapine
  - Moderate: Paliperidone, quetiapine, risperidone
  - Lower: Asenapine, brexpiprazole
  - Least weight gain: Aripiprazole, lurasidone, ziprasidone, most first-generation antipsychotics (eg, haloperidol, perphenazine)
- *Sedation:*
  - Most sedating: Clozapine, olanzapine, quetiapine (note that sedation can sometimes be beneficial for agitated, anxious, or manic patients)
  - Moderately sedating: Asenapine, cariprazine, lurasidone, risperidone, ziprasidone
  - Least sedating: Aripiprazole, brexpiprazole
- *Cardiac issues (primarily prolonged QT interval):*
  - Most issues: Thioridazine, ziprasidone
  - Moderate: Chlorpromazine, haloperidol, iloperidone, paliperidone, quetiapine
  - Fewest issues: Aripiprazole, asenapine, brexpiprazole, cariprazine, clozapine, loxapine, lurasidone, olanzapine, risperidone
- *EPS:*
  - Most EPS: Fluphenazine, haloperidol, paliperidone, risperidone
  - Most akathisia: Aripiprazole, brexpiprazole
  - Moderate: Asenapine, cariprazine, perphenazine
  - Least EPS: Chlorpromazine, clozapine, iloperidone, olanzapine, quetiapine, ziprasidone

Antipsychotics

Discontinuing Antipsychotics

Patients may elect to stop their antipsychotics for a variety of reasons, such as noxious side effects, a feeling of stigma, or simply a desire to see how their lives go when they're off meds. Here are some potential issues to watch out for:

- *Supersensitivity psychosis.* We know that relapse to mood or psychotic symptoms is more likely when patients stop medications. Med withdrawal psychosis might be "supersensitivity" psychosis—which is theoretically caused by an upregulation in the number or sensitivity of dopamine receptors due to chronic exposure to antipsychotics. Because antipsychotics block dopamine receptors, the brain responds by creating more receptors to "harvest" the missing dopamine. But once you remove those receptor blockers (by stopping the medication), suddenly there are many more receptors to accept dopamine, potentially worsening psychosis. According to this mechanism, withdrawal psychosis would then be more severe and more sudden than you'd otherwise predict. There's not much you can do to prevent this, but you might want to let patients know about the risk, and taper meds more slowly if it has occurred before.

- *Withdrawal dyskinesia.* Withdrawal dyskinesia occurs when stopping or reducing the dose of an antipsychotic; it causes symptoms that look like tardive dyskinesia (such as lip puckering, tongue movements, hand or foot movements, and others). It sometimes goes away after a few weeks, but other times it persists and may require reintroducing an antipsychotic at low doses in order to quiet the movements.

- *Cholinergic rebound.* Antipsychotics such as clozapine and olanzapine are particularly anticholinergic. This can lead to cholinergic supersensitivity, so that when these meds are stopped (or when you switch a patient to a less anticholinergic drug), symptoms of the parasympathetic nervous system can result. Many of us remember these symptoms with the medical mnemonic SLUD: salivation, lacrimation, urination, defecation. These are more commonly described as nausea, vomiting, diarrhea, headache, sweating, and insomnia. Rarely, cholinergic symptoms can even cause delirium and psychosis—which can be easily confused with relapse of psychotic symptoms. Cholinergic rebound is more likely when anticholinergic antipsychotics like clozapine, olanzapine, or chlorpromazine are discontinued too suddenly, or when accompanying benztropine is stopped suddenly.

Switching Antipsychotics: Abrupt or Gradual?

We often switch antipsychotics due to side effects or lack of efficacy. There are two types of switches: immediate and cross-tapering. In the cross-taper, you gradually taper the old drug while gradually titrating up the dose of the new drug. We've likely all seen at least a case or two where an intended cross-taper stalled and resulted in unintended long-term polypharmacy.

Anecdotally, it appears that most clinicians use the cross-tapering strategy, because it seems like the more cautious and reasonable approach. However, a recent study indicates that immediate switches are just as effective. This was a meta-analysis of nine randomized controlled trials that involved more than 1,400 patients. There was no clear benefit of gradual switching, and immediate switching was generally tolerated well. These trials covered discontinuation of the following agents: risperidone, olanzapine, ziprasidone, aripiprazole, iloperidone, and clozapine (Takeuchi H et al, *Schiz Bull* 2017;43(4):862–871).

What about switching from oral antipsychotics to long-acting injectables (LAIs)? Please see the fact sheet on LAIs for guidance on this topic.

Cost

As of this writing, the following second-generation antipsychotics are available as generics, rendering them relatively inexpensive: aripiprazole, asenapine (sublingual), clozapine, olanzapine, paliperidone, quetiapine, risperidone, and ziprasidone.

On the other hand, the following antipsychotics are brand-name only and are often ridiculously expensive (up to, or even over, $1,000 per month): asenapine (Secuado transdermal), brexpiprazole (Rexulti), cariprazine (Vraylar), iloperidone (Fanapt), lumateperone (Caplyta), and lurasidone (Latuda).

Class Warnings

All of the second-generation antipsychotics carry the same FDA class warnings. Rather than repeating these concerns on each fact sheet, we will mention them here:

- In 2003, the FDA required all manufacturers of second-generation antipsychotics to revise their package labeling to reflect the potential risks for weight gain, hyperglycemia, new-onset or worsening diabetes, and hyperlipidemias. While this has become a class warning, it's clear that there are a handful of really bad actors here: Clozapine and olanzapine are the worst, quetiapine and risperidone relatively less so but still problematic for many.

- Patient-specific factors may also play a role. In general, the incidence and severity of weight gain and metabolic effects appear to be greater in the pediatric population.

- A black box warning for all agents in this class suggests a substantially *higher mortality rate in geriatric patients with dementia-related psychosis* receiving second-generation antipsychotics (4.5%) compared with those receiving placebo (2.6%). Although most fatalities resulted from cardiac-related events (eg, heart failure, sudden death) or infections (mostly pneumonia) as opposed to a clearly direct effect of medication, second-generation antipsychotics are *not* approved for the treatment of dementia-related psychosis, and such use should be avoided or minimized when possible.

- *Adverse cerebrovascular events* (eg, stroke, TIA), sometimes fatal, have been reported in geriatric patients (ages 73–97) with dementia-related psychosis. The FDA has issued a black box warning on second-generation antipsychotics to reflect this risk; several studies have shown that cerebrovascular event risk is elevated with first-generation antipsychotics, as well.

A 2004 consensus statement from the American Psychiatric Association and American Diabetes Association recommends the following monitoring protocol for patients on second-generation agents (Table 7). These are the minimum recommendations for monitoring; some patients—for example, individuals with elevated triglycerides or blood sugar—may necessitate more frequent monitoring.

Table 7: **Metabolic Monitoring Recommendations for Patients on Second-Generation Antipsychotics**

Personal/Family History[1]	Baseline, Annually
Weight (BMI)	Baseline, every 4 weeks for the first 12 weeks, then every 3 months
Waist circumference	Baseline, annually
Blood pressure, pulse, fasting blood glucose, HgA1c, fasting lipids	Baseline, at 12 weeks, then annually

[1]Personal or family history of obesity, diabetes, hypertension, or cardiovascular disease

BMI = body mass index

Adapted from: The American Diabetes Association, from *Diabetes Care* 2004;27(2), and *The American Psychiatric Association Practice Guideline for the Treatment of Patients With Schizophrenia,* Third Edition (September 2020)

Other warnings that should be considered for all antipsychotic agents (first and second generation) include the following:

- *Neuroleptic malignant syndrome (NMS),* a potentially fatal syndrome characterized by fever, severe muscle rigidity, and autonomic instability, has been reported in patients receiving antipsychotic agents. Treatment requires immediate discontinuation of the drug and intensive symptomatic treatment in a hospital setting.

- *Tardive dyskinesia (TD),* a syndrome of potentially irreversible, involuntary dyskinetic movements, has been reported. TD is more common with first-generation antipsychotics than with second-generation agents.

- *Extrapyramidal and withdrawal symptoms* in newborns have been reported with maternal use of first-generation antipsychotics during the third trimester of pregnancy. Symptoms may include agitation, feeding disorder, hypertonia or hypotonia, respiratory distress, and somnolence. These effects vary in severity and may be self-limiting (subsiding within hours or days) or, in rare cases, require hospitalization.

Psychosis Treatment Algorithm

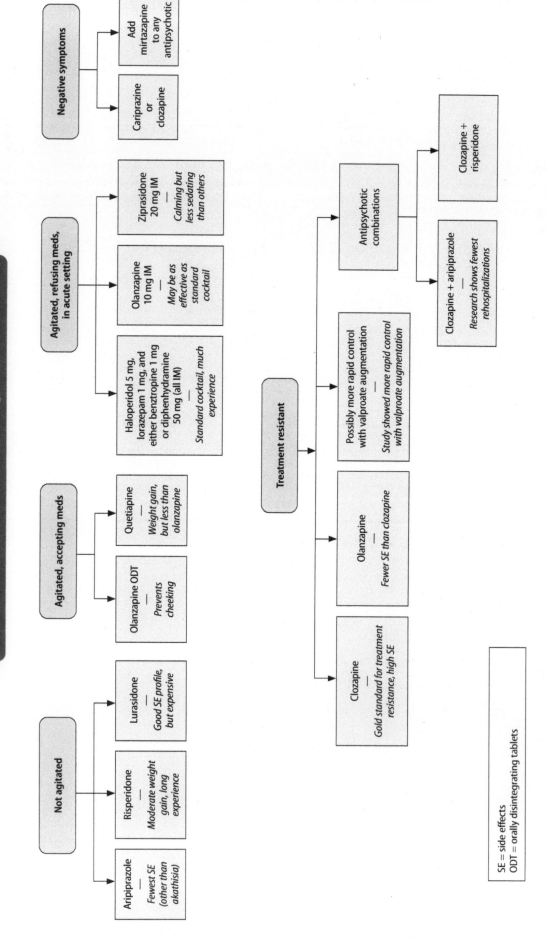

Negative symptoms
- Cariprazine or clozapine
- Add mirtazapine to any antipsychotic

Agitated, refusing meds, in acute setting
- Haloperidol 5 mg, lorazepam 1 mg, and either benztropine 1 mg or diphenhydramine 50 mg (all IM)
  Standard cocktail, much experience
- Olanzapine 10 mg IM
  May be as effective as standard cocktail
- Ziprasidone 20 mg IM
  Calming but less sedating than others

Agitated, accepting meds
- Olanzapine ODT
  Prevents cheeking
- Quetiapine
  Weight gain, but less than olanzapine

Not agitated
- Aripiprazole
  Fewest SE (other than akathisia)
- Risperidone
  Moderate weight gain, long experience
- Lurasidone
  Good SE profile, but expensive

Treatment resistant
- Clozapine
  Gold standard for treatment resistance, high SE
- Olanzapine
  Fewer SE than clozapine
- Possibly more rapid control with valproate augmentation
  Study showed more rapid control with valproate augmentation
- Antipsychotic combinations
  - Clozapine + aripiprazole
    Research shows fewest rehospitalizations
  - Clozapine + risperidone

SE = side effects
ODT = orally disintegrating tablets

Table 8: **First-Generation Antipsychotics**

Generic Name (Brand Name) Year FDA Approved [G] denotes generic availability	Relevant FDA Indication(s)	Available Strengths (mg)	Dosage Equivalents	Usual Dosage Range (starting–max) (mg)	Notes
Chlorpromazine [G] (Thorazine[1]) 1957	Psychosis, mania, nausea/vomiting	Tablet: 10, 25, 50, 100, 200 Liquid: 30 mg/mL, 100 mg/mL IM injection: 25 mg/mL	100	50–600	Injectable available; photosensitivity
Fluphenazine [G] (Prolixin[1], Prolixin Decanoate[1]) 1960	Psychosis	Tablet: 1, 2.5, 5, 10 Liquid: 2.5 mg/5 mL, 5 mg/mL IM injection: 2.5 mg/mL LAI: Decanoate (see fact sheet)	2	2–20	Oral solution; injectables (short and LAI) available
Haloperidol [G] (Haldol, Haldol Decanoate) 1967	Psychosis, Tourette's disorder	Tablet: 0.5, 1, 2, 5, 10, 20 Liquid: 2 mg/mL IM injection: 5 mg/mL LAI: Decanoate (see fact sheet)	2	2–20	Oral solution; injectables (short and LAI) available
Loxapine [G] (Adasuve, Loxitane[1]) 1975	Schizophrenia	Capsule: 5, 10, 25, 50 Inhaler: 10	10	20–100	10 mg oral inhalation powder available as Adasuve since 2012; available only in enrolled health care facilities
Molindone [G] (Moban[1]) 1974	Schizophrenia	Tablet: 5, 10, 25	10	50–100	Less weight gain than others
Perphenazine [G] (Trilafon[1]) 1957	Schizophrenia (12+), severe nausea/vomiting	Tablet: 2, 4, 8, 16	8	8–64	Mid-potency agent studied and compared to second-generation agents in CATIE (see fact sheet)
Thioridazine [G] (Mellaril[1]) 1962	Schizophrenia	Tablet: 10, 25, 50, 100	100	50–600	QT prolongation; irreversible retinal pigmentation at >800 mg/day
Thiothixene [G] (Navane[1]) 1967	Schizophrenia	Capsule: 1, 2, 5, 10	4	6–40	High-potency agent
Trifluoperazine [G] (Stelazine[1]) 1959	Schizophrenia, nonpsychotic anxiety	Tablet: 1, 2, 5, 10	5	4–40	High-potency agent

[1]Brand discontinued; no longer available as brand

IM = intramuscular

Antipsychotics

Table 9: Second-Generation Antipsychotics

Generic Name (Brand Name) Year FDA Approved [G] denotes generic availability	Relevant FDA Indication(s) (pediatric ages specified where relevant)	Available Strengths (mg)	Usual Dosage Range (starting–max) (mg)[1]	Notes
Aripiprazole [G] (Abilify, Abilify Discmelt) 2002	Schizophrenia (13+) Bipolar mania, monotherapy and adjunctive (10+) Bipolar maintenance, monotherapy and adjunctive Depression adjunct Irritability in autism (6–17) Tourette's disorder (6–18) Agitation in schizophrenia or bipolar (IM only) Acute schizophrenia relapse (LAI Maintena only)	Tablet: 2, 5, 10, 15, 20, 30 ODT: 10, 15, 20, 30 Liquid: 1 mg/mL LAI: Maintena, Initio, Aristada (see fact sheet)	10–30 QD	Probably most "activating," though higher doses can be sedating
Asenapine [G] (Saphris, Secuado) 2009 Generic not available for patch	Schizophrenia Bipolar mania, monotherapy and adjunctive (10+)	SL tablet: 2.5, 5, 10 Patch: 3.8, 5.7, 7.6/24 h	SL: 5–10 BID TD: 3.8–7.6 QD	Avoid food or drink for 10 minutes after taking SL; sedating
Brexpiprazole (Rexulti) 2015	Schizophrenia (13+) Depression adjunct	Tablet: 0.25, 0.5, 1, 2, 3, 4	1–4 QD	Newer agent with limited data; weight gain and akathisia most common adverse effects
Cariprazine (Vraylar) 2015	Schizophrenia Bipolar I depression Bipolar mania and mixed episodes	Capsule: 1.5, 3, 4.5, 6	1.5–6 QD	Newest agent with limited data; possible negative symptom efficacy
Clozapine [G] (Clozaril, FazaClo, Versacloz) 1989 Generic not available for oral suspension	Treatment-resistant schizophrenia Recurrent suicidal behavior in schizophrenia or schizoaffective disorders	Tablet: 25, 50, 100, 200 ODT: 12.5, 25, 100, 150, 200 Oral suspension: 50 mg/mL	12.5–450 BID	Probably most effective antipsychotic
Iloperidone (Fanapt) 2009	Schizophrenia	Tablet: 1, 2, 4, 6, 8, 10, 12	2–12 BID	Orthostatic dizziness; must be titrated
Lumateperone (Caplyta) 2019	Schizophrenia Bipolar I or II depression	Capsule: 10.5, 21, 42	42 QD	Take with dinner
Lurasidone (Latuda) 2010	Schizophrenia (13+) Bipolar I depression (10+)	Tablet: 20, 40, 60, 80, 120	40–160 QD	Sedating; must take with food
Olanzapine [G] (Zyprexa, Zyprexa Zydis) 1996 Generic not available for LAI	Schizophrenia (13+) Bipolar mania, monotherapy and adjunctive (13+) Bipolar maintenance, monotherapy Bipolar I depression (with fluoxetine) (10+) Treatment-resistant depression (with fluoxetine) Agitation in schizophrenia or bipolar (IM only)	Tablet: 2.5, 5, 7.5, 10, 15, 20 ODT: 5, 10, 15, 20 IM injection: 10 mg/vial LAI: Relprevv (see fact sheet)	10–20 QD	Greatest weight gain
Olanzapine/samidorphan (Lybalvi) 2021	Schizophrenia Bipolar mania monotherapy and adjunctive Bipolar maintenance	Tablet: 5/10, 10/10, 15/10, 20/10	10/10–20/10 QD	Less weight gain than olanzapine alone but still moderate weight gain; avoid in patients taking opioids
Paliperidone [G] (Invega) 2006 Generic not available for LAI	Schizophrenia (12+) Schizoaffective disorder	ER tablet: 1.5, 3, 6, 9 LAI: Sustenna, Trinza, Hafyera (see fact sheet)	6–12 QD	Good for those with hepatic impairment; increases prolactin

ODT = orally disintegrating tablet, LAI = long-acting injectable ER, XR = extended release, IM = intramuscular, SL = sublingual, TD = transdermal

[1] For schizophrenia indication

Generic Name (Brand Name) Year FDA Approved [G] denotes generic availability	Relevant FDA Indication(s) (pediatric ages specified where relevant)	Available Strengths (mg)	Usual Dosage Range (starting–max) (mg)[1]	Notes
Pimavanserin (Nuplazid) 2016	Parkinson's disease psychosis	Tablet: 10 Capsule: 34	34 QD	No data in schizophrenia
Quetiapine [G] (Seroquel) (Seroquel XR) 1997	Schizophrenia (13+) Bipolar mania, monotherapy and adjunctive (10+) Bipolar disorder maintenance Bipolar I or II depression Depression adjunct (approved in ER form)	Tablet: 25, 50, 100, 200, 300, 400 ER tablet: 50, 150, 200, 300, 400	50–800 divided BID to TID; 300–800 QHS for XR	Sedating
Risperidone [G] (Risperdal, Risperdal M-Tab) 1993 Generic not available for LAI	Schizophrenia (13+) Bipolar mania, monotherapy and adjunctive (10+) Irritability in autism (5–16)	Tablet: 0.25, 0.5, 1, 2, 3, 4 ODT: 0.25, 0.5, 1, 2, 3, 4 Liquid: 1 mg/mL LAI: Consta, Perseris (see fact sheet)	2–6 divided QD to BID	Increases prolactin
Ziprasidone [G] (Geodon) 2001	Schizophrenia Bipolar mania, monotherapy Bipolar maintenance, adjunctive Agitation in schizophrenia (IM injection)	Capsule: 20, 40, 60, 80 IM injection: 20 mg/mL	20–80 BID	Take with food

ODT = orally disintegrating tablet, LAI = long-acting injectable ER, XR = extended release, IM = intramuscular, SL = sublingual, TD = transdermal

[1]For schizophrenia indication

Antipsychotics

Table 10: Comparison of Relative Side Effects Among Antipsychotics

	Wt/ Metabolic	Sedation	QT Prolongation	Orthostasis	Akathisia	EPS (Park/ Dyst)	TD	Prolactin	Anti-cholinergic	Seizures
First Generation										
Chlorpromazine	+	+++	++++	+++	+	+	+++	+	+++	++
Fluphenazine	+	+	++	+	+++	+++	+++	+++	+	+
Haloperidol	+	+	++	+	+++	+++	+++	+++	+	+
Loxapine	+	++	++	++	++	++	++	++	++	+
Molindone	0/+	++	++	+	++	++	++	++	+	+
Perphenazine	+	++	++	++	++	++	++	++	++	+
Thioridazine	+	+++	++++	+++	+	+	++	++	+++	++
Thiothixene	+	+	++	+	+++	+++	+++	+++	+	+++
Trifluoperazine	+	+	++	+	++	++	++	++	++	+
Second Generation										
Aripiprazole	0/+	+	0/+	+	+++	+	+	+	+	+
Asenapine	++	++	++	++	++	+	++	++	+	+
Brexpiprazole	0/+	+	++	+	+++	+	+	+	+	+
Cariprazine	++	++	++	+	++	+	+	+	++	+
Clozapine	+++	+++	++	+++	0/+	0/+	0/+	+	+++	+++
Iloperidone	++	++	+++	+++	+	+	+	++	+	+
Lumateperone	+	+	+	++	+	+	+	+	+	+
Lurasidone	+	++	+	+	++	++	++	+	+	+
Olanzapine	+++	+++	++	++	++	++	+	++	++	++
Olanzapine/ samidorphan	++	+++	++	++	++	++	+	++	++	++
Paliperidone	++	+	++	++	++	++	++	+++	+	+
Pimavanserin (Parkinson's psychosis only)	+	+	++	+	0	0	0	0	0	+
Quetiapine	++	+++	++	++	0/+	0/+	+	+	++	++
Risperidone	++	++	++	++	++	++	++	+++	+	+
Ziprasidone	0/+	++	+++	++	++	+	+	++	+	+

Adapted from *The American Psychiatric Association Practice Guideline for the Treatment of Patients With Schizophrenia,* Third Edition (September 2020).

ARIPIPRAZOLE (Abilify) Fact Sheet [G]

Bottom Line:
Aripiprazole is a good choice for minimizing risk of weight gain and metabolic side effects, but beware of akathisia. Large number of indications and reports of success at a variety of doses make it difficult to predict dosing for individual patients.

FDA Indications:
Schizophrenia (adults, adolescents 13–17 years); **bipolar disorder,** acute treatment of manic and mixed episodes (adults, children 10–17 years); **bipolar disorder, maintenance treatment** (adults); **major depression,** as adjunct (adults); **irritability in autism** (children 6–17 years); **Tourette's disorder** (children 6–18 years).

Off-Label Uses:
Bipolar depression; behavioral disturbances.

Dosage Forms:
- **Tablets (G):** 2 mg, 5 mg, 10 mg, 15 mg, 20 mg, 30 mg.
- **Orally disintegrating tablets (G):** 10 mg, 15 mg, 20 mg, 30 mg.
- **Oral liquid (G):** 1 mg/mL.
- **IM depot: Abilify Maintena:** 300 mg and 400 mg; **Aristada:** 441 mg, 662 mg, 882 mg, 1064 mg; **Aristada Initio:** 675 mg (see LAI fact sheet and table).
- **Tablet with sensor (Abilify MyCite):** 2 mg, 5 mg, 10 mg, 15 mg, 20 mg, 30 mg.

Dosage Guidance:
- Schizophrenia and bipolar disorder: Adults: Start and target dose 10–15 mg/day; max 30 mg/day. Children: Start 2 mg/day, increase on third day to 5 mg/day; may increase further by 5 mg/day increments weekly to target dose 10 mg/day, max 30 mg/day.
- Irritability in autism (children): Start 2 mg/day, ↑ to 5 mg/day in weekly increments to target dose 5–10 mg/day, max 15 mg/day.
- Depression: Start 2–5 mg/day, ↑ to usual dose 5–10 mg/day, as adjunct. Titrate gradually to prevent agitation/akathisia (max 15 mg/day).
- Tourette's: Start 2 mg/day, ↑ to target 5 mg/day, max 10 mg/day (<50 kg); 10 mg/day, max 20 mg/day (>50 kg).
- Depot: After oral dose tolerated, start Abilify Maintena 400 mg/four weeks (continue oral aripiprazole for first 14 days), target dose 300–400 mg/four weeks. For Aristada: Start 441 mg, 662 mg, or 882 mg monthly—corresponds to 300 mg, 450 mg, and 600 mg of aripiprazole, respectively. Or, start 882 mg dose every six weeks or 1064 mg dose every two months. For all Aristada regimens, continue oral aripiprazole for first 21 days unless using concurrent Initio dose.
- Liquid dosing: Oral solution equivalent to tablet dose up to 25 mg; for 30 mg tablets, give 25 mg oral solution.
- Orally disintegrating tablet: Same as regular tablet dosing.
- Dose timing: Can be taken in the morning or at night; may unpredictably cause drowsiness or insomnia.

Monitoring: Fasting glucose, lipids.

Cost: $; ODT, liquid: $$$$

Side Effects:
- Most common: Akathisia, anxiety, insomnia, sedation, tremors.
- Serious but rare: Rare reports of reversible pathologic gambling and other impulse control problems (eating, spending, sexual).

Mechanism, Pharmacokinetics, and Drug Interactions:
- Dopamine D2 and serotonin 5-HT1A receptor partial agonist and serotonin 5-HT2A receptor antagonist.
- Metabolized by CYP2D6 and 3A4; t ½: 3–6 days.
- Use ½ usual dose in presence of 2D6 or 3A4 inhibitors or in known 2D6 poor metabolizers; ¼ dose if both 2D6 inhibitor/poor metabolizer and 3A4 inhibitor; double dose if also using 3A4 inducer.

Clinical Pearls:
- Some prescribers use low-dose aripiprazole to counteract antipsychotic-induced prolactinemia, given its partial agonist properties.
- In November 2017 FDA approved Abilify MyCite, which is aripiprazole with an embedded ingestible sensor to track adherence. After a "limited initial launch" in August 2018, the system is only available through a specialty pharmacy.

Fun Fact:
After aripiprazole's generic launch, Otsuka followed up with brexpiprazole (see fact sheet), another dopamine partial agonist, approved for schizophrenia and depression (as adjunct) and in clinical trials for ADHD.

ASENAPINE (Saphris, Secuado) Fact Sheet [G]

Bottom Line:

Asenapine's claim to fame is its availability in both sublingual and skin patch formulations, so it's a good choice for patients who can't or don't want to swallow a pill. Mouth numbness (Saphris), sedation, dizziness, akathisia, weight gain, and potential for allergic reaction are significant liabilities. Not recommended for first-line use.

FDA Indications:

Schizophrenia; bipolar disorder, acute and maintenance treatment of manic or mixed episodes (adults, children 10–17 years).

Off-Label Uses:

Bipolar depression; behavioral disturbances; impulse control disorders.

Dosage Forms:

- **SL tablets (G):** 2.5 mg, 5 mg, 10 mg. (Must be taken sublingually because if swallowed, too much medication is metabolized by the liver during first-pass metabolism.)
- **Transdermal patch (Secuado):** 3.8 mg, 5.7 mg, 7.6 mg/24 hour patch.

Dosage Guidance:

- Schizophrenia: Start 5 mg SL BID, may ↑ after one week to max dose of 10 mg SL BID.
- Bipolar (adults): Same dosing as schizophrenia.
- Bipolar (children): Start 2.5 mg SL BID, increase as needed up to 10 mg SL BID.
- Do not swallow tablets. Avoid food or drink for 10 minutes after taking (they significantly reduce absorption and bioavailability).
- For patch: Start 3.8 mg/24 hours, may ↑ after one week to 5.7 mg/24 hours or to max dose of 7.6 mg/24 hours after one more week. Patch should be applied to hip, abdomen, upper arm, or upper back area.

Monitoring: Fasting glucose, lipids.

Cost: SL: $$$$; patch: $$$$$

Side Effects:

- Most common: Akathisia (seems to be dose-related), oral hypoesthesia (numbing of the tongue or decreased oral sensitivity), somnolence, dizziness, EPS, weight gain.
- Serious but rare: Hypersensitivity reactions including anaphylaxis, angioedema, low blood pressure, rapid heart rate, swollen tongue, difficulty breathing, wheezing, or rash; orthostatic hypotension and syncope, particularly early in treatment (FDA warning, September 2011).

Mechanism, Pharmacokinetics, and Drug Interactions:

- Dopamine D2 and serotonin 5-HT2A receptor antagonist.
- Metabolized by glucuronidation and CYP1A2; t ½: 24 hours. Inhibitor of 2D6; may double paroxetine levels. Smoking may induce metabolism and may lower levels of asenapine via 1A2 induction; adjust dosing. CYP1A2 inhibitors (eg, fluvoxamine) may increase levels of asenapine; adjust dose.
- Caution with antihypertensive agents and other drugs that can cause additive hypotension or bradycardia.

Clinical Pearls:

- Has a receptor-binding profile similar to clozapine, although asenapine has very little anticholinergic activity.
- Weight gain seems to be a problem in many patients.
- Contraindicated in patients with severe hepatic impairment due to seven-fold higher levels.
- Most useful for patients who don't like swallowing pills.
- Steady state with patch is achieved in 72 hours. Patch daily dose equivalence of 3.8 mg is 5 mg SL BID and 7.6 mg is 10 mg SL BID.
- Mnemonic for remembering the brand name: The first two letters of asenapine are A-S, or Asenapine-Saphris.

Fun Fact:

Black cherry flavor was developed after patients complained about original tablets.

BREXPIPRAZOLE (Rexulti) Fact Sheet

Bottom Line:

Brexpiprazole is a cousin of aripiprazole and is also a partial dopamine agonist. It has a very similar efficacy profile (including efficacy for depression) and similar side effect profile, but is much more expensive. We recommend choosing the cheaper, generic aripiprazole.

FDA Indications:

Schizophrenia (adults, adolescents 13–17 years); **depression adjunct.**

Off-Label Uses:

Dementia-related psychosis; borderline personality disorder.

Dosage Forms:

Tablets: 0.25 mg, 0.5 mg, 1 mg, 2 mg, 3 mg, 4 mg.

Dosage Guidance:

- Schizophrenia: Start 1 mg/day on days one through four; ↑ to 2 mg/day on days five through seven; then up to max 4 mg/day based on patient response. Usual dose 2–4 mg/day. Children: Start 0.5 mg/day, increase on fifth day to 1 mg/day and 2 mg/day on eighth day; may increase further by 1 mg/day increments weekly to target dose of 2-4 mg/day
- Depression adjunct: Start 0.5–1 mg/day, ↑ at weekly intervals up to target 2 mg/day, max 3 mg/day.
- Dose timing: Like aripiprazole, can be taken in the morning or at night; may unpredictably cause drowsiness or insomnia.

Monitoring: Fasting glucose, lipids.

Cost: $$$$

Side Effects:

- Most common: Weight gain, akathisia, somnolence.
- Serious but rare: Rare reports of reversible pathologic gambling and other impulse control problems (eating, spending, sexual).

Mechanism, Pharmacokinetics, and Drug Interactions:

- Dopamine D2 and serotonin 5-HT1A receptor partial agonist and serotonin 5-HT2A receptor antagonist.
- Metabolized by CYP2D6 and CYP3A4; t ½: 91 hours.
- Use ½ usual dose in presence of 2D6 or 3A4 inhibitors or in known 2D6 poor metabolizers; ¼ dose if both 2D6 inhibitor/poor metabolizer and 3A4 inhibitor; double dose if also using 3A4 inducer.

Clinical Pearls:

- As the name suggests, brexpiprazole is chemically and structurally related to its manufacturer's previous blockbuster aripiprazole (Abilify).
- Although the FDA-approved target dose for schizophrenia is 2–4 mg/day, 2 mg/day was no better than placebo in one of two preclinical registration studies.
- Unlike aripiprazole, brexpiprazole may not be effective in bipolar mania. It was no better than placebo at reducing symptoms in about 650 patients enrolled in two studies in acute mania. One study compared weight gain from brexpiprazole to aripiprazole and found a similar increase of about 5–10 pounds over a year.
- Once-a-day dosing with no regard to meals makes this an easy-to-use option.
- Generic/brand name mnemonic: "Brex is Rex" (thanks to Dr. Raj Mago).

Fun Fact:

Plan on seeing more trial results with Rexulti in the future, including those in patients with ADHD, PTSD, and agitation associated with Alzheimer's dementia.

Antipsychotics

CARIPRAZINE (Vraylar) Fact Sheet

Bottom Line:

Cariprazine, like aripiprazole and brexpiprazole, is a partial dopamine agonist. Some preliminary data imply that it might be effective for negative symptoms, but it's too soon to tell. Beyond that, it appears similar to the other two partial dopamine agonists, with a high rate of EPS and akathisia but minimal weight gain. It is available as a brand name only and is therefore very expensive (as opposed to aripiprazole, which has gone generic).

FDA Indications:

Schizophrenia; acute treatment of **bipolar disorder (manic or mixed episodes); bipolar I depression.**

Off-Label Uses:

Negative symptoms of schizophrenia; major depression.

Dosage Forms:

Capsules: 1.5 mg, 3 mg, 4.5 mg, 6 mg.

Dosage Guidance:

- Schizophrenia and bipolar disorder: Start 1.5 mg/day, may ↑ to 3 mg/day as early as second day. Adjust by 1.5–3 mg/day increments to usual dose 1.5–6 mg/day in schizophrenia and 3–6 mg/day in bipolar disorder.
- Bipolar depression: Start 1.5 mg QD, may ↑ to 3 mg QD after two weeks or longer; max dose 3 mg/day.
- Dose timing: Either morning or night; some patients experience restlessness that can interfere with sleep, in which case morning is preferred.

Monitoring: Fasting glucose, lipids.

Cost: $$$$$

Side Effects:

- Most common: EPS, akathisia, weight gain, sedation.
- Serious but rare: See class warnings in chapter introduction.

Mechanism, Pharmacokinetics, and Drug Interactions:

- Dopamine D2 and D3 and serotonin 5-HT1A receptor partial agonist; serotonin 5-HT2A receptor antagonist.
- Metabolized primarily by CYP3A4; t ½: 2–4 days for cariprazine (1–3 weeks for active metabolites).
- Caution with CYP3A4 inhibitors; 50% dose reduction may be necessary. Avoid use with 3A4 inducers.

Clinical Pearls:

- Most closely similar to aripiprazole with partial D2 agonism.
- Manufacturer and very early data suggest D3 activity may result in negative symptom improvement.
- While cariprazine showed enough efficacy to gain an indication for bipolar depression, this was only true in patients with bipolar type I. In trials with bipolar II patients, it was no better than placebo.

Fun Fact:

Cariprazine was developed by a Hungarian pharmaceutical company, Gedeon Richter, which was founded in 1901 by a pharmacist. Gedeon Richter initially processed extracts from plants to produce herbal drugs.

CHLORPROMAZINE (Thorazine) Fact Sheet [G]

Bottom Line:

Chlorpromazine was the first antipsychotic to be developed. Its long track record and good sedative properties make it popular for certain populations, especially patients with chronic psychosis, agitation, and mania, particularly when they are hospitalized. Its availability as an IM injection is an advantage for treating acute agitation. As a low-potency agent, it is less likely to cause EPS or TD than many other antipsychotics.

FDA Indications:

Psychosis; mania; severe behavioral disorders (6 months–17 years); nausea and vomiting; intractable hiccups.

Off-Label Uses:

Bipolar disorder; behavioral disturbances; impulse control disorders.

Dosage Forms:

- **Tablets (G):** 10 mg, 25 mg, 50 mg, 100 mg, 200 mg.
- **Oral concentrate (G):** 30 mg/mL, 100 mg/mL.
- **Injectable (G):** 25 mg/mL.

Dosage Guidance:

- Schizophrenia: Start 10–25 mg TID; ↑ by 20–50 mg/day increments every three to four days to lowest effective dose. Dose range 200–600 mg/day in divided doses; max FDA-approved dose 1000 mg/day.
- IM for agitation: Usual dose is 25–50 mg; may repeat after one hour, with maximum dose of 200 mg/day.

Monitoring: ECG if cardiac disease.

Cost: $$–$$$$ (depending on dose); oral concentrate: $$$$$

Side Effects:

- Most common: Sedation, orthostasis, tachycardia, drowsiness, dry mouth, constipation, blurred vision, prolactin elevation (sexual side effects, amenorrhea, galactorrhea).
- Serious but rare: Skin pigmentation and ocular changes (both dose related); jaundice; QT prolongation; seizure.

Mechanism, Pharmacokinetics, and Drug Interactions:

- Dopamine D2 receptor antagonist.
- Metabolized primarily by CYP2D6, also CYP1A2 and CYP3A4. Patients who are poor metabolizers of CYP2D6 metabolize the drug more slowly, potentially increasing its effects; t ½: 23–37 hours.
- CYP2D6 inhibitors (eg, fluoxetine, paroxetine, quinidine) may increase chlorpromazine levels.

Clinical Pearls:

- Chlorpromazine is a low-potency first-generation antipsychotic; this leads to less EPS compared to high-potency agents (eg, haloperidol, fluphenazine) and to more anticholinergic side effects compared to mid- and high-potency agents (eg, perphenazine and haloperidol, respectively).
- Extremely sedating agent and often used for this effect. Dosing limited by orthostasis and sedation.

Fun Fact:

Thorazine was developed by a French surgeon in 1948 to induce relaxation and indifference in surgical patients.

CLOZAPINE (Clozaril, FazaClo, Versacloz) Fact Sheet [G]

Bottom Line:

Clozapine is the only drug with convincing evidence of superior efficacy over other antipsychotics for treatment-resistant schizophrenia. Consider using it after two failed trials of other antipsychotics. Side effects can be a real challenge, including severe weight gain, constipation, drooling, sedation, and the potential for neutropenia.

FDA Indications:

Treatment-resistant schizophrenia; reduction in risk of suicide in schizophrenia and schizoaffective disorder.

Off-Label Uses:

Treatment-resistant bipolar disorder; treatment-resistant aggression and violence.

Dosage Forms:

• **Tablets (Clozaril):** 25 mg (scored), 100 mg (scored).
• **Tablets (G):** 25 mg (scored), 50 mg (scored), 100 mg (scored), 200 mg (scored).
• **Orally disintegrating tablets (FazaClo, [G]):** 12.5 mg, 25 mg, 100 mg, 150 mg, 200 mg.
• **Oral suspension (Versacloz):** 50 mg/mL.

Dosage Guidance:

• Start 12.5 mg once or twice daily; ↑ gradually, in increments of 25–50 mg/day to target dose 300–450 mg/day by end of two weeks; may ↑ further in increments ≤100 mg and no more frequently than once or twice weekly. May require doses as high as 600–900 mg/day; max 900 mg/day (usually in two or three divided doses). May take four to six weeks, or as long as three to six months, for response.
• If dosing is interrupted for ≥48 hours, must be re-titrated from 12.5–25 mg/day; may be increased more rapidly than initial titration, as tolerated.
• Dose timing: Although it can be sedating, many patients develop tolerance and can take it twice daily without significant daytime fatigue.

Monitoring:

• Fasting glucose, lipids.
• Before starting clozapine, ensure absolute neutrophil count (ANC) >1500; for benign ethnic neutropenia population, ensure two baseline ANCs ≥1000. Repeat ANC weekly for first six months, then every two weeks from months six to 12, then monthly after 12 months. If ANC falls below 1500, guidelines become complex depending on how low the value is; consult clozapine Risk Evaluation and Mitigation Strategy (REMS) (http://b.link/clozapine-rems) for advice.
• Serum level monitoring can be useful; therapeutic response generally occurs at 350–450 ng/mL, though some patients may show response at lower levels. Upper limit is not well defined; increased risk of toxic effects at levels above 700 ng/mL.

Cost: $$; oral suspension, ODT: $$$$$

Side Effects (see Table 11 for more detailed information):

• Most common: Sedation, orthostatic hypotension, hypersalivation (place towel on pillow), weight gain (15–30 pound average weight gain after one year), constipation (risk of toxic megacolon if untreated), tachycardia (can treat with propranolol).
• Serious but rare: Potentially life-threatening neutropenia (1%–2%); periodic ANC testing must occur (as above, see prescribing information for monitoring details).

Mechanism, Pharmacokinetics, and Drug Interactions:

• Dopamine D2 and serotonin 5-HT2A receptor antagonist.
• Metabolized primarily by CYP4501A2, also CYP2D6 and CYP3A4; t ½: 12 hours.
• Avoid use with drugs that may cause bone marrow suppression (eg, carbamazepine, antineoplastics), lower seizure threshold, or have additive anticholinergic effects. Collapse, respiratory arrest, and cardiac arrest reported during initial clozapine treatment in patients taking benzodiazepines. Caution with P450 inhibitors and inducers. Smoking increases clozapine clearance by 30%–50%.

Clinical Pearls:

• Risk of neutropenia greatest within first six months, then incidence declines but can still occur.
• Divided doses may minimize some adverse effects (eg, hypotension, seizures).
• A growing number of case reports have been published linking very high clozapine levels to infection. Monitor levels and symptoms of toxicity closely, especially in patients hospitalized for infection.
• FDA-mandated REMS program requires prescribers to be certified to prescribe clozapine (see www.clozapinerems.com for details).

Fun Fact:

The Quiet Room is a compelling memoir written by patient Lori Schiller, who was an early user of clozapine.

Table 11: Monitoring and Managing Patients on Clozapine

Side Effects	Occurrence	Management	Comments
Constipation/hypomotility	Constipation 60%; obstruction 33%; ileus 1%–2%	• Routinely monitor bowel function (frequency of bowel movements, abdominal pain or distension, absent bowel sounds, diarrhea due to overflow constipation, vomiting) • Encourage hydration, exercise, prune juice • For chronic constipation, use polyethylene glycol 17 g QD–TID or lactulose 10–40 g QD; bisacodyl or senna are second-line options • For immediate response, use magnesium citrate, glycerin suppository, or sodium phosphate enema • Discontinue anticholinergic agents	• Risk factors: higher dose, concomitant anticholinergics or opioids • In severe cases, potentially life threatening • Necrosis, bowel obstruction, GI perforation, sepsis, and death have occurred • Avoid bulk-forming laxatives such as psyllium as they may increase risk of perforation in slow-transit constipation
Hypotension/orthostasis	9%	• Follow dosing titration guidelines • Adjust to slower titration if hypotension occurs	• Highest risk during initial dose titration, particularly if rapid or large dose increases • If patient misses >48 hours of clozapine, re-titrate to minimize orthostasis • Rarely, syncope may occur
Myocarditis/cardiomyopathy	<1%	• Early signs are nonspecific and include tachycardia, malaise, chest pain • If suspected, check cardiac enzymes (troponin, C-reactive protein), ECG, chest x-ray • If myocarditis, discontinue clozapine, give supportive care (diuretics, beta blockers, ACE inhibitors used) • Rechallenge in confirmed myocarditis is controversial; use clinical judgment based on risk/benefit	• Myocarditis typically occurs early in therapy (first 8 weeks) • Cardiomyopathy may develop after 6 months and may be a consequence of persistent tachycardia • Detecting early can prevent serious outcomes including death in 12%–24% of cases
Neutropenia/agranulocytosis	Neutropenia 3%–4%; agranulocytosis <1%	• Check baseline and weekly ANC; if normal, can reduce frequency to every 2 weeks after 6 months and then monthly after another 6 months • See Table 11A (immediately below) for details	• Risk is greatest in first 18 weeks • Not dose related • "Do not rechallenge" list has been eliminated; if patient experiences severe neutropenia (ANC <500), continuation is based on clinical judgment
Nocturnal enuresis	21%	• Lower dose or slow titration schedule • Divide dose into BID–TID to lower dose burden at night	• Common particularly early in dosing titration
Sedation/somnolence	40%	• Lower dose or slow titration schedule • Consolidate dosing to all at bedtime if tolerated	• Early side effects for which many patients develop tolerance
Seizures	1%–5% depending on dose	• Lower dose if clinically appropriate • Add anticonvulsant for prophylaxis at higher doses (>600 mg/day). valproate often preferred; avoid carbamazepine due to additive risk for neutropenia	• Dose related: 1%–2% at <300 mg/day, 3%–4% at 300–600 mg/day, 5%+ at >600 mg/day
Sialorrhea	Rates of 30%–90% reported	• Nonpharmacologic: chew sugarless gum (assists with swallowing saliva, reduces pooling and drooling), use towel on pillow at night • Atropine 1% ophthalmic drops (1–6 drops SL divided QD–TID): limited evidence, effect may not be sustained • Benztropine 0.5–2 mg/day in divided doses: limited evidence, caution additive anticholinergic effects	• More common and severe at night • May impact medication adherence • May increase risk for aspiration pneumonia • May be due to parotid gland inflammation and impaired swallowing

	Occurrence	Management	Comments
Tachycardia	25%	• Reduce dose or slow titration • Consider propranolol 10–20 mg QD–TID	• Dose related and reversible • Usually associated with initial dose titration and transient in many patients • Persistent tachycardia may increase risk for cardiomyopathy
Weight gain, hyperlipidemia, hyperglycemia	Very common	• Educate regarding diet, exercise • Use lowest effective dose • Monitor weight, waist circumference, glucose, HgA1c, lipids regularly • Consider metformin and topiramate for weight gain	• Dose dependent • Non-obese patients may gain more weight • Monitor for signs of hyperglycemia (polyphagia, polydipsia, polyuria)
Therapeutic Drug Monitoring			
• Order "clozapine, norclozapine, total level" • Draw at trough (generally in the morning, 12 hours after nighttime dose but before morning dose)	N/A	• Target clozapine level is >350 ng/mL • Target clozapine to norclozapine ratio is 1.5:1 to 2:1 • Side effects and toxicity generally appear >750 ng/mL	• Check in patients not responding to usual doses, or having side effects, or when non-adherence is suspected • Wait a minimum of 3 full days at a new dosage before checking serum level to ensure steady state is reached • Norclozapine generally associated with adverse effects; hence achieving target ratio of clozapine:norclozapine is associated with better clinical response and fewer side effects • If ratio <1.5:1, consider fluvoxamine 25–50 mg

Table 11A: ANC Monitoring for Clozapine Treatment

ANC (in /uL)	Treatment Recommendation[1]	ANC Monitoring
Baseline to initiate clozapine ≥1500 (BEN population: ≥1000)	Obtain 1 baseline ANC, then initiate treatment	Weekly for first 6 months; every 2 weeks for months 6–12; monthly after 12 months
Mild neutropenia: 1000–1499	Continue treatment	3 times weekly until ANC ≥1500, then return to previous usual monitoring interval
Moderate neutropenia: 500–999	Hematology consult; hold clozapine; resume when ANC ≥1000	Daily until ANC ≥1000, then 3 times weekly until ANC ≥1500, then weekly for 4 weeks, then return to previous usual interval
Severe neutropenia: <500	Hematology consult; discontinue clozapine; do not rechallenge unless benefits outweigh risks	Daily until ANC ≥1000; 3 times weekly until ANC ≥1500; if rechallenge, resume as new patient

[1]Note: 25%–50% of Black individuals have benign ethnic neutropenia (BEN) and their clozapine monitoring protocol is modified; see https://www.clozapinerems.com/CpmgClozapineUI/rems/pdf/resources/ANC_Table.pdf

FLUPHENAZINE (Prolixin) Fact Sheet [G]

Bottom Line:

Fluphenazine is an effective, inexpensive first-generation antipsychotic with a long history of experience and use, but clinical utility is limited in some patients due to EPS.

FDA Indications:

Psychosis.

Off-Label Uses:

Bipolar disorder; behavioral disturbances; impulse control disorders.

Dosage Forms:

- **Tablets (G):** 1 mg, 2.5 mg, 5 mg, 10 mg.
- **Oral liquid (G):** 2.5 mg/5 mL.
- **Oral concentrate (G):** 5 mg/mL.
- **Injection (G):** 2.5 mg/mL.
- **Long-acting injection (G):** 25 mg/mL (see LAI fact sheet and table).

Dosage Guidance:

Start 1–2.5 mg BID (5 mg BID for hospitalized patients); adjust to lowest effective dose. Dose range 2.5–20 mg/day divided BID; max FDA-approved dose is 40 mg/day, but doses >20 mg/day are difficult to tolerate and rarely more effective.

Monitoring: No routine monitoring recommended unless clinical picture warrants.

Cost: $$

Side Effects:

- Most common: EPS, headache, drowsiness, dry mouth, prolactin elevation (sexual side effects, amenorrhea, galactorrhea).
- Serious but rare: See class warnings in chapter introduction.

Mechanism, Pharmacokinetics, and Drug Interactions:

- Dopamine D2 receptor antagonist.
- Metabolized primarily by CYP2D6; t ½: 15 hours. Poor metabolizers of CYP2D6 metabolize the drug more slowly; may have increased effects.
- CYP2D6 inhibitors (eg, fluoxetine, paroxetine, quinidine) may increase fluphenazine levels.

Clinical Pearls:

- Fluphenazine is a high-potency first-generation antipsychotic; this leads to more EPS compared to mid- or low-potency agents (eg, perphenazine or chlorpromazine, respectively) and to less sedation, less orthostasis, and fewer anticholinergic side effects compared to low-potency agents (eg, chlorpromazine).
- Relatively lower seizure side effect risk compared to lower-potency agents. Long-acting injectable decanoate formulation allows option for patients who don't take oral formation reliably.
- Availability of short-acting injectable and oral liquid formulations also allows for more flexibility in administration.
- Oral concentrate liquid must be diluted with at least two ounces of a liquid such as milk, tomato juice, fruit juice (but not apple juice), or a soft drink that does not contain caffeine.

Fun Fact:

Prolixin is the most well-known brand of fluphenazine, but there was also a branded fluphenazine on the market under the name Permitil.

HALOPERIDOL (Haldol) Fact Sheet [G]

Bottom Line:

Haloperidol is an effective, inexpensive first-generation antipsychotic with low weight gain potential and a long history of experience and use, but clinical utility is limited due to EPS and potential for TD. It's favored by many clinicians for treatment of acute agitation, especially when given in an IM "cocktail" with lorazepam and diphenhydramine.

FDA Indications:

Psychosis (adults, 3–17 years); **Tourette's disorder** (adults, 3–17 years); **severe behavioral disorders** (3–17 years).

Off-Label Uses:

Bipolar disorder; behavioral disturbances; impulse control disorders; delirium.

Dosage Forms:

- **Tablets (G):** 0.5 mg (scored), 1 mg (scored), 2 mg (scored), 5 mg (scored), 10 mg (scored), 20 mg (scored).
- **Oral concentrate (G):** 2 mg/mL.
- **Injection (G):** 5 mg/mL.
- **Long-acting injection (G):** 50 mg/mL and 100 mg/mL (see LAI fact sheet and table).

Dosage Guidance:

- Schizophrenia: Start 1–2 mg BID (5 mg BID for hospitalized patients); adjust to lowest effective dose. Usual dose range is 5–20 mg/day. Max FDA-approved dose is 100 mg/day, but doses >20 mg/day are rarely used.
- IM for agitation: 2.5–10 mg IM, often combined with lorazepam 1 mg IM and diphenhydramine 50 mg IM; maximum 20 mg/day.
- IV for severe agitation (generally in the ICU setting): 2.5–10 mg IV Q4–8 hours; maximum 20 mg/day.

Monitoring: No routine monitoring recommended unless clinical picture warrants. Monitor ECG with IV use due to increased risk for QT prolongation.

Cost: $

Side Effects:

- Most common: EPS, headache, drowsiness, dry mouth, prolactin elevation (sexual side effects, amenorrhea, galactorrhea).
- Serious but rare: See class warnings in chapter introduction.

Mechanism, Pharmacokinetics, and Drug Interactions:

- Dopamine D2 receptor antagonist.
- Metabolized primarily by CYP2D6 and CYP3A4; t ½: 21–24 hours. Patients who are poor metabolizers of CYP2D6 metabolize the drug more slowly; may have increased effects.
- CYP2D6 inhibitors (eg, fluoxetine, paroxetine, quinidine) may increase haloperidol levels. May inhibit CYP2D6; caution with substrates of 2D6 as haloperidol may increase their levels and effects.

Clinical Pearls:

- Haloperidol is a high-potency first-generation antipsychotic; this leads to more EPS compared to mid- or low-potency agents (eg, perphenazine or chlorpromazine, respectively) and to less sedation, less orthostasis, and fewer anticholinergic side effects compared to low-potency agents (eg, chlorpromazine).
- Relatively lower seizure side effect risk compared to lower-potency agents.
- Short-acting injectable and oral liquid formulations allow for more flexibility in administration.
- Long-acting injectable decanoate formulation allows option for patients who don't take oral formation reliably.

Fun Fact:

Haldol was discovered in 1958 by Paul Janssen, the founder of Belgian pharmaceutical company Janssen Pharmaceutica.

ILOPERIDONE (Fanapt) Fact Sheet

Bottom Line:

Iloperidone is not recommended as a first-choice agent due to twice-daily dosing, need for titration, QT prolongation (comparable to ziprasidone), dizziness, moderate weight gain, and increases in blood sugar; and because it appears less efficacious than other antipsychotics.

FDA Indications:

Schizophrenia.

Off-Label Uses:

Bipolar disorder; major depression; behavioral disturbances; impulse control disorders.

Dosage Forms:

Tablets: 1 mg, 2 mg, 4 mg, 6 mg, 8 mg, 10 mg, 12 mg.

Dosage Guidance:

Start 1 mg BID; ↑ to 2 mg BID on day two and then daily by 4 mg/day to a target dose of 6–12 mg BID daily; max 12 mg BID.

Monitoring: Fasting glucose, lipids.

Cost: $$$$$

Side Effects:

- Most common: Dizziness (dose-related), dry mouth, fatigue, nasal congestion, orthostatic hypotension (can minimize by gradual dose titration), somnolence, tachycardia (dose-related), moderate weight gain.
- Serious but rare: Relatively moderate to high risk of QTc prolongation (risk is increased in patients taking potent CYP2D6 or CYP3A4 inhibitors, or at higher doses); avoid use in patients with bradycardia, history of MI, hypokalemia, hypomagnesemia, or concomitant use of other drugs that prolong QTc. Priapism reported rarely.

Mechanism, Pharmacokinetics, and Drug Interactions:

- Dopamine D2 and serotonin 5-HT2A receptor antagonist.
- Metabolized primarily through CYP2D6, also CYP3A4; t ½: 18 hours (33 hours in poor metabolizers).
- Avoid concomitant use of other drugs known to prolong the QTc interval.
- Potent inhibitors of CYP2D6 (eg, paroxetine, fluoxetine, quinidine) or CYP3A4 (eg, ketoconazole, clarithromycin) may increase iloperidone levels; in such cases, decrease iloperidone dose by 50%.

Clinical Pearls:

- Must follow initial titration schedule if treatment has been interrupted for more than three days.
- Minimal data regarding long-term use in schizophrenia and uses other than schizophrenia.
- Avoid use in patients with severe hepatic impairment due to potential for elevated levels leading to QT interval prolongation.
- A network meta-analysis of 212 studies involving more than 43,000 patients found that olanzapine and risperidone improved core symptoms more than other second-generation antipsychotics, and that paliperidone improved core illness symptoms more than lurasidone and iloperidone (*American Psychiatric Association Practice Guideline for the Treatment of Patients With Schizophrenia*, September 2020).

Fun Fact:

Iloperidone was initially on track for FDA approval in 2002, but its approval was delayed to 2009 due to multiple company mergers and out-licensing deals as well as the FDA's request for more data.

Antipsychotics

LOXAPINE (Adasuve, Loxitane) Fact Sheet [G]

Bottom Line:

Loxapine is being rediscovered as a well-tolerated first-generation antipsychotic—it is of medium potency, and causes minimal EPS or weight gain. An oldy-but-goody alternative to second-generation antipsychotics.

FDA Indications:

Schizophrenia; acute agitation associated with schizophrenia or acute bipolar mania.

Off-Label Uses:

Bipolar disorder; behavioral disturbances; impulse control disorders.

Dosage Forms:

- **Capsules (G):** 5 mg, 10 mg, 25 mg, 50 mg.
- **Single-use disposable inhaler (Adasuve),** for acute agitation: 10 mg as inhalation powder.

Dosage Guidance:

- Schizophrenia: Start 10 mg BID; ↑ by 10 mg/day increments weekly and adjust to lowest effective dose. Dose range 60–100 mg divided BID–TID; max FDA-approved dose is 250 mg/day, but doses >100 mg/day rarely used.
- Acute agitation (oral inhalation): Give one puff every 24 hours as needed (must be given by health care professional).

Monitoring: No routine monitoring recommended unless clinical picture warrants.

Cost: Capsule: $; inhalation: $$$

Side Effects:

- Most common: EPS, headache, drowsiness, dry mouth, prolactin elevation (sexual side effects, amenorrhea, galactorrhea), throat irritation (Adasuve).
- Serious but rare: See class warnings in chapter introduction.

Mechanism, Pharmacokinetics, and Drug Interactions:

- Dopamine D2 and serotonin 5-HT2A receptor antagonist.
- Metabolized primarily by CYP2D6 and CYP3A4; t ½: 4–8 hours.
- Caution with inhibitors of CYP2D6 and CYP3A4 and inducers of CYP3A4; adjust dose.

Clinical Pearls:

- Loxapine is an intermediate-potency first-generation antipsychotic; this leads to less EPS compared to high-potency agents (eg, haloperidol, fluphenazine) and to less sedation, less orthostasis, and fewer anticholinergic side effects compared to low-potency agents (eg, chlorpromazine).
- Loxapine belongs to the dibenzoxazepine class of antipsychotics and is structurally related to clozapine (which belongs to the chemically akin class of dibenzodiazepines). Some have argued that loxapine may behave as a second-generation antipsychotic.
- The newer Adasuve oral inhalation version has the advantage of treating agitation quickly without the need for swallowing or a shot. But the risks of bronchospasm and respiratory arrest, along with the contraindication in patients with asthma, COPD, or other lung disease, make this formulation rather unappealing overall.

Fun Fact:

Loxapine is metabolized to the tetracyclic antidepressant amoxapine.

LUMATEPERONE (Caplyta) Fact Sheet

Bottom Line:
Lumateperone is the newest second-generation antipsychotic, approved to treat adults with schizophrenia or bipolar disorder. It appears to have a good tolerability profile and the convenience of once-daily dosing and no titration. But for now, cost relegates it to second-line use.

FDA Indications:
Schizophrenia; bipolar I or II depression.

Off-Label Uses:
Unipolar depression.

Dosage Forms:
Capsules: 10.5 mg, 21 mg, 42 mg.

Dosage Guidance:
Start, target, and max dose of 42 mg QD with food; no titration needed.

Monitoring: No routine monitoring recommended unless clinical picture warrants.

Cost: $$$$$

Side Effects:
- Most common: Somnolence, sedation, dry mouth, nausea, dizziness.
- Serious but rare: See class warnings in chapter introduction.

Mechanism, Pharmacokinetics, and Drug Interactions:
- Dopamine D2 and serotonin 5-HT2A receptor antagonist.
- Metabolized primarily by UGT 1A1, 1A4, 2B15 and CYP3A4, CYP2C8, CYP1A2; t ½: 18 hours.
- Avoid use with potent inhibitors and inducers of CYP3A4.

Clinical Pearls:
- Lumateperone may be better tolerated if taken at dinner due to sedating effects.
- New indication for depression associated with bipolar I and bipolar II followed original schizophrenia indication. It is also currently being studied for unipolar depression with mixed features.
- Lower affinity at D2 receptors means relatively lower risk for EPS.
- In studies to date, lumateperone appears to have low levels of akathisia, weight gain, metabolic side effects, and prolactin elevation.
- New lower dose capsules to be used for patients with moderate or severe hepatic impairment or those taking potent CYP3A4 inhibitors.
- A long-acting injectable of lumateperone is currently in development.

Fun Fact:
This antipsychotic was expected to be approved a couple of years earlier, but a Phase 3 study in 2016 in nearly 700 patients showed no difference from placebo at both 20 mg and 60 mg. This may have been a "failed trial" with a high placebo response rate, and risperidone also failed to separate from placebo in this study.

Antipsychotics

LURASIDONE (Latuda) Fact Sheet

Bottom Line:

Lurasidone offers some advantages, including no need for titration, once-daily dosing, relatively low-moderate metabolic profile, and relatively low QTc prolongation risk. It is also one of three antipsychotics approved for bipolar depression (along with cariprazine and quetiapine). However, its use is limited by the need to administer with at least 350 calories of food, potential for drug interactions, and side effects including sedation, akathisia, and EPS. In clinical practice, you might lump lurasidone with the other second-generation antipsychotics that cause little weight gain, such as aripiprazole and ziprasidone.

FDA Indications:

Schizophrenia (adults, adolescents 13–17); **bipolar I depression** (as monotherapy and adjunct; adults, children 10–17).

Off-Label Uses:

Mixed depression; treatment-resistant depression; impulse control disorders.

Dosage Forms:

Tablets: 20 mg, 40 mg, 60 mg, 80 mg, 120 mg.

Dosage Guidance:

- Schizophrenia (adolescents and adults): Start 40 mg QD, with food (at least 350 calories); no titration required. Usual dose 40–120 mg/day. Max dose 160 mg QD (80 mg/day for adolescents).
- Bipolar depression (adults and children): Start 20 mg QD, with food (at least 350 calories); no titration required. Usual dose 20–120 mg/day (20–40 mg/day in kids). Max dose 120 mg QD (80 mg/day in kids), although doses >80 mg/day rarely more effective.

Monitoring: Fasting glucose, lipids.

Cost: $$$$$

Side Effects:

- Most common: Sedation (dose-related), akathisia (dose-related), nausea, parkinsonism, agitation.
- Serious but rare: Orthostatic hypotension and syncope reported (rarely).

Mechanism, Pharmacokinetics, and Drug Interactions:

- Dopamine D2 and serotonin 5-HT2A and 5-HT7 antagonist; serotonin 5-HT1A partial agonist.
- Metabolized primarily through CYP3A4; t ½: 18 hours.
- Avoid use with medications that cause orthostasis, potent CYP3A4 inhibitors (eg, ketoconazole, clarithromycin), or inducers (eg, rifampin, St. John's wort, carbamazepine). Exercise caution/monitor when using in combination with moderate 3A4 inhibitors (eg, diltiazem); decrease lurasidone dose by 50% in patients taking moderate CYP3A4 inhibitors.

Clinical Pearls:

- Administration with food (at least 350 calories) increases bioavailability two-fold and peak serum levels roughly three-fold; fat content of meal is not important.
- Appears to be relatively weight-neutral, and cardiometabolic parameters were little affected in company-sponsored trials, although post-marketing observations have been limited. In kids, weight gain was a common side effect in studies.
- A network meta-analysis of 10 RCTs with 3,336 adults with schizophrenia found that 40 mg, 80 mg, 120 mg, and 160 mg of lurasidone were effective but not 20 mg. The 160 mg dose was best for PANSS score reduction. Side effects, especially sedation and EPS, increased as dose went up. A good target may be 80 mg, which produced efficacy in 50% of patients. If patients still symptomatic but tolerating, increase to 120–160 mg.
- While using lurasidone in bipolar depression has not been associated with increase in the development of mania, its efficacy in treating manic episodes has not been established, so its use should be reserved for depressive episodes.

Fun Fact:

One unique feature of Latuda is its high affinity for the 5-HT7 receptor, which has been linked to depression, learning/memory, cognition, anxiety, and pain. Unfortunately, to date, Latuda has shown no clear benefit over other second-generation antipsychotics on these measures.

MOLINDONE (Moban) Fact Sheet [G]

Bottom Line:
Molindone is an effective, well-tolerated first-generation antipsychotic of medium potency—a solid medication that some clinicians have gained experience with and favor for select patients. Recently it has been reintroduced into the market, and is still generic and inexpensive.

FDA Indications:
Schizophrenia.

Off-Label Uses:
Bipolar disorder; behavioral disturbances; impulse control disorders.

Dosage Forms:
Tablets (G): 5 mg, 10 mg, 25 mg.

Dosage Guidance:
Start 50–75 mg/day divided BID–QID; ↑ to 100 mg/day in three or four days. Max dose 225 mg/day divided TID–QID.

Monitoring: No routine monitoring recommended unless clinical picture warrants.

Cost: $$$$

Side Effects:
- Most common: Sedation (dose-related), EPS, agitation.
- Serious but rare: Rare reports of leukopenia and leukocytosis.

Mechanism, Pharmacokinetics, and Drug Interactions:
- Dopamine D2 antagonist.
- Metabolized primarily through CYP2D6; t ½: 1.5 hours.

Clinical Pearls:
- Molindone is an intermediate-potency first-generation antipsychotic; this leads to less EPS compared to high-potency agents (eg, haloperidol, fluphenazine) and to less sedation, less orthostasis, and fewer anticholinergic side effects compared to low-potency agents (eg, chlorpromazine).
- Unlike most antipsychotics, molindone has been shown to reduce weight in some patients.

Fun Fact:

In 2010, the only manufacturer of molindone in the US (as brand Moban), Endo Pharmaceuticals, announced that they would be discontinuing production because of poor sales. In December 2015, Core Pharma launched a new generic version, bringing molindone back to life.

OLANZAPINE (Lybalvi, Symbyax, Zyprexa) Fact Sheet [G]

Bottom Line:

Many consider olanzapine to be more effective than other antipsychotics and just below clozapine in effectiveness. Its high efficacy along with its once-daily dosing and low risk of QT interval prolongation are appealing. However, olanzapine's high risk for weight gain and metabolic complications make it a second-line choice for many. The newly approved Lybalvi combines olanzapine with samidorphan to minimize weight gain—but it's only moderately successful.

FDA Indications:

Schizophrenia (adults and children ≥13 years); **acute or mixed bipolar** I manic episodes, as monotherapy or adjunct (adults and children ≥13 years); **maintenance treatment of bipolar disorder**; **bipolar I depression** (with fluoxetine, sold as Symbyax, adults and children ≥10 years); **treatment-resistant unipolar depression** (with fluoxetine); **acute agitation** in schizophrenia and bipolar mania (injectable form).

Off-Label Uses:

Behavioral disturbances; impulse control disorders; reduce weight gain in patients on olanzapine (as Lybalvi).

Dosage Forms:

- **Tablets (G):** 2.5 mg, 5 mg, 7.5 mg, 10 mg, 15 mg, 20 mg.
- **Orally disintegrating tablets (Zyprexa Zydis, [G]):** 5 mg, 10 mg, 15 mg, 20 mg.
- **IM injection (G):** 10 mg.
- **Long-acting injection (Zyprexa Relprevv):** 210 mg, 300 mg, 405 mg (see LAI fact sheet and table).
- **Fixed-combination capsules with fluoxetine (Symbyax, [G]):** 3/25 mg, 6/25 mg, 12/25 mg, 6/50 mg, 12/50 mg olanzapine/fluoxetine.
- **Fixed-combination tablets with samidorphan (Lybalvi):** 5/10 mg, 10/10 mg, 15/10 mg, 20/10 mg olanzapine/samidorphan.

Dosage Guidance:

- Schizophrenia, bipolar disorder, depression (adults): Start most patients at 5–10 mg QD; may ↑ by 5 mg QD, in weekly increments, to target dose 10–20 mg QD.
- Acute mania (adults): Start 10–15 mg QD; may ↑ by 5 mg daily, in 24-hour increments, to target dose 10–20 mg QD.
- Max approved dose: 20 mg/day, although doses 30–50 mg/day have been used.
- For Lybalvi: Dose as above, using Lybalvi dose with equivalent olanzapine component. Do not divide or combine Lybalvi strengths.
- Bipolar depression (Symbyax, adults): Start 6/25 mg QPM, ↑ as indicated to target dose 6–12/25–50 mg olanzapine/fluoxetine.
- IM for agitation: Usual dose of 2.5–10 mg IM; maximum dose of 30 mg/day. Avoid concomitant use with IM benzodiazepines because of potential for excessive sedation and cardiorespiratory depression.

Monitoring: Fasting glucose, lipids.

Cost: $; combination with fluoxetine: $$; Lybalvi: $$$$$

Side Effects:

- Most common: Somnolence (dose related), dry mouth (dose related), constipation, weight gain (up to 40% incidence; may be substantial; 10–30 pounds weight gain is common), increased appetite, EPS (dose related).
- Serious but rare: Rare but potentially fatal drug reaction with eosinophilia and systemic symptoms (DRESS) possible; often starts as rash that may spread, fever, swollen lymph nodes, and elevated eosinophils.

Mechanism, Pharmacokinetics, and Drug Interactions:

- Dopamine D2 and serotonin 5-HT2A receptor antagonist.
- Metabolized primarily by CYP1A2, also CYP2D6 (minor), and direct glucuronidation; t ½: 1–2 days.
- CYP1A2 inducers (eg, carbamazepine, ritonavir, smoking) may reduce olanzapine levels by 50%; CYP1A2 inhibitors (eg, fluvoxamine) may increase olanzapine bioavailability by 50%–100%. Adjust olanzapine dosing in presence of 1A2 inducers or inhibitors.

Clinical Pearls:

- Use in children and adolescents may result in increased weight gain and sedation, as well as greater increases in LDL cholesterol, total cholesterol, triglycerides, prolactin, and liver transaminase levels when compared to adults.
- Newly approved combination with opioid antagonist samidorphan reduces risk of weight gain, but patients are still at moderate risk. In a 24-week study, 17.8% experienced ≥10% weight gain (vs 29.8% on olanzapine alone) and 27.5% experienced ≥7% weight gain (vs 42.7% on olanzapine alone).
- Avoid using samidorphan combination product in patients taking opioids who may experience withdrawal effects or inadvertently take a high dose of opioid in order to overcome samidorphan's opioid receptor blockade, leading to increased risk for overdose.

Fun Fact:

Olanzapine has been studied and is used for chemotherapy-induced nausea and vomiting.

PALIPERIDONE (Invega) Fact Sheet [G]

Bottom Line:
Paliperidone is the active metabolite of risperidone. In comparison with its parent compound, paliperidone has the advantages of no drug-drug interactions, an easy transition to several long-acting injectable formulations, and a unique FDA indication for schizoaffective disorder. Disadvantages include more QT interval prolongation than risperidone, more tachycardia, possibly more EPS, and the same amount of hyperprolactinemia.

FDA Indications:
Schizophrenia in adults and children ≥12 years; **schizoaffective disorder.**

Off-Label Uses:
Bipolar disorder; behavioral disturbances; impulse control disorders.

Dosage Forms (see LAI fact sheet and table for long-acting injections):
• **Controlled-release tablets (G):** 1.5 mg, 3 mg, 6 mg, 9 mg (not breakable).
• **Monthly long-acting injection (Invega Sustenna):** 39 mg, 78 mg, 117 mg, 156 mg, 234 mg.
• **Every-three-month long-acting injection (Invega Trinza):** 273 mg, 410 mg, 546 mg, 819 mg.
• **Every-six-month long-acting injection (Invega Hafyera):** 1,092 mg, 1,560 mg.

Dosage Guidance:
• Schizophrenia/schizoaffective disorder (adults): Start 6 mg QAM, which may be the effective dose; if required, may ↑ by 3 mg/day at intervals of greater than five days to max 12 mg/day.
• Schizophrenia (adolescents): Start 3 mg QAM, ↑ by 3 mg/day at intervals of >5 days to max 6 mg/day (<51 kg) or 12 mg/day (≥51 kg).
• Paliperidone 3 mg, 6 mg, 9 mg, and 12 mg roughly equivalent to 1–2 mg, 2–4 mg, 4–6 mg, and 6–8 mg risperidone, respectively.
• Dose timing: The manufacturer recommends taking it in the morning; however, some patients experience drowsiness and should try nighttime dosing.

Monitoring: Fasting glucose, lipids; prolactin if symptoms.

Cost: $$$

Side Effects:
• Most common: Akathisia, EPS (dose-related), tremor, tachycardia, insomnia, somnolence (especially adolescents), weight gain, orthostatic hypotension, headache, prolactin elevation.
• Serious but rare: Modest increase in QTc interval. Orthostatic hypotension and syncope reported. Rarely, controlled-release tablet may get caught in GI tract and cause obstructive symptoms in patients with known strictures; avoid use in patients with severe, preexisting GI narrowing (either pathologic or iatrogenic). Esophageal dysmotility and aspiration possible; use caution in patients at risk for aspiration pneumonia (eg, those with advanced Alzheimer's dementia).

Mechanism, Pharmacokinetics, and Drug Interactions:
• Dopamine D2 and serotonin 5-HT2A receptor antagonist.
• Not metabolized by liver; t ½: 23 hours.
• Avoid use with drugs known to prolong the QTc interval or to cause orthostasis. Paliperidone is the principal active metabolite of risperidone; therefore, avoid use with risperidone. Minimal drug interactions.

Clinical Pearls:
• Warn your patients that they may find what looks like intact capsules in their stool. These are actually empty "ghost pills." They appear because Invega is an extended-release tablet based on the OROS osmotic delivery system (as is Concerta; see fact sheet in ADHD chapter). Water from the GI tract enters through a semipermeable membrane coating the tablet, causing the drug to be expelled through laser-drilled holes in the coating. The shell is nonabsorbable and will be expelled in the stool, but the drug itself is absorbed.
• Swallow whole, with fluids; do not chew, divide, or crush.
• Adjust dose in patients with renal impairment.
• Studies suggest paliperidone is not highly effective in acute mania, either as monotherapy or in combination with lithium or valproate.
• Along with risperidone, causes the most EPS and hyperprolactinemia of all the second-generation antipsychotics.

Fun Fact:
First drug with FDA approval for schizoaffective disorder, allowing Janssen to carve out a marketing niche and separate this drug from its competitors (at least from a commercial and marketing perspective).

Antipsychotics

PERPHENAZINE (Trilafon) Fact Sheet [G]

Bottom Line:

Perphenazine, first introduced in 1957, is an older first-generation agent that enjoyed a big boost in popularity after the 2005 CATIE trial found it to be as effective as most second-generation agents with minimal weight gain or metabolic problems. It has become a favorite go-to antipsychotic for many clinicians—an effective, well-tolerated, and inexpensive alternative to second-generation antipsychotics.

FDA Indications:

Schizophrenia (children ≥12 years); severe nausea and vomiting.

Off-Label Uses:

Bipolar disorder; behavioral disturbances; impulse control disorders.

Dosage Forms:

Tablets (G): 2 mg, 4 mg, 8 mg, 16 mg.

Dosage Guidance:

- Schizophrenia: Start 4–8 mg TID (8–16 mg BID–QID for hospitalized patients); adjust to lowest effective dose. Dose range 8–16 mg BID–QID; max FDA-approved dose for non-hospitalized patients is 24 mg/day, but hospitalized psychotic patients may be dosed up to 64 mg/day.
- Dose timing: Most patients take perphenazine BID, and the usual strategy is to give a larger amount at night due to sedation. If needed, you can dose it all at HS.

Monitoring: No routine monitoring recommended unless clinical picture warrants.

Cost: $

Side Effects:

- Most common: EPS, headache, drowsiness, dry mouth, prolactin elevation (sexual side effects, amenorrhea, galactorrhea).
- Serious but rare: Tachycardia (especially with sudden marked increase in dose).

Mechanism, Pharmacokinetics, and Drug Interactions:

- Dopamine D2 receptor antagonist.
- Metabolized primarily by CYP2D6; t ½: 9–12 hours. May inhibit CYP2D6. Poor metabolizers of CYP2D6 metabolize the drug more slowly; may have increased effects.
- CYP2D6 inhibitors (eg, fluoxetine, paroxetine, quinidine) may increase perphenazine levels. Caution with substrates of 2D6 as perphenazine may increase their levels and effects.

Clinical Pearls:

- Perphenazine is an intermediate-potency first-generation antipsychotic; this leads to less EPS compared to high-potency agents (eg, haloperidol, fluphenazine) and to less sedation, less orthostasis, and fewer anticholinergic side effects compared to low-potency agents (eg, chlorpromazine).
- Fewer metabolic effects (weight gain, glucose, lipids) than some antipsychotics.
- Based on an 18-month randomized trial of 1,493 patients with schizophrenia (CATIE trial), perphenazine appears similar in efficacy and EPS compared to second-generation antipsychotics (olanzapine, quetiapine, risperidone, ziprasidone).

Fun Fact:

Perphenazine has long been available in a formulation with amitriptyline (a tricyclic antidepressant) called Triavil. This combination antipsychotic/antidepressant was first available in 1965, foreshadowing the next such combination drug (Symbyax) by 38 years.

PIMAVANSERIN (Nuplazid) Fact Sheet

Bottom Line:
Pimavanserin is the only antipsychotic with virtually no effect on dopamine receptors. It is the only approved medication for psychosis in Parkinson's disease, but we do not yet know if it has any efficacy advantages over quetiapine, which has generally been the go-to antipsychotic for this syndrome. Its lack of weight gain is a side effect advantage, but there are some concerns about increases in hospitalization and higher mortality in patients with Parkinson's disease psychosis.

FDA Indications:
Hallucinations and delusions associated with Parkinson's disease psychosis.

Off-Label Uses:
Depression.

Dosage Forms:
- **Tablets:** 10 mg.
- **Capsules:** 34 mg.

Dosage Guidance:
Start and continue with 34 mg once daily (no titration). Use 10 mg tablet in patients taking concurrent CYP3A4 inhibitors.

Monitoring: Fasting glucose, lipids.

Cost: $$$$$

Side Effects:
- Most common: Nausea, peripheral edema, confusion.
- Serious but rare: QT prolongation (dose related; mean prolongation of 5–8 msec at usual dose); class warning regarding increased mortality in elderly.

Mechanism, Pharmacokinetics, and Drug Interactions:
- Second-generation antipsychotic with combination of inverse agonist and antagonist activity at 5-HT2A and, less so, at 5-HT2C receptors.
- Metabolized by CYP3A4 and CYP3A5; t ½: 57 hours (200 hours for active metabolite).
- Caution with potent inhibitors or inducers of CYP3A4 (adjust dose per above). Avoid use with other medications that may increase QT interval.

Clinical Pearls:
- FDA approval based on a six-week placebo-controlled outpatient study of 185 patients that showed only modest (but statistically significant) improvement in hallucinations and delusions compared to placebo.
- The study didn't find any difference (improvement or worsening) in motor function between those who received Nuplazid or placebo.
- All in all, though, pimavanserin did not show statistically significant benefit in three out of four pre-approval clinical studies.
- Reports of post-marketing deaths in patients who had taken Nuplazid have sparked investigation and controversy, though we still don't know if it's any more dangerous than clozapine or quetiapine use in Parkinson's.
- Preliminary data have shown antidepressant efficacy when pimavanserin is added to an SSRI or SNRI in patients with inadequate response.

Fun Fact:
The FDA rejected an indication bid for dementia-related psychosis due to lack of significantly meaningful effect in some subgroups of patients.

QUETIAPINE (Seroquel, Seroquel XR) Fact Sheet [G]

Bottom Line:

Quetiapine's low risk for EPS and broad spectrum of efficacy make it an appealing first-choice agent. However, sedation, weight gain, and orthostasis may limit use. Dosing at bedtime, or switching to XR, may help reduce daytime sedation.

FDA Indications:

Schizophrenia (adults and children ≥13 years); **bipolar,** manic/mixed (adults and children ≥10 years); **bipolar I or II depression; maintenance treatment for bipolar; major depression,** as adjunct.

Off-Label Uses:

Insomnia; anxiety disorders; behavioral disturbances; impulse control disorders.

Dosage Forms:

- **Tablets (G):** 25 mg, 50 mg, 100 mg, 200 mg, 300 mg, 400 mg.
- **XR tablets (G):** 50 mg, 150 mg, 200 mg, 300 mg, 400 mg.

Dosage Guidance:

- Schizophrenia (adults): Start 25 mg BID or 300 mg XR QHS. Target dose: 400–800 mg/day.
- Bipolar (adults): Start 50 mg BID or 300 mg XR QHS. Target dose: 400–800 mg/day (mania, maintenance), 300 mg/day (depression).
- Adolescents: Start 25 mg BID or 50 mg XR QHS, increase to 100 mg/day (IR divided BID, XR taken QHS) on day two, then increase by 100 mg/day daily to target dose 400–600 mg/day (mania) or 400–600 mg/day (schizophrenia).
- Depression: Start 50 mg IR/XR QHS. Target dose: 150–300 mg/day.
- For all indications: May ↑ dose by 50–100 mg/day increments, given in divided doses, every one to four days (or as much as 300 mg/day XR increments in intervals of greater than one day) to target dose.
- Max daily dose in adults: 800 mg/day.
- Consider dosing slower and lower in pediatric, elderly, or debilitated patients.
- Dose timing: Usually dosed at bedtime due to sedation, but the XR formulation has been shown to be less sedating than IR and is often tolerated with morning dosing.

Monitoring: Fasting glucose, lipids.

Cost: $

Side Effects:

- Most common: Somnolence, hypotension, dry mouth, dizziness, constipation, weight gain, fatigue.
- Serious but rare: Orthostatic hypotension, particularly at high dose or with rapid titration.

Mechanism, Pharmacokinetics, and Drug Interactions:

- Dopamine D2 and serotonin 5-HT2A receptor antagonist.
- Metabolized by CYP3A4; t ½: 6 hours (XR: 7 hours).
- Avoid or use caution with agents that may cause additional orthostasis. CYP3A4 inducers (eg, carbamazepine) may lower quetiapine levels; CYP3A4 inhibitors (eg, erythromycin, ketoconazole) may increase quetiapine levels. Adjust quetiapine dose in presence of CYP3A4 inducers or inhibitors.

Clinical Pearls:

- Swallow XR tablet whole; do not break, crush, or chew; switch between IR and XR at the same total daily dose; dose adjustments may be necessary based on response and tolerability.
- If patient discontinues drug for more than one week, re-titrate dose as with initial therapy.
- Quetiapine abuse has been reported, particularly in incarcerated populations.

Fun Fact:

Cataracts developed in initial studies with beagle dogs; human studies have not shown an association. However, the label still recommends a slit-lamp exam every six months.

RISPERIDONE (Risperdal) Fact Sheet [G]

Bottom Line:
Tried and true, risperidone's moderate side effect profile has led to its wide use, and many clinicians consider it their antipsychotic of choice for first-episode psychotic disorders. Just be cautious when dosing higher than 4 mg daily, since akathisia and other side effects are more common. Hyperprolactinemia is fairly common, so be vigilant for symptoms such as lowered libido, amenorrhea, gynecomastia, and galactorrhea.

FDA Indications:
Schizophrenia (adults and children ≥13 years); **bipolar disorder, manic/mixed** (adults and children ≥10 years); **irritability symptoms of autism** (children ≥5 years).

Off-Label Uses:
Bipolar depression; behavioral disturbances; impulse control disorders; Tourette's syndrome.

Dosage Forms (see LAI fact sheet and table for long-acting injections):
- **Tablets (G):** 0.25 mg, 0.5 mg, 1 mg, 2 mg, 3 mg, 4 mg.
- **Oral solution (G):** 1 mg/mL.
- **Orally disintegrating tablets (Risperdal M-Tab, [G]):** 0.25 mg, 0.5 mg, 1 mg, 2 mg, 3 mg, 4 mg.
- **Long-acting IM injection (Risperdal Consta):** 12.5 mg, 25 mg, 37.5 mg, 50 mg.
- **Long-acting SQ injection (Perseris):** 90 mg, 120 mg.

Dosage Guidance:
- Schizophrenia, bipolar (adults): Start 1 mg BID; may ↑ by 1–2 mg/day at intervals ≥24 hours to a recommended dosage range of 4–6 mg/day; may be given as a single daily dose once maintenance dose achieved. Max approved dose is 16 mg/day, but daily dosages >6 mg provide no additional benefit, only higher risk for EPS, which is dose dependent.
- Children, elderly, first-episode psychosis: Lower initial dosages (eg, 0.5–1 mg daily) and slower titration to initial target dose of 2 mg daily.
- Autism (children ≥5 years): If <15 kg (33 lbs), use with caution. For 15–20 kg (33–44 lbs), start 0.25 mg/day, ↑ to 0.5 mg/day after at least four days. If response insufficient, may ↑ by 0.25 mg/day in at least two-week intervals; give QD or BID. For ≥20 kg (44 lbs), start 0.5 mg/day; may ↑ to 1 mg/day after at least four days. If response insufficient, may ↑ dose by 0.5 mg/day in at least two-week intervals; give QD or BID.
- Bipolar mania or schizophrenia (children): Start 0.5 mg QD; ↑ in increments of 0.5–1 mg/day at intervals ≥24 hours to target dose of 2–3 mg/day; doses >3 mg/day do not confer additional benefit and are associated with increased side effects.
- Dose timing: Usually well tolerated whether taken in the morning or night.

Monitoring: Fasting glucose, lipids; prolactin if symptoms.

Cost: $

Side Effects:
- Most common: EPS, somnolence (particularly in children), anxiety, constipation, nausea, dyspepsia, dizziness, rhinitis, prolactin elevation, weight gain.
- Serious but rare: Orthostatic hypotension may occur, particularly at higher doses or with rapid titration. Hyperprolactinemia with clinical symptoms (sexual side effects, galactorrhea, amenorrhea).

Mechanism, Pharmacokinetics, and Drug Interactions:
- Dopamine D2 and serotonin 5-HT2A receptor antagonist.
- Metabolized primarily by CYP2D6; t ½: 20 hours.
- CYP2D6 inhibitors (eg, fluoxetine, paroxetine, quinidine) may increase effects of risperidone; reduce risperidone dose. Carbamazepine reduces levels and effects of risperidone; may need to double risperidone dose.

Clinical Pearls:
- Along with paliperidone, causes the most EPS and hyperprolactinemia of all the second-generation antipsychotics.
- When reinitiating after discontinuation, initial titration schedule should be followed.
- An ultra-long-acting extended-release weekly oral formulation of risperidone is in development to help address medication non-adherence in roughly 50% of patients with schizophrenia, without a needle.

Fun Fact:
Risperdal M-Tabs are marketed in other countries as Risperdal Quicklets.

THIORIDAZINE (Mellaril) Fact Sheet [G]

Bottom Line:

Thioridazine prolongs the cardiac QT interval more than any other antipsychotic, rendering it too risky to use for the majority of patients.

FDA Indications:

Schizophrenia (not for first-line use).

Off-Label Uses:

Anxiety, insomnia.

Dosage Forms:

Tablets (G): 10 mg, 25 mg, 50 mg, 100 mg.

Dosage Guidance:

Start 50–100 mg TID; ↑ by 50–100 mg/day increments every three to seven days and adjust to lowest effective dose. Dose range 200–800 mg/day divided BID–QID; max FDA-approved dose is 800 mg/day due to ocular pigmentation at high doses.

Monitoring: ECG if cardiac disease.

Cost: $

Side Effects:

- Most common: EPS, headache, sedation, drowsiness, dry mouth, constipation, blurred vision, dizziness, prolactin elevation (sexual side effects, amenorrhea, galactorrhea).
- Serious but rare: QT prolongation and torsades de pointes (highest risk of all antipsychotics); ocular pigmentation and degenerative retinopathies.

Mechanism, Pharmacokinetics, and Drug Interactions:

- Dopamine D2 receptor antagonist.
- Metabolized primarily by CYP2D6; t ½: 24 hours. May inhibit CYP2D6. Poor metabolizers of CYP2D6 metabolize the drug more slowly; may have increased effects.
- CYP2D6 inhibitors (eg, fluoxetine, paroxetine, quinidine) may increase thioridazine levels. Caution with substrates of CYP2D6 as thioridazine may increase their levels and effects.

Clinical Pearls:

- Thioridazine is a low-potency first-generation antipsychotic; this leads to less EPS and to more sedation, orthostasis, and anticholinergic side effects compared to high-potency agents (eg, haloperidol, fluphenazine).
- Efficacy has not been studied in refractory schizophrenia, but thioridazine is indicated only for and should be reserved for use only in patients who have failed to respond to other medications. This is due to the significant risks associated with thioridazine, particularly QT prolongation.

Fun Fact:

Thioridazine can kill antibiotic-resistant bacteria such as *Staphylococcus aureus* (including MRSA) and extensively drug-resistant *Mycobacterium tuberculosis*. Researchers are studying how thioridazine does this (latest studies show a weakening of bacterial cell walls) in order to develop drugs that can target resistant bacteria.

THIOTHIXENE (Navane) Fact Sheet [G]

Bottom Line:

Thiothixene is one of the original high-potency first-generation antipsychotics—but most clinicians would opt for haloperidol or fluphenazine because of their greater familiarity and range of formulation options (eg, liquid, injectable, long-acting).

FDA Indications:
Schizophrenia.

Off-Label Uses:
Bipolar disorder; behavioral disturbances; impulse control disorders.

Dosage Forms:
Capsules (G): 1 mg, 2 mg, 5 mg, 10 mg.

Dosage Guidance:
Start 2 mg TID–5 mg BID; ↑ by 2–5 mg/day increments every three to seven days and adjust to lowest effective dose. Usual dose range 20–30 mg/day divided BID–TID; max FDA-approved dose is 60 mg/day, but doses >40 mg/day are rarely used.

Monitoring: No routine monitoring recommended unless clinical picture warrants.

Cost: $

Side Effects:
- Most common: EPS, headache, drowsiness, dry mouth, prolactin elevation (sexual side effects, amenorrhea, galactorrhea).
- Serious but rare: See class warnings in chapter introduction.

Mechanism, Pharmacokinetics, and Drug Interactions:
- Dopamine D2 receptor antagonist.
- Metabolized primarily by CYP1A2; t ½: 34 hours.
- Smoking status may affect thiothixene metabolism as smoking is a potent CYP1A2 inducer; smokers may need higher doses.

Clinical Pearl:

Thiothixene is a high-potency first-generation antipsychotic; this leads to more EPS compared to mid- and low-potency agents (eg, perphenazine or chlorpromazine, respectively) and to less sedation, less orthostasis, and fewer anticholinergic side effects compared to low-potency agents (eg, chlorpromazine).

Fun Fact:

Pfizer developed thiothixene in the 1960s, and the drug was found to be an effective antidepressant, as well as an antipsychotic. For commercial reasons, the company chose to market it for schizophrenia rather than depression.

TRIFLUOPERAZINE (Stelazine) Fact Sheet [G]

Bottom Line:

Trifluoperazine, like thiothixene (Navane), is an effective older agent with similar potency to haloperidol or fluphenazine; however, given all our antipsychotic options, it sees only rare use these days.

FDA Indications:

Schizophrenia; nonpsychotic anxiety.

Off-Label Uses:

Bipolar disorder; behavioral disturbances; impulse control disorders.

Dosage Forms:

Tablets (G): 1 mg, 2 mg, 5 mg, 10 mg.

Dosage Guidance:

Schizophrenia: Start 1–2 mg BID; ↑ by 2–5 mg/day increments every three to seven days and adjust to lowest effective dose. Usual dose range 5–10 mg BID; max FDA-approved dose 40 mg/day.

Monitoring: No routine monitoring recommended unless clinical picture warrants.

Cost: $

Side Effects:

- Most common: EPS, headache, drowsiness, dry mouth, prolactin elevation (sexual side effects, amenorrhea, galactorrhea).
- Serious but rare: See class warnings in chapter introduction.

Mechanism, Pharmacokinetics, and Drug Interactions:

- Dopamine D2 receptor antagonist.
- Metabolized primarily by CYP1A2; t ½: 18 hours.
- Smoking status may affect trifluoperazine metabolism as smoking is a potent CYP1A2 inducer; smokers may need higher doses.

Clinical Pearls:

- Trifluoperazine is a high-potency first-generation antipsychotic; this leads to more EPS compared to mid- and low-potency agents (eg, perphenazine or chlorpromazine, respectively) and to less sedation, less orthostasis, and fewer anticholinergic side effects compared to low-potency agents (eg, chlorpromazine).
- Trifluoperazine was FDA approved for nonpsychotic anxiety at doses of no more than 6 mg/day used for no more than 12 weeks, but it is no longer used for this indication.

Fun Fact:

Stelazine was marketed with the tagline "Calm, but still alert."

ZIPRASIDONE (Geodon) Fact Sheet [G]

Bottom Line:
Ziprasidone has an appealing weight and metabolic profile, but many clinicians get scared off by its reputation for lengthening the QT interval. This risk is overblown, and it should probably be prescribed more.

FDA Indications:
Schizophrenia; bipolar disorder, acute treatment of manic/mixed episodes; maintenance treatment of bipolar disorder as adjunct; **acute agitation** in patients with schizophrenia (IM only).

Off-Label Uses:
Bipolar disorder; behavioral disturbances; impulse control disorders.

Dosage Forms:
- **Capsules (G):** 20 mg, 40 mg, 60 mg, 80 mg.
- **Injection (G):** 20 mg/mL.

Dosage Guidance:
- Schizophrenia, bipolar disorder: Start 20 mg BID (40 mg BID for acute mania) with meals for two to three days; ↑ by 40 mg/day increments; can usually ↑ rather quickly to target dose 60–80 mg BID. Max approved dose is 160 mg/day, though can go higher in some patients; there are some safety data for doses up to 320 mg/day.
- Schizophrenia, acute agitation (IM injection): 10 mg Q2 hours or 20 mg Q4 hours; max 40 mg/day. Replace with oral therapy as soon as possible.

Monitoring: Fasting glucose, lipids; ECG if cardiac disease.

Cost: $

Side Effects:
- Most common: Somnolence, dizziness, akathisia, rash (5%).
- Serious but rare: May result in minor QTc prolongation (dose related; 10 msec at 160 mg/day). Clinically relevant prolongation (>500 msec) rare (0.06%) and less than placebo (0.23%). Avoid in patients with hypokalemia, hypomagnesemia, bradycardia, persistent QTc intervals >500 msec, or those receiving other drugs that prolong QTc interval. Drug reaction with eosinophilia and systemic symptoms (DRESS) has been reported with ziprasidone exposure. DRESS begins as a rash that can spread all over the body; it may also include swollen lymph nodes, fever, and damage to organs such as the heart, liver, pancreas, or kidneys, and is sometimes fatal; discontinue ziprasidone if DRESS is suspected.

Mechanism, Pharmacokinetics, and Drug Interactions:
- Dopamine D2 and serotonin 5-HT2A receptor antagonist.
- Metabolized in liver principally by aldehyde oxidase; less than one-third of clearance mediated by CYP3A4 and CYP1A2; t ½: 7 hours.
- Avoid use with other drugs that prolong QTc interval.

Clinical Pearls:
- Administer twice daily, ideally with meals; ingestion of several hundred calories is necessary to increase absorption up to two-fold.
- Causes less weight gain than clozapine, olanzapine, quetiapine, or risperidone.
- Average increase in QTc is greater than any other second-generation antipsychotics, although not much more than for quetiapine. Post-marketing surveillance has shown one or two instances of torsades de pointes possibly related to ziprasidone use.

Fun Fact:
The brand name Geodon has been suggested to bring to mind the phrase "down (don) to earth (geo)," referring to the goals of the medication.

Antipsychotics

LONG-ACTING INJECTABLE (LAI) ANTIPSYCHOTICS

INTRODUCTION: DO LAIs WORK?

These formulations used to be known as "depot" antipsychotics, but the newer term "long-acting injectables" (LAIs) helps to remove some of the stigma associated with their use.

The potential advantages of LAIs are numerous and include the following:

- LAIs ensure that otherwise non-adherent patients have robust serum levels of antipsychotics

- Serum levels are more consistent over time than they are with oral meds

- Both families and clinicians spend less time struggling with patients about medication adherence

- LAIs present a lower risk of overdose because you aren't providing your patient with large quantities of pills

Studies attempting to demonstrate advantages of LAIs have been mixed. One large meta-analysis found no difference between LAIs and oral meds in relapse rates, with the exception of first-generation LAIs in older studies (Kishimoto T et al, *Schiz Bull* 2014;40(1):192–213). But a meta-analysis of 25 naturalistic observational studies, involving 5,940 patients, found that switching these patients to LAIs strongly decreased the number of hospitalizations (Kishimoto T et al, *J Clin Psychiatry* 2013;74(10):957–965).

The bottom line is that patients who do poorly on pills because of non-adherence are likely to do better on LAIs—if you can get them to agree to an injection.

DECIDING AMONG THE LAIs

General Notes on LAIs

- It's best to choose an LAI version of an oral medication that your patient has already taken, so that you can be more confident about the agent's effectiveness and tolerability.

- Insurance coverage still often dictates the choice of good old haloperidol decanoate. Even when a patient's insurance supposedly covers newer agents, the patient co-pay may be prohibitive, whereas haloperidol decanoate is almost always an affordable option.

- Paliperidone has become the go-to for many clinicians because of a number of factors, including the lack of required oral overlap and the availability of every-three-month (Trinza) and every-six-month (Hafyera) formulations.

- Be patient. The full therapeutic effect of LAIs can take longer than orals—ie, several months. Don't adjust the LAI dose prematurely.

- Consider oral overlap. LAIs differ in how quickly the full dose is absorbed. Many formulations say in their package insert that no oral overlap is required, and you'll see that guidance in our LAI table. This means that, at least theoretically, on the day of the injection your patient's serum level of the medication will immediately approximate a therapeutic level. In other cases, such as haloperidol decanoate or risperidone Consta, serum levels will take days to ramp up, and you will need to temporarily supplement with an overlapping oral dose. In the real world, even in "no oral overlap" meds, some patients will need additional oral doses to prevent breakthrough psychosis. This is a matter of clinical judgment and experience.

- *Never* initiate an LAI on a patient who has a history of neuroleptic malignant syndrome (NMS) on any antipsychotic. That's just asking for trouble.

LAI Options

There's a pretty comprehensive table on the following pages that reports, for each LAI, the **FDA indication(s), medication names, costs, available strengths, dosing information,** and **pharmacokinetics** (need for oral overlap and dosing interval). But here, we'll give you a shorthand version of the most relevant clinical pearls:

First-generation antipsychotics

- **Fluphenazine (Prolixin Decanoate)**—Dosed every two to three weeks. Injections are painful. Cheap, but relatively high risk of EPS and TD. Oral overlap required.

- **Haloperidol (Haldol Decanoate)**—Dosed monthly. As cheap as Prolixin, and since it's dosed less often and has more predictable pharmacokinetics, it's generally the better choice between the first-generation LAI antipsychotics. Oral overlap required, although some use a "loading dose" method (20 times oral dose, followed by 10–15 times oral dose in subsequent months) that requires no oral overlap (Ereshefsky L et al, *Hosp Community Psychiatry* 1993;44(12):1155–1161).

Second-generation antipsychotics

- **Aripiprazole (Abilify Maintena)**—Dosed monthly. Comes in two strengths (300 and 400 mg). Oral overlap required for 14 days. Deltoid or gluteal injection. Expensive, but a good side effect profile.

- **Aripiprazole lauroxil (Aristada)**—Dosed monthly, every six weeks, or every two months. Comes in four strengths. Smallest dose (441 mg monthly) may be given deltoid or gluteal; other doses must be given gluteal. Dosing interval flexibility makes this formulation appealing, although oral overlap is required for 21 days. You can forgo the oral overlap if you give your patient a dose of **Aristada Initio** 675 mg plus 30 mg oral aripiprazole on the same day as your first dose of Aristada. First dose of Aristada may be delayed up to 10 days after Initio. Expensive, but a good side effect profile.

- **Olanzapine (Zyprexa Relprevv)**—Dosed either every two weeks or monthly, depending on the dose needed. Comes in three doses. Gluteal injection only. No oral overlap. May be the worst choice among all LAIs for multiple reasons. High potential for weight gain. There's a small risk of a post-injection delirium/sedation syndrome, occurring in less than 1% of patients, caused by accidental intravascular injection. For this reason, you have to give the injection at a registered health care facility where patients can be continuously monitored for at least three hours after the injection. Restricted use requires physician and facility registration, and additional paperwork with Eli Lilly's program. High cost, restriction of use, monitoring requirement, and risk of adverse outcome all limit use severely. Expensive.

- **Paliperidone palmitate, monthly (Invega Sustenna)**—Monthly dosing. Comes in five doses. First two doses deltoid; subsequent doses may be deltoid or gluteal. No oral overlap. Less painful injection than risperidone Consta or olanzapine Relprevv. Expensive, but appealing features include no oral overlap and potential to transition to every-three-month and every-six-month formulations.

- **Paliperidone palmitate, every three months (Invega Trinza)**—Dosed every three months, but your patient must have done well on monthly injections of Sustenna for at least four months before switching to Trinza. Deltoid or gluteal injection. Must shake syringe vigorously for at least 15 seconds to ensure uniform suspension of long-acting particles and prevent clogging in needle. Expensive.

- **Paliperidone palmitate, every six months (Invega Hafyera)**—Dosed every six months, but your patient must have done well on monthly injections of Sustenna for at least four months or on Trinza for at least one three-month cycle. Gluteal injection. Switching from lower doses of Sustenna (39, 78, 117 mg) or Trinza (273, 410 mg) was not studied so not recommended. Must shake syringe vigorously for at least 30 seconds to ensure uniform suspension and prevent clogging in needle. Expensive.

- **Risperidone (Risperdal Consta)**—Dosed every two weeks. Comes in four doses. Deltoid or gluteal injection. A three-week oral overlap and the need for a refrigerated solution make this LAI more cumbersome to use than some of its competitors. Painful injection. Must shake for at least 10 seconds to ensure uniform suspension of microspheres. Expensive.

- **Risperidone (Perseris)**—Monthly dosing option for risperidone, an improvement over the every-two-week dosing of Consta. Comes in two doses. No oral overlap. It's the first LAI to be dosed subcutaneously (into the abdomen) rather than a deep and more painful IM injection. Note that the highest dose of Perseris is equivalent to 4 mg/day of oral risperidone, so this isn't a good option for patients on higher doses. Expensive.

General Notes on Administration of LAIs

(Note: While it's rare for prescribing clinicians to administer LAI injections, it may be useful for you to know what both nurses and patients have to be aware of when it comes time for your patients to actually get their shots!)

- Most LAIs are administered by deep IM injection (the exception is risperidone Perseris, which is administered subcutaneously). To ensure medication is delivered effectively into deep muscle and not subcutaneous fatty tissue (which would delay absorption significantly), administer to the ventrogluteal muscle (of the hip). This muscle is easily located and relatively free of major blood vessels and nerves.

- Z-track technique should be used when administering fluphenazine or haloperidol decanoate to gluteal muscle. To do this, stretch and displace the skin by pulling it laterally away from the intended point of injection. Insert the needle into the site at a 90-degree angle; aspirate by pulling back on the plunger for five seconds, allowing time for any blood to travel from a penetrated vessel up the bore of the needle. If blood is aspirated, withdraw the needle and seal the wound; repeat at another site with new needle. If no blood is aspirated, give the injection, wait 10 seconds, and then withdraw the needle and release the skin, allowing the displaced tissue to seal the needle track.

You can use the Z-track technique with other agents also to ensure deep IM administration and minimize or prevent drug leakage.

- In general, women tend to have more fatty tissue in the gluteal area, especially in the dorsogluteal muscle, and this should be considered when choosing needle length. Longer needles should also be used in obese patients. When medication is delivered into fatty tissue inadvertently, the patient is at increased risk for granuloma, sterile abscess, redness and swelling, ulceration, or fat necrosis.

- Maximum recommended volume to be administered:
  - Gluteal: 3 mL
  - Deltoid: 2 mL

- Aspiration to ensure needle tip has not accidentally punctured a blood vessel is generally good practice. However, it is not possible with prefilled syringe formulations of Abilify Maintena, Aristada, or Aristada Initio due to the syringe design.

- Administer dose immediately after suspending and/or shaking to avoid settling or needle occlusion. See product information for specific details on preparation and administration.

- **Do not massage the injection site** (and advise patients not to massage the site) because this can promote dispersal into fatty tissue.

Table 12: Long-Acting Injectable Antipsychotics

Generic Name (Brand Name) Year FDA Approved [G] denotes generic availability	Relevant FDA Indication(s)	Available Strengths	Oral Overlap	Dosing Interval	Initial Dosing	Maintenance Dose*	Cost for Monthly Supply at Average Dose (November 2021)
First-Generation Antipsychotics							
Fluphenazine decanoate [G] (Prolixin Decanoate[1]) 1972	Schizophrenia	25 mg/mL	Continue total oral dose for 2–3 days, then ↓ by 50% increments every 2–3 days until discontinued (by next injection)	2–3 weeks	1.25× total daily oral dose Q2–3 weeks (eg, 10 mg/day oral ~ 12.5 mg IM Q2–3 weeks)	Increase in increments of 12.5 mg; do not exceed 100 mg per dose; usual dose 6.25–25 mg Q2–3 weeks	$ [G]
Haloperidol decanoate [G] (Haldol Decanoate) 1986	Schizophrenia	50 mg/mL and 100 mg/mL	Decrease oral dose by 50% after first injection, then discontinue after second injection (third for some patients); alternatively, no oral overlap if loading dose of 20× oral given	4 weeks	10–15× total oral daily dose (eg, 10 mg/day oral ~ 100–150 mg IM). Alternatively, 20× total oral daily dose if loading dose with no oral overlap (eg, 10 mg/day oral ~ 200 mg IM). First dose should be ≤100 mg; if higher dose needed, give remainder in 1–2 weeks.	Continue 10–15× total oral daily dose Q4 weeks with either method (eg, 10 mg/day ~ 100–150 mg IM Q4 weeks)	$ [G] $$$ Haldol Dec
Second-Generation Antipsychotics							
Aripiprazole (Abilify Maintena) 2013	Schizophrenia Bipolar disorder	300 mg and 400 mg vials and prefilled syringes	For 14 days	4 weeks	400 mg Q4 weeks	400 mg Q4 weeks; decrease to 300 mg Q4 weeks if side effects (estimated equivalence is 20 mg/day oral ~ 300 mg IM monthly and 30 mg/day oral ~ 400 mg IM monthly)	$$$$$
Aripiprazole lauroxil (Aristada) 2015	Schizophrenia	441, 662, 882, 1064 mg	For 21 days	Monthly, every 6 weeks, or every 2 months	441, 662, or 882 mg monthly (equivalent to 10, 15, and 20 mg/day); or 882 mg every 6 weeks (15 mg/day); or 1064 mg every 2 months (15 mg/day)	Continue initial dosing or adjust based on clinical response	$$$$$
Aripiprazole lauroxil (Aristada Initio) 2018	Schizophrenia	675 mg syringes	Aripiprazole 30 mg PO ×1 dose	See Aristada above	To be given as single initial dose, in conjunction with Aristada as above (on same day or within 10 days of Initio)	See above	$$$$$

[1]Brand discontinued; available as generic only

*Reducing the dosing interval may be preferable to dosage increase for patients who lose some efficacy prior to next scheduled dose

Generic Name (Brand Name) Year FDA Approved [G] denotes generic availability	Relevant FDA Indication(s)	Available Strengths	Oral Overlap	Dosing Interval	Initial Dosing	Maintenance Dose*	Cost for Monthly Supply at Average Dose (November 2021)
Olanzapine (Zyprexa Relprevv) 2009	Schizophrenia	210, 300, 405 mg vials	No overlap	2–4 weeks	10 mg/day oral: 210 mg Q2 weeks ×4 doses or 405 mg Q4 weeks ×2 doses / 15 mg/day oral: 300 mg Q2 weeks ×4 doses / 20 mg/day oral: 300 mg Q2 weeks	10 mg/day oral: 150 mg Q2 weeks or 300 mg Q4 weeks / 15 mg/day oral: 210 mg Q2 weeks or 405 mg Q4 weeks / 20 mg/day oral: 300 mg Q2 weeks / Maximum dose: 300 mg Q2 weeks or 405 mg Q4 weeks	$$$$$
Paliperidone palmitate (Invega Sustenna) 2009	Schizophrenia Schizoaffective disorder (monotherapy or adjunct)	39, 78, 117, 156, 234 mg in prefilled syringes	No overlap	4 weeks	234 mg IM in deltoid, then 156 mg 1 week later	117 mg 3 weeks after second dose then Qmonth; may adjust monthly dose (maintenance given deltoid or gluteal). Approx. equivalence: 3 mg oral: 39–78 mg / 6 mg oral: 117 mg / 12 mg oral: 234 mg	$$$$$
Paliperidone palmitate (Invega Trinza) 2015	Schizophrenia (only after at least 4 months of adequate treatment on Invega Sustenna)	273, 410, 546, 819 mg in prefilled syringes	No overlap	3 months	Based on previous monthly Invega Sustenna dose: For 78 mg, give 273 mg Trinza / For 117 mg, give 410 mg Trinza / For 156 mg, give 546 mg Trinza / For 234 mg, give 819 mg Trinza	Give same conversion dose of Trinza every 3 months; adjust if necessary per patient response	$$$$$
Paliperidone palmitate (Invega Hafyera) 2021	Schizophrenia (only after at least 4 months of adequate treatment on Sustenna or 3 months on Trinza)	1,092, 1,560 mg in prefilled syringes	No overlap	6 months	Based on previous monthly Sustenna dose: For 156 mg, give 1,092 mg Hafyera / For 234 mg, give 1,560 mg Hafyera / Or 3-month Trinza dose: For 546 mg, give 1,092 mg Hafyera / For 819 mg, give 1,560 mg Hafyera	Give same conversion dose of Hafyera every 6 months; adjust if necessary per patient response	$$$$$
Risperidone (Perseris) 2018	Schizophrenia	90, 120 mg	No overlap	Monthly	Start 90 or 120 mg SQ to abdomen monthly	Approx. equivalence: 90 mg monthly: 3 mg/day oral / 120 mg monthly: 4 mg/day oral	$$$$$
Risperidone (Risperdal Consta) 2003	Schizophrenia Bipolar, manic/mixed (monotherapy or adjunct)	12.5, 25, 37.5, 50 mg vials	With usual oral dose for 21 days	2 weeks	Start at 25 mg Q2 weeks; adjust dose no more frequently than Q4 weeks as needed for response	Approx. equivalence: <4 mg/day oral: 25 mg / 4–6 mg/day oral: 37.5 mg / >6 mg/day oral: 50 mg / Maximum dose: 50 mg Q2 weeks	$$$$$

¹Brand discontinued; available as generic only

*Reducing the dosing interval may be preferable to dosage increase for patients who lose some efficacy prior to next scheduled dose

Anxiolytic and Hypnotic Medications

GENERAL PRESCRIBING TIPS FOR ANXIOLYTICS

Although antidepressants are arguably the most effective medications for anxiety disorder, in this chapter we focus on benzodiazepines and other drugs used specifically for symptoms of anxiety or anxiety disorders.

Psychiatry has long had a love/hate relationship with benzodiazepines. They work quickly and predictably, but they often lead to misuse or dependence. That said, a history of substance use disorder doesn't absolutely rule out prescribing a benzo—it just makes it more important to monitor use closely, including limiting the number of refills and consistently inquiring about substance use over the course of treatment.

Here's a reasonable approach to deciding on which anxiolytic medication to prescribe:

1. Start with a long-acting medication such as clonazepam. It's somewhat less likely to lead to misuse because its onset and offset are more gradual.

2. Reserve short-acting benzos, like alprazolam or lorazepam, for patients who have occasional anxiety, and prescribe these on an as-needed basis.

3. If you are starting patients on an SSRI for an anxiety disorder, it's good practice to simultaneously start a short course of a benzodiazepine. Tell them that in two weeks they will be able to stop taking the benzo because the antidepressant will have kicked in.

4. Give buspirone a chance, especially for generalized anxiety disorder. It may not work as reliably as benzos, but it lacks risk for misuse, dependence, and withdrawal.

5. Don't forget propranolol, which can be very effective for patients who have strong somatic symptoms of anxiety, such as pounding heart and shortness of breath.

6. Alpha-2 agonist clonidine and alpha-1 antagonist prazosin are often helpful for both anxiety and insomnia; prazosin may be especially effective in patients with PTSD, though evidence is mixed.

7. Hydroxyzine may be a particularly good option in patients who want an immediate ("as needed") effect but have a substance use disorder history or risk.

8. There are lots of other options for anxiety/insomnia, many of which are off-label. See the anxiety treatment algorithm for a handy graphical display of your choices.

GENERAL PRESCRIBING TIPS FOR HYPNOTICS

The preferred way to treat insomnia is to treat the underlying cause, as opposed to reflexively writing scripts for hypnotics. There are plenty of reasons for our patients to lose sleep, including depression and anxiety, stressful life circumstances, and medication side effects. A common scenario, for example, is the patient who presents with major depression with insomnia as one of the depressive symptoms. In this case, we recommend either prescribing an antidepressant alone, or an antidepressant plus a two-week prescription for a hypnotic. In most cases, the antidepressant will have kicked in around the two-week point, and your patient will no longer need the hypnotic.

In addition to treating the underlying disorder, get into the habit of discussing sleep hygiene techniques with your patients. The key elements of sleep hygiene are:

• Avoid or reduce the use of substances that interfere with sleep, such as nicotine, caffeine, and alcohol.

• Get more exercise.

• Make the bedroom more conducive to sleep—eg, keep the lighting dim, reduce screen time, get comfortable sheets, and reserve the bed for sleeping and sex.

• Practice basic sleep restriction, which means reducing the time in bed to sleep time only.

• Do some relaxation exercises, such as deep breathing, meditation, or progressive muscle relaxation.

Another nonpharmacological intervention is cognitive behavioral therapy for insomnia (CBT-I), which is generally more effective than medications, especially for those with chronic insomnia. CBT-I decreases insomnia by about 50%, and unlike medications, 50%–70% of patients maintain their clinical gains after it is discontinued. Unfortunately, it may be challenging to find a local therapist who is skilled in the techniques involved. If you are interested in becoming trained yourself, check out www.med.upenn.edu/cbti/cont_ed.html and www.med.upenn.edu/cbti.

Assuming that you and your patient have resigned yourselves to a hypnotic, there's a pretty long menu of reasonable offerings. The options below are not listed in any particular order, because we don't have any specific recommendations one way or another. We tend to pick and choose among them, which often requires trials of more than one before hitting on the sleep ambrosia for a particular patient.

- **"Z-drugs"** (eszopiclone, zaleplon, zolpidem) bind selectively to specific subunits of the GABA receptors that induce sleep, but they don't have the same relaxation effects of benzos and are probably somewhat less addictive. Zolpidem 5–10 mg has become an old standard. For patients who wake up in the middle of the night, use zaleplon instead because of its very short duration of action.

- **Antihistamines** (diphenhydramine, doxylamine, hydroxyzine) are over-the-counter agents that induce sedation by blocking histamine H1 receptors. Start with diphenhydramine 25 mg QHS and increase to 50 mg if needed. The older the patient, the less appropriate this option, as antihistamines can cause confusion when used chronically. While this can occur with anyone, it's more common in the elderly.

- **Benzodiazepines** do present the danger of tolerance; however, some patients take a small dose of one of the benzos every night and seem to suffer no ill effects, and there is often no dosage creep over many years or even decades. Use more caution in the elderly, whose risk for falls is increased.

- **Melatonin** is a natural compound secreted from the pineal gland in a 24-hour circadian rhythm, with levels naturally peaking in the middle of the night. Giving it exogenously as a supplement helps some people sleep, though the effect is not dramatic.

- **Ramelteon** is a melatonin agonist.

- **Lemborexant and suvorexant** are in a new class of agents called **dual orexin (OX1 and OX2) receptor antagonists,** or DORAs for short.

- **Doxepin** (Silenor) was approved by the FDA for use as a hypnotic. It is an old drug in new clothing—a tricyclic antidepressant being used for its antihistamine properties. Because it is still expensive as a generic, we suggest using a low dose of generic doxepin to achieve the same effects as Silenor. This may entail prescribing the liquid version in order to get to doses in the 3 mg range.

- **Trazodone,** another antidepressant, is commonly used for insomnia at a dose of 25–50 mg QHS. You can find the fact sheet for trazodone in the Antidepressants chapter.

- **Mirtazapine** is a sedating antidepressant, and is quite effective for insomnia but causes weight gain.

- **Quetiapine** is the classic sedating antipsychotic, which is commonly prescribed at 25 mg and is quite popular as a non-addictive alternative for substance users.

Potential Side Effects of Most Hypnotics

Although taken by millions, hypnotics are a high-risk class of medications, especially for the elderly, who are at greater risk for confusion, memory problems, and gait disturbances (sometimes leading to falls). Therefore, try to avoid hypnotics in the elderly, and when you do use them, use the lowest effective dose for the shortest duration of time possible.

Certain precautions apply to most hypnotics, and we'll list them below to minimize repetition in the fact sheets:

- *Daytime grogginess or hangover effect.* This effect is most likely to occur with antihistamines or with longer-acting benzodiazepines or extended-release zolpidem.

- *Anterograde amnesia.* This is most likely to occur with benzodiazepines and Z-drugs. Among benzos, triazolam (Halcion) has a particularly bad rep. Just avoid triazolam—there's no need to prescribe it given the wealth of alternatives.

- *CNS depression.* Hypnotics may impair physical or mental abilities and alertness; advise patients to use caution when performing tasks that require alertness (eg, driving).

- *Respiratory depression.* Benzodiazepines in particular may depress respiration; avoid in patients at risk, including those with COPD or sleep apnea, or those taking other depressants such as opiates. In fact, the FDA issued a black box warning about the dangers of combining benzodiazepines with opiates due to a concerning incidence of serious side effects with the combination, including profound sedation, respiratory depression, coma, and death (see the following page for more details on this warning).

- *Paradoxical reactions.* Reports include hyperactive or aggressive behavior, and these reactions are particularly seen with benzodiazepines. Younger patients, the elderly, and those with head injury or organic brain syndromes are at greatest risk.

- *Tolerance.* Patients generally develop tolerance to the sedating effects of benzodiazepines after several weeks of continuous use (one-third of patients will experience tolerance after four weeks of use). Tolerance to anxiolytic effects occurs more slowly, and to anti-seizure effects very little or not at all. Psychological and physical dependence occurs with prolonged use.

- *Discontinuation syndrome.* Withdrawal effects occur with most hypnotics and include rebound insomnia, agitation, anxiety, and malaise. Discontinuation syndromes from benzodiazepines are most severe with longer-term use, higher doses, and shorter-acting agents; in severe cases, discontinuation may include seizures. Hypnotics should not be abruptly discontinued; doses should be tapered gradually.

- *Recreational use and misuse.* This is a risk with many hypnotics, particularly the benzodiazepines. Avoid or minimize use in patients who have addiction risk or when abuse is suspected. Note that the FDA updated its class warning for all benzodiazepines in 2020 with a boxed warning (its most prominent warning) to emphasize the "risks of abuse, misuse, addiction, withdrawal, and physical dependence." They felt the previous prescribing information did not adequately convey these risks and the potential harm of these medications.

- *Complex sleep-related behaviors.* Sleep driving, sleep eating, sleep texting, and sleep sex have all been reported. Although these behaviors can occur when using benzodiazepines or Z-drugs alone and at usual therapeutic doses, they often occur with high-dose use or in combination with other CNS depressants, including alcohol. Typically, these events occur when the individual is not fully awake, and often there will be no memory of the behavior. In 2019, the FDA added a black box warning specifying that these behaviors can lead to injury and death, and recommended against prescribing them to anyone who has experienced complex sleep-related behaviors in the past.

Class Warnings Specific to Benzodiazepines

- *Combining benzodiazepines with opiates.* The FDA has issued a black box warning about the dangers of combining benzodiazepines with opiates due to the risks of profound sedation, respiratory depression, coma, and death. The FDA stipulates reserving the benzo/opioid combination for patients who have unsuccessfully tried alternative options, minimizing the dosage and duration of treatment, and monitoring patients closely for sedation and respiratory depression.

- *Sleep architecture.* Benzodiazepines affect sleep architecture; thus, long-term use is discouraged.

- *Use in elderly patients.* We worry about two potential risks when using benzodiazepines in the elderly: falls and cognitive impairment. A number of meta-analyses have reported about a 1.5-fold increased risk of falls in the elderly who are taking a benzo. Fall risk is greatest during the first two weeks of treatment, so use particular caution during this time. Lower doses reduce fall risk, but the data are conflicting as to whether short- or long-acting benzos are more dangerous. As for cognition, several earlier studies had hinted at a relationship between benzos and dementia, but a recent larger study with superior methodology did not support this connection—in fact, it found a *lower* risk of dementia within two years after benzos or Z-drugs were prescribed (Osler M and Jorgensen MB, *Am J Psych* 2020;177(6):497–505).

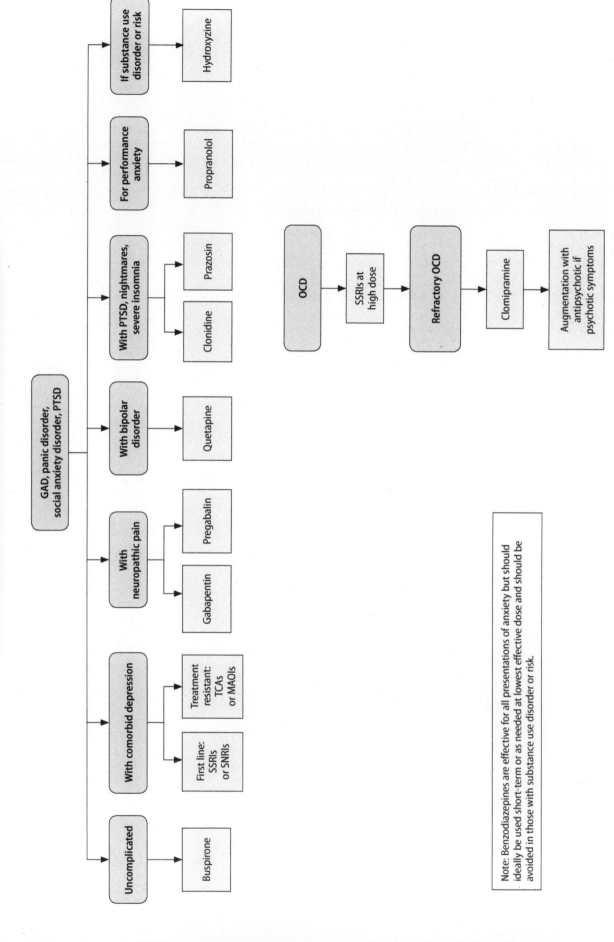

Anxiety Treatment Algorithm

GAD, panic disorder, social anxiety disorder, PTSD

Uncomplicated
→ Buspirone

With comorbid depression
→ First line: SSRIs or SNRIs
→ Treatment resistant: TCAs or MAOIs

With neuropathic pain
→ Gabapentin
→ Pregabalin

With bipolar disorder
→ Quetiapine

With PTSD, nightmares, severe insomnia
→ Clonidine
→ Prazosin

For performance anxiety
→ Propranolol

If substance use disorder or risk
→ Hydroxyzine

OCD → SSRIs at high dose → **Refractory OCD** → Clomipramine → Augmentation with antipsychotic if psychotic symptoms

Note: Benzodiazepines are effective for all presentations of anxiety but should ideally be used short-term or as needed at lowest effective dose and should be avoided in those with substance use disorder or risk.

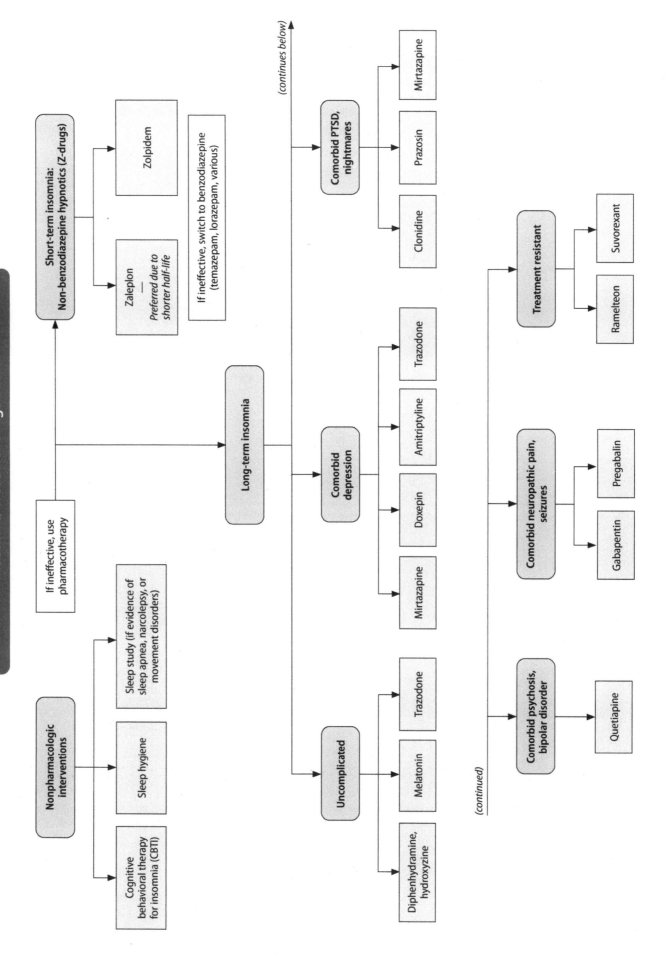

Insomnia Treatment Algorithm

Nonpharmacologic interventions
- Cognitive behavioral therapy for insomnia (CBTI)
- Sleep hygiene
- Sleep study (if evidence of sleep apnea, narcolepsy, or movement disorders)

If ineffective, use pharmacotherapy

Short-term insomnia: Non-benzodiazepine hypnotics (Z-drugs)
- Zaleplon — *Preferred due to shorter half-life*
- Zolpidem

If ineffective, switch to benzodiazepine (temazepam, lorazepam, various)

Long-term insomnia

Uncomplicated
- Diphenhydramine, hydroxyzine
- Melatonin
- Trazodone

Comorbid depression
- Mirtazapine
- Doxepin
- Amitriptyline
- Trazodone

Comorbid PTSD, nightmares
- Clonidine
- Prazosin
- Mirtazapine

Comorbid psychosis, bipolar disorder
- Quetiapine

Comorbid neuropathic pain, seizures
- Gabapentin
- Pregabalin

Treatment resistant
- Ramelteon
- Suvorexant

(continued)

(continues below)

Table 13: **Anxiolytic and Hypnotic Medications**

Generic Name (Brand Name) Year FDA Approved [G] denotes generic availability	Relevant FDA Indication(s)	Available Strengths (mg)	Onset of Action (oral)	Half-Life (hours)	Duration of Action (hours)	Usual Dosage Range (starting–max) (mg)
Antihistamines						
Diphenhydramine [G] (Benadryl, others) 1946 Available OTC and Rx	Insomnia (adults and children 12+ years)	Capsule: 25, 50 Tablet: 25 Liquid: 12.5 mg/mL	1 hour	3.5–9	4–6	25–50 QHS
Doxepin [G] (Silenor) 2010/1969	Insomnia (sleep maintenance)	Tablet: 3, 6 Capsule: 10, 25, 50, 75, 100, 150 Liquid: 10 mg/mL	1 hour	15	4–6	3–6 QHS
Doxylamine [G] (Unisom, others) 1978 Available OTC and Rx	Insomnia	Tablet: 25	1 hour	10	4–6	25–50 QHS
Hydroxyzine [G] (Atarax, Vistaril) 1956	GAD	Capsule: 25, 50, 100 Tablet: 10, 25, 50 Liquid: 10 mg/5 mL Injection: 25 mg/mL, 50 mg/mL	30 min	7–10	4–6	25–50 Q4–6H PRN or up to 25–100 QID
Benzodiazepines						
Alprazolam [G] (Xanax, Xanax XR) 1981	GAD Panic disorder	Tablet: 0.25, 0.5, 1, 2 ER tablet: 0.5, 1, 2, 3 ODT: 0.25, 0.5, 1, 2 Liquid: 1 mg/mL	30 min (IR, ODT) 1–2 hours (XR)	11–16	3–4 (IR) 10 (XR)	0.25–2 TID 0.5–3 QD (XR)
Clonazepam [G] (Klonopin, Klonopin Wafers[1]) 1975	Panic disorder Insomnia (off-label)	Tablet: 0.5, 1, 2 ODT: 0.125, 0.25, 0.5, 1, 2	1 hour	20–80	4–8	0.5 BID–2 TID 0.25–1 QHS
Diazepam [G] (Valium) 1963	GAD Alcohol withdrawal	Tablet: 2, 5, 10 Liquid: 5 mg/5 mL, 5 mg/mL Injection: 5 mg/mL	30 min	>100	4–6	2 BID–10 QID
Flurazepam [G] (Dalmane[1]) 1970	Insomnia (short term)	Capsule: 15, 30	30–60 min	40–100	7–8	15–30 QHS
Lorazepam [G] (Ativan, Loreev XR) 1977	GAD Insomnia (off-label)	Tablet: 0.5, 1, 2 ER capsule: 1, 2, 3 Liquid: 2 mg/mL Injection: 2 mg/mL, 4 mg/mL	30–60 min	10–20	4–6	1–5 BID (QD for XR) 1–4 QHS
Temazepam [G] (Restoril) 1981	Insomnia (short term)	Capsule: 7.5, 15, 22.5, 30	30–60 min	9–18	4–6	15–30 QHS
Triazolam [G] (Halcion) 1982	Insomnia (short term)	Tablet: 0.125, 0.25	15–30 min	1.5–5.5	Unknown	0.25–0.5 QHS
Dual Orexin Receptor Antagonists (DORA)						
Lemborexant (Dayvigo) 2019	Insomnia (sleep onset and sleep maintenance)	Tablet: 5, 10	30–60 min	17–19	6–8	5–10 QHS
Suvorexant (Belsomra) 2014	Insomnia (sleep onset and sleep maintenance)	Tablet: 5, 10, 15, 20	30–60 min	12	6–8	10–20 QHS
Z-Hypnotics						
Eszopiclone [G] (Lunesta) 2004	Insomnia (sleep onset and sleep maintenance)	Tablet: 1, 2, 3	30 min	6	6–8	1–3 QHS
Zaleplon [G] (Sonata) 1999	Insomnia (short term, sleep onset)	Capsule: 5, 10	30 min	1	4	10–20 QHS

Generic Name (Brand Name) Year FDA Approved [G] denotes generic availability	Relevant FDA Indication(s)	Available Strengths (mg)	Onset of Action (oral)	Half-Life (hours)	Duration of Action (hours)	Usual Dosage Range (starting–max) (mg)
Zolpidem [G] (Ambien, Ambien CR, Edluar, Zolpimist) 1992 Generic not available for Edluar or Zolpimist SL	Insomnia (IR: short term, sleep onset; CR: sleep onset and maintenance)	Tablet: 5, 10 ER tablet: 6.25, 12.5 SL tablet: 5, 10 Oral spray: 5 mg/spray	30 min	2.5–3	6–8	10, 12.5 CR (5, 6.25 in women)
Zolpidem low dose [G] (Intermezzo) 2011	Difficulty falling asleep after middle-of-the-night awakening	SL tablet: 1.75, 3.5	30 min	2.5	4	1.75 women; 3.5 men
Others						
Buspirone [G] (BuSpar[1]) 1986	GAD	Tablet: 5, 7.5, 10, 15, 30	1–2 weeks+	2–3	N/A	5–20 TID
Clonidine (Catapres, Kapvay) 1974	Anxiety (off-label)	Tablet: 0.1, 0.2, 0.3 ER tablet: 0.1, 0.2 Patch: 0.1 mg/day, 0.2 mg/day, 0.3 mg/day	30–60 min (oral) 1–2 days (patch)	6–13	8–12 (IR) 8–24 (patch)	0.1–0.2 Q4–6H PRN (IR) 0.1–0.2 QD–BID
Gabapentin [G] (Neurontin) 1993	Anxiety (off-label)	Capsule: 100, 300, 400 Tablet: 600, 800 Oral solution: 50 mg/mL ER tablet: 300, 600	1-2 hours	5–7	5–8	100 QHS–1200 TID
Prazosin [G] (Minipress) 1976	PTSD (off-label)	Capsule: 1, 2, 5	1–2 hours	2–3	4–6	1–10 mg/day QHS or divided BID
Pregabalin [G] (Lyrica) 2004	Anxiety (off-label)	Capsule: 25, 50, 75, 100, 200, 225, 300 Oral solution: 20 mg/mL	1–2 hours	6	8–12	75–300 BID
Propranolol [G] (Inderal) 1973	Performance anxiety (off-label)	Tablet: 10, 20, 40, 60, 80	60 min	3–6	4–6	10–40 PRN
Ramelteon [G] (Rozerem) 2005	Insomnia (sleep onset)	Tablet: 8	30 min	1–2.6	Unknown	8 QHS
Trazodone [G] (Desyrel[1], Oleptro[1]) 1981/2010	Depression Insomnia (off-label)	Tablet: 50, 100, 150, 300 ER tablet: 150, 300	1 hour	7–10	Unknown	25–200 QHS

[1]Brand discontinued; available as generic only

Table 13A: **Benzodiazepine Dosage Equivalencies**

Benzodiazepine	Approximate Equivalent Dosage (mg)
Alprazolam (Xanax)	0.5
Chlordiazepoxide (Librium)	25
Clonazepam (Klonopin)	0.25–0.5
Clorazepate (Tranxene)	7.5
Diazepam (Valium)	5
Estazolam (ProSom)	1
Flurazepam (Dalmane)	15
Lorazepam (Ativan)	1
Oxazepam (Serax)	15
Quazepam (Doral)	15
Temazepam (Restoril)	15
Triazolam (Halcion)	0.25

Anxiolytic and Hypnotic Medications

ALPRAZOLAM (Xanax) Fact Sheet [G]

Bottom Line:

Alprazolam is fast acting and effective for GAD and panic disorder, but its short duration of action may contribute to breakthrough symptoms between doses and make withdrawal more difficult.

FDA Indications:

Generalized anxiety disorder (GAD); panic disorder.

Off-Label Uses:

Other anxiety disorders; insomnia; acute mania or psychosis; catatonia.

Dosage Forms:

- **Tablets (G):** 0.25 (scored), 0.5 mg (scored), 1 mg (scored), 2 mg (scored).
- **ER tablets (Xanax XR, [G]):** 0.5 mg, 1 mg, 2 mg, 3 mg.
- **Orally disintegrating tablets (G):** 0.25 mg, 0.5 mg, 1 mg, 2 mg.
- **Oral concentrate (G):** 1 mg/mL.

Dosage Guidance:

- GAD: Start 0.25–0.5 mg TID; ↑ by 0.25–0.5 mg/day increments every three to four days as needed and tolerated to max dose 4 mg/day divided TID–QID.
- Panic disorder: Start 0.5 mg TID; ↑ by increments of no more than 1 mg/day every three to four days as needed to target dose 4–6 mg/day divided TID–QID. Max dose 10 mg/day.
- Panic disorder using XR: Start 0.5–1 mg QD; ↑ by increments of no more than 1 mg/day at intervals of three to four days to target dose 3–6 mg QD.

Monitoring: No routine monitoring recommended unless clinical picture warrants.

Cost: $

Side Effects:

- Most common: Sedation, somnolence, memory impairment, slurred speech, incoordination, dependence.
- Serious but rare: Anterograde amnesia, increased fall risk, paradoxical reaction (irritability, agitation), respiratory depression (avoid in patients with sleep apnea or on opioids).

Mechanism, Pharmacokinetics, and Drug Interactions:

- Binds to benzodiazepine receptors to enhance GABA effects.
- Metabolized primarily through CYP3A4; t ½: 11–16 hours.
- Avoid use with other CNS depressants, including alcohol and opioids (additive effects). Potent CYP3A4 inhibitors (eg, fluvoxamine, erythromycin) may increase alprazolam levels; CYP3A4 inducers (eg, carbamazepine) may decrease alprazolam levels.

Clinical Pearls:

- Schedule IV controlled substance.
- Benzodiazepines are very effective immediately for GAD and panic disorder, particularly in the early weeks of SSRI therapy while awaiting onset of therapeutic effect.
- Paradoxical reaction of aggression, agitation, and combativeness is more likely to occur in the elderly or those with brain injury.
- While benzodiazepines are highly abusable, patients with panic disorder rarely self-increase their dose when treated adequately, indicating that tolerance to anxiolytic effects does not occur.

Fun Fact:

There are many slang terms for alprazolam; some of the more common ones are bars, Z-bars, zannies, footballs, blues, or blue footballs.

ANTIHISTAMINES (Diphenhydramine, others) Fact Sheet [G]

Bottom Line:

Antihistamines can be very effective sleep aids for many patients, although some patients may experience too much grogginess ("hangover") in the morning. They are good first-line agents due to a low risk of drug tolerance, dependence, or abuse, but exercise caution in the elderly, who are more sensitive to cognitive and peripheral effects.

FDA Indications:

Insomnia (adults, children 12–17 years); allergies; motion sickness; **antiparkinsonism.**

Off-Label Uses:

Extrapyramidal symptoms; nausea and vomiting (morning sickness).

Dosage Forms:

- **Tablets, chewable tablets, caplets, capsules, and oral solutions, varies by brand:** 25 mg, 50 mg.
- **Common brand names:**
  - **Diphenhydramine:** Benadryl, Compoz, Nytol, Simply Sleep, Sleep-Eze, Sominex, Unisom SleepGels, Unisom SleepMelts, and generic.
  - **Doxylamine:** NyQuil, Unisom SleepTabs, and generic.
  - **Hydroxyzine:** Vistaril, Atarax, and generic (see fact sheet).

Dosage Guidance:

Insomnia: Start 25 mg, 30 minutes before bedtime. The dose required to induce sleep can be as low as 6.25 mg, but usual dose is 25 mg. Some patients may require 50 mg at bedtime.

Monitoring: No routine monitoring recommended unless clinical picture warrants.

Cost: $

Side Effects:

- Most common: Dry mouth, ataxia, urinary retention, constipation, drowsiness, memory problems.
- Serious but rare: Blurred vision, tachycardia.

Mechanism, Pharmacokinetics, and Drug Interactions:

- Histamine H1 antagonist.
- Metabolized by liver, primarily CYP2D6; t ½: for diphenhydramine, 3.5–9 hours; for doxylamine, 10 hours (12–15 in elderly).
- Avoid use with other antihistamines or anticholinergics (additive effects).

Clinical Pearls:

- These antihistamines non-selectively antagonize central and peripheral histamine H1 receptors. They also have secondary anticholinergic effects, which can cause side effects including dry mouth and urinary retention, as well as cognitive impairment in susceptible populations.
- Be aware that anticholinergic drugs are often used to treat or prevent EPS in patients taking antipsychotics; diphenhydramine is often chosen and dosed at night to take advantage of its sedative effect.
- Antihistamines can be helpful for some patients with anxiety. See hydroxyzine fact sheet.

Fun Fact:

The name NyQuil is a portmanteau of "night" and "tranquil."

BUSPIRONE (BuSpar) Fact Sheet [G]

Bottom Line:
Buspirone is a reasonable option in patients for whom benzodiazepines are not appropriate. Don't expect as robust a response, and make sure patients know it may take a week or two to kick in.

FDA Indications:
Generalized anxiety disorder (GAD).

Off-Label Uses:
Treatment-resistant depression; anxiety symptoms in depression.

Dosage Forms:
Tablets (G): 5 mg (scored), 7.5 mg (scored), 10 mg (scored), 15 mg (scored), 30 mg (scored).

Dosage Guidance:
Start 7.5 mg BID or 5 mg TID; ↑ by increments of 5 mg/day every two to three days to target dose 20–30 mg/day divided BID–TID; max 20 mg TID.

Monitoring: No routine monitoring recommended unless clinical picture warrants.

Cost: $

Side Effects:
Most common: Dizziness, nervousness, nausea, headache, jitteriness.

Mechanism, Pharmacokinetics, and Drug Interactions:
- Serotonin 5-HT1A receptor partial agonist.
- Metabolized primarily through CYP3A4; t ½: 2–3 hours.
- Avoid use with MAOIs; caution with serotonergic agents due to additive effects and risk for serotonin syndrome. Caution with CYP3A4 inhibitors or inducers as they may affect buspirone serum levels; adjust dose.

Clinical Pearls:
- Similar to antidepressants, buspirone requires one or two weeks for onset of therapeutic effects, with full effects occurring over several weeks, and offers no "as-needed" benefits.
- Non-sedating, non-habit-forming alternative to benzodiazepines for anxiety. May be less effective or ineffective in patients who have previously responded to benzos.
- Has only shown efficacy in GAD, not in other anxiety disorders (PTSD, OCD, panic disorder).
- May potentiate antidepressant effects when used in combination with SSRIs in refractory depression.

Fun Fact:
Psychotropic agents with 5-HT1A partial agonist effects include aripiprazole, ziprasidone, and vilazodone, among others.

CLONAZEPAM (Klonopin) Fact Sheet [G]

Bottom Line:

Due to its longer half-life, clonazepam causes fewer breakthrough symptoms compared to alprazolam when used for anxiety. May also work as a good short-term hypnotic, although development of dependence and long half-life limit this use.

FDA Indications:

Seizure disorders; **panic disorder.**

Off-Label Uses:

Other anxiety disorders; insomnia; acute mania or psychosis; catatonia.

Dosage Forms:

- **Tablets (G):** 0.5 mg (scored), 1 mg (scored), 2 mg (scored).
- **Orally disintegrating tablets (G):** 0.125 mg, 0.25 mg, 0.5 mg, 1 mg, 2 mg.

Dosage Guidance:

- Dose varies based on patient characteristics (eg, age) and tolerance to benzodiazepines.
- Anxiety: Start 0.5 mg BID; ↑ by 0.5–1 mg/day increments every two to four days to max 6 mg/day divided BID–TID.
- Insomnia (off-label use): Start 0.25–0.5 mg QHS as needed for insomnia. Max 2 mg at bedtime.
- Use lower doses for elderly.

Monitoring: No routine monitoring recommended unless clinical picture warrants.

Cost: $

Side Effects:

- Most common: Somnolence, daytime grogginess, confusion, ataxia.
- Serious but rare: Anterograde amnesia, increased fall risk, paradoxical reaction (irritability, agitation), respiratory depression (avoid in patients with sleep apnea or on opioids).

Mechanism, Pharmacokinetics, and Drug Interactions:

- Binds to benzodiazepine receptors to enhance GABA effects.
- Metabolized primarily through CYP3A4; t ½: 20–80 hours.
- Avoid concomitant use with other CNS depressants, including alcohol and opioids (additive effects). Potent CYP3A4 inhibitors (eg, fluvoxamine, erythromycin) may increase clonazepam levels; CYP3A4 inducers (eg, carbamazepine) may decrease clonazepam levels.

Clinical Pearls:

- Schedule IV controlled substance.
- High-potency, long-acting benzodiazepine with active metabolites that may accumulate.
- Withdrawal effects may not be seen until three to five days after abrupt discontinuation and may last 10–14 days due to long half-life and active metabolites of clonazepam.
- Full effects of a particular dose may not be evident for a few days since active metabolites will accumulate with continual use (versus PRN use). Wait several days before increasing dose if patient is taking clonazepam regularly.

Fun Fact:

Klonopin tablets (or "K-pins") have a street value of $2–$5 per tablet, depending on dose and geographic region.

DIAZEPAM (Valium) Fact Sheet [G]

Bottom Line:

Diazepam has a long history of use with good efficacy for anxiety. Its long half-life makes it a particularly effective anxiolytic for some patients, and it is a good alternative to chlordiazepoxide for alcohol withdrawal.

FDA Indications:

Generalized anxiety disorder; alcohol withdrawal; seizures; muscle spasms.

Off-Label Uses:

Other anxiety disorders; insomnia; acute mania or psychosis; catatonia.

Dosage Forms:

- **Tablets (G):** 2 mg (scored), 5 mg (scored), 10 mg (scored).
- **Oral liquid (G):** 5 mg/5 mL, 5 mg/1 mL.
- **Injection (G):** 5 mg/1 mL.
- **Rectal gel (Diastat, [G]):** 2.5 mg, 10 mg, 20 mg per applicator.

Dosage Guidance:

Anxiety: Start 2–5 mg BID; ↑ by 2–5 mg/day increments every two to four days to max 40 mg/day divided BID–QID.

Monitoring: No routine monitoring recommended unless clinical picture warrants.

Cost: $

Side Effects:

- Most common: Somnolence, daytime grogginess, confusion, ataxia.
- Serious but rare: Anterograde amnesia, increased fall risk, paradoxical reaction (irritability, agitation), respiratory depression (avoid in patients with sleep apnea or on opioids).

Mechanism, Pharmacokinetics, and Drug Interactions:

- Binds to benzodiazepine receptors to enhance GABA effects.
- Metabolized primarily through CYP3A4 and CYP2C19; t ½: >100 hours.
- Avoid concomitant use with other CNS depressants, including alcohol and opioids (additive effects).

Clinical Pearls:

- Schedule IV controlled substance.
- Long-acting benzodiazepine with active metabolites that may accumulate.
- Tolerance to sedative effect may develop more rapidly (within two to four weeks of use) than tolerance to anti-anxiety effect.
- Withdrawal effects may not be seen until three to five days after abrupt discontinuation and may last 10–14 days due to long half-life and active metabolites of diazepam.
- Diazepam has the highest lipid solubility of all benzos, which means very rapid distribution into and out of the CNS, resulting in the greatest "rush" felt by patients using in a single-dose manner. This feature makes diazepam an especially abusable benzo.

Fun Fact:

Valium has been glorified in music more than once. The Rolling Stones' "little yellow pill" in "Mother's Little Helper" and Lou Reed's "Walk on the Wild Side" ("Jackie is just speeding away/Thought she was James Dean for a day/Then I guess she had to crash/Valium would have helped that bash") are two good examples.

DOXEPIN (Silenor) Fact Sheet [G]

Bottom Line:
Doxepin may be a good agent to put in your arsenal, particularly for those patients in whom you want to avoid benzodiazepines or Z-drugs. Now that the low-dose (3 and 6 mg) generic version of Silenor is available, price is no longer a limitation.

FDA Indications:
Insomnia (sleep maintenance). Generic doxepin (at higher doses) approved for **depression, anxiety disorders.**

Off-Label Uses:
Headache; neuropathic pain; fibromyalgia.

Dosage Forms:
- **Tablets (Silenor, [G]):** 3 mg, 6 mg.
- **Capsules (G):** 10 mg, 25 mg, 50 mg, 75 mg, 100 mg, 150 mg.
- **Oral concentrate (G):** 10 mg/mL.

Dosage Guidance:
Insomnia:
- Silenor: Start, target, and max dose 6 mg QHS, taken within 30 minutes of bedtime. Use 3 mg/day in elderly. Avoid meals within three hours of taking Silenor.
- Doxepin: Start 10 mg capsule, or achieve a lower dose by using the oral concentrate or by opening the 10 mg capsule, dissolving it in a cup of juice, and drinking a portion of the juice.

Monitoring: No routine monitoring recommended unless clinical picture warrants.

Cost: Generic 10 mg and up: $; Silenor, generic 3 and 6 mg: $$$

Side Effects:
- Most common: Somnolence, nausea, dry mouth, constipation.
- Serious but rare: Orthostasis (more likely at higher doses).

Mechanism, Pharmacokinetics, and Drug Interactions:
- Tricyclic antidepressant with norepinephrine and serotonin reuptake inhibition and histamine H1 antagonism.
- Metabolized primarily through CYP2C19 and CYP2D6 (also CYP1A2 and CYP2C9 to lesser extent); t ½: 15 hours.
- Clinically significant drug interactions not likely at the low doses used for hypnotic effects.

Clinical Pearls:
- Silenor is a branded version of generic doxepin, but available in lower doses.
- Taking within three hours of eating delays therapeutic effect by up to three hours. For faster onset and to minimize next-day effects, don't take within three hours of a meal.

Fun Fact:
Somaxon Pharmaceuticals, the original but fledgling manufacturer of Silenor, was acquired by Pernix, which hopes to eventually pursue over-the-counter approval.

ESZOPICLONE (Lunesta) Fact Sheet [G]

Bottom Line:

Like other Z-drugs, eszopiclone is an effective hypnotic with less potential for dependence than the benzodiazepines. Dosing is simple and, apart from the bitter aftertaste, its rapid onset and long duration of action make it well accepted among patients. As with all sedatives/hypnotics, nightly use should be discouraged.

FDA Indications:

Insomnia (sleep onset and sleep maintenance).

Dosage Forms:

Tablets (G): 1 mg, 2 mg, 3 mg.

Dosage Guidance:

Start 1 mg QHS; may ↑ to max 3 mg QHS. Use lower doses in elderly (max 2 mg QHS). Take immediately before falling asleep and at least seven to eight hours before planned awakening time. Avoid administering with a high-fat meal (delays onset of effect).

Monitoring: No routine monitoring recommended unless clinical picture warrants.

Cost: $

Side Effects:

- Most common: Somnolence, headache, unpleasant taste, dizziness, dry mouth.
- Serious but rare: Anaphylaxis, complex sleep-related behavior (sleep driving, cooking, eating, phone calls).

Mechanism, Pharmacokinetics, and Drug Interactions:

- Selective GABA-A alpha-1 subunit agonist.
- Metabolized primarily through CYP3A4 and CYP2E1; t ½: 6 hours (9 hours in elderly).
- Avoid concomitant use with other CNS depressants, including alcohol (additive effects). Potent CYP3A4 inhibitors (eg, fluvoxamine, erythromycin) may increase effects of eszopiclone significantly, whereas CYP3A4 inducers (eg, carbamazepine) may decrease eszopiclone levels; adjust eszopiclone dosing.

Clinical Pearls:

- Schedule IV controlled substance.
- Non-benzodiazepine in structure, but binds to the GABA-benzodiazepine receptor complex like benzodiazepines do; selective for the alpha receptor subtype (causing hypnotic effects but none of the other pharmacologic effects of benzodiazepines); one of the Z-drugs. Eszopiclone is the s-enantiomer of zopiclone (a hypnotic agent available in other countries).
- Unlike benzodiazepines, eszopiclone does not disrupt sleep architecture (stages).
- Taking after a large, high-fat meal will delay its onset of action (by about an hour). Because of its rapid onset of action, eszopiclone should be taken immediately before bedtime or once difficulty falling asleep has occurred.
- Higher doses increase next-day impairment of driving and alertness.

Fun Fact:

Sepracor, the manufacturer, tried to get Lunesta approved in Europe under the brand name Lunivia, but the European agency determined that eszopiclone was too similar to the already-marketed zopiclone to qualify as a patentable product. Sepracor, realizing that it might encounter future generic competition, withdrew its application.

FLURAZEPAM (Dalmane) Fact Sheet [G]

Bottom Line:
Flurazepam is an older benzodiazepine that has fallen out of favor due to its very long half-life and its active metabolites. It is not our first choice of benzodiazepines for insomnia; we prefer temazepam or lorazepam instead.

FDA Indications:
Insomnia (short term).

Off-Label Uses:
Anxiety disorders; acute mania or psychosis; catatonia.

Dosage Forms:
Capsules (G): 15 mg, 30 mg.

Dosage Guidance:
Start 15 mg QHS. Max 30 mg nightly. Use lower doses in elderly.

Monitoring: No routine monitoring recommended unless clinical picture warrants.

Cost: $

Side Effects:
- Most common: Somnolence, dizziness, weakness, ataxia.
- Serious but rare: Anterograde amnesia, increased fall risk, paradoxical reaction (irritability, agitation), respiratory depression (avoid in patients with sleep apnea or on opioids).

Mechanism, Pharmacokinetics, and Drug Interactions:
- Binds to benzodiazepine receptors to enhance GABA effects.
- Metabolized primarily through CYP3A4; t ½: 40–100 hours.
- Avoid concomitant use with other CNS depressants, including alcohol and opioids (additive effects). Avoid use with potent CYP3A4 inhibitors (eg, erythromycin, ketoconazole, fluvoxamine) as they may increase flurazepam levels significantly, whereas CYP3A4 inducers (eg, carbamazepine) may decrease flurazepam levels; adjust flurazepam dosing.

Clinical Pearls:
- Schedule IV controlled substance.
- Flurazepam is less favored than temazepam because of active metabolites, long half-life, potential for accumulation, and next-day grogginess.
- Tolerance to sedative effect may develop within two to four weeks of use, and benzodiazepines affect sleep architecture; thus, long-term use is discouraged.

Fun Fact:
Advertising for Dalmane in the 1970s featured a nightgown-clad woman trapped inside a giant eyeball sphere, trying to get out. The tagline: "One less concern for your patient with insomnia."

HYDROXYZINE (Atarax, Vistaril) Fact Sheet [G]

Bottom Line:

Hydroxyzine is an antihistamine that is a good non-addictive option when your patient needs a rapid-acting anxiolytic. But beware of its anticholinergic effects, especially in patients who take many doses throughout the day.

FDA Indications:

Generalized anxiety disorder (GAD); pruritis; pre-anesthetic sedative.

Off-Label Uses:

Other anxiety disorders; insomnia; anxiety and agitation related to opioid withdrawal.

Dosage Forms:

• **Hydroxyzine pamoate capsules (Vistaril, [G]):** 25 mg, 50 mg, 100 mg.
• **Hydroxyzine hydrochloride tablets (Atarax, [G]):** 10 mg, 25 mg, 50 mg.
• **Hydroxyzine hydrochloride oral liquid (G):** 10 mg/5 mL.
• **Hydroxyzine hydrochloride injection (G):** 25 mg/1 mL, 50 mg/1 mL.

Dosage Guidance:

• Anxiety: Start 25 mg Q4H or Q6H PRN; ↑ by 25 mg/day increments every three to five days to max 100 mg Q6H PRN. May also be used with scheduled dosing, divided TID–QID. Max dose 400 mg/day.
• Insomnia: Start 25 mg QHS; may ↑ by 25 mg/day increments every three to seven days to usual dosage range of 25–100 mg QHS.

Monitoring: No routine monitoring recommended unless clinical picture warrants.

Cost: $

Side Effects:

• Most common: Sedation, somnolence, daytime grogginess, dry mouth, constipation.
• Serious but rare: QT prolongation.

Mechanism, Pharmacokinetics, and Drug Interactions:

• Histamine H1 antagonist.
• Metabolized primarily through liver, CYP enzymes unknown; t ½: 7–20 hours.
• Avoid concomitant use with other antihistamines or anticholinergics (additive effects).

Clinical Pearls:

• Technically, the 1956 FDA indication is for "symptomatic relief of anxiety and tension associated with psychoneurosis and as an adjunct in organic disease states in which anxiety is manifested," which likely is closest to what we'd consider GAD today.
• Hydroxyzine's anticholinergic effects might raise concerns about memory problems, especially in the elderly, but it was tested against lorazepam and was found to be much more favorable in terms of both cognition and balance.
• May be useful as a "PRN" med but generally considered second line in anxiety disorders due to side effects and, unlike first-line SSRIs and SNRIs, lack of efficacy for usual comorbid disorders such as depression.

Fun Fact:

Confusingly, there are two versions of hydroxyzine: hydroxyzine hydrochloride tablets, oral liquid, and injection (Atarax) and hydroxyzine pamoate capsules (Vistaril). Popular opinion is that the pamoate salt (Vistaril) may have greater solubility or lipophilicity, thereby making it better for anxiety and sedation while Atarax is better for itching, but this is a myth. Essentially, it doesn't matter which you use.

LEMBOREXANT (Dayvigo) Fact Sheet

Bottom Line:

Like the first agent in this class, Lemborexant is an orexin receptor antagonist. It is no more effective than benzos or Z-drugs, and it has a similar abuse liability. We're concerned that next-day impairment is a potential side effect at the highest approved dose of 10 mg, particularly since sleepless patients may decide on their own to take even higher doses. It's not a first-line hypnotic.

FDA Indications:

Insomnia (sleep onset and sleep maintenance).

Dosage Forms:

Tablets: 5 mg, 10 mg.

Dosage Guidance:

Start 5 mg QHS, 30 minutes before bedtime and at least seven hours before planned awakening time. If tolerated but not effective, may increase to max 10 mg QHS. For more rapid onset, patients should wait at least an hour after a meal before taking it. Avoid administering within an hour of a high-fat meal (delays therapeutic effect by about 1.5 hours).

Monitoring: No routine monitoring recommended unless clinical picture warrants.

Cost: $$$$

Side Effects:

* Most common: Somnolence, headache, abnormal dreams, dry mouth.
* Serious but rare: Impaired alertness and motor coordination, including impaired driving; worsening depression or suicidal ideation; sleep paralysis (inability to speak or move for up to a few minutes during the sleep-wake transition), hypnagogic/hypnopompic hallucinations (including vivid and disturbing perceptions), and cataplexy-like symptoms (leg weakness for seconds up to a few minutes both in the nighttime and the daytime) reported, especially at higher doses.

Mechanism, Pharmacokinetics, and Drug Interactions:

* "DORA" or dual orexin (OX1 and OX2) receptor antagonist.
* Metabolized primarily through CYP3A4, with minor contribution from CYP3A5; t ½: 17–19 hours.
* Caution with CYP3A4 inhibitors and inducers; lemborexant dose adjustment recommended. Caution with alcohol and other CNS depressants.

Clinical Pearls:

* Schedule IV controlled substance. Data in recreational drug users found they "liked" lemborexant more than placebo and as much as zolpidem and suvorexant.
* Lemborexant is contraindicated in patients with narcolepsy.
* Incidence of suicidal ideation or behavior was 0.3% (10 mg) and 0.4% (5 mg) compared to 0.2% in patients taking placebo. Closely monitor and assess patients for suicidality, especially those with depression.
* Lemborexant has a unique mechanism of action. Unlike other hypnotics, it does not act by stimulating GABA or melatonin receptors or by blocking histamine. Instead, lemborexant blocks orexin receptors (orexins are neurotransmitters that promote wakefulness).
* Risk of next-day impairment increases with dose; caution patients taking 10 mg against next-day driving and other activities requiring mental alertness.

Fun Fact:

Eisai, the drug company that pursued FDA approval and now markets Dayvigo, bought the rights to this medication in 2015 from Purdue Pharma, the company that brought us OxyContin and pleaded guilty to criminal charges related to the opioid epidemic.

LORAZEPAM (Ativan, Loreev XR) Fact Sheet [G]

Bottom Line:
When a benzodiazepine is appropriate for use (short-term; minimal risk of abuse), we consider lorazepam to be a first-line agent.

FDA Indications:
Generalized anxiety disorder; status epilepticus (IV route).

Off-Label Uses:
Other anxiety disorders; insomnia; acute mania or psychosis; catatonia; pre-operative sedation; chemotherapy related nausea and vomiting.

Dosage Forms:
- **Tablets (G):** 0.5 mg (scored), 1 mg (scored), 2 mg (scored).
- **ER capsules (Loreev XR):** 1 mg, 2 mg, 3 mg.
- **Oral concentrate (G):** 2 mg/mL.
- **Injection (G):** 2 mg/mL, 4 mg/mL.

Dosage Guidance:
- Anxiety: Start 1 mg BID; ↑ by 0.5–1 mg/day increments every two to four days up to 6 mg/day divided BID–TID. Max 10 mg/day divided BID–TID.
- ER capsules for patients taking stable, evenly divided TID dosing with IR; to be taken once daily in morning.
- Insomnia (off-label use): Start 0.5–1 mg QHS, 20–30 minutes before bedtime; max 4 mg nightly.
- Use lower doses in elderly.

Monitoring: No routine monitoring recommended unless clinical picture warrants.

Cost: $; Loreev XR: $$$$

Side Effects:
- Most common: Somnolence, dizziness, weakness, ataxia.
- Serious but rare: Anterograde amnesia, increased fall risk, paradoxical reaction (irritability, agitation), respiratory depression (avoid in patients with sleep apnea or on opioids).

Mechanism, Pharmacokinetics, and Drug Interactions:
- Binds to benzodiazepine receptors to enhance GABA effects.
- Metabolism primarily hepatic (non-CYP450) to inactive compounds; t ½: 10–20 hours.
- Avoid concomitant use with other CNS depressants, including alcohol and opioids (additive effects). No risk for CYP450 drug interactions.

Clinical Pearls:
- Schedule IV controlled substance.
- Lorazepam does not have a long half-life or active metabolites that could accumulate, and poses no CYP450 drug interaction risk.
- Withdrawal symptoms are usually seen on the first day after abrupt discontinuation and last five to seven days in patients receiving benzodiazepines with short to intermediate half-lives, such as lorazepam. A gradual taper is highly recommended, particularly if the patient is receiving prolonged treatment on a high dose.
- Tolerance to sedative effect may develop within two to four weeks of use, and benzodiazepines affect sleep architecture; thus, long-term use is discouraged.

Fun Fact:
Early Ativan marketing efforts included clever direct-to-consumer advertising campaigns. These included "Now it can be yours—the Ativan experience" in 1977 and "In a world where certainties are few... no wonder Ativan is prescribed by so many caring clinicians" in 1987.

PRAZOSIN (Minipress) Fact Sheet [G]

Bottom Line:
Prazosin is an alpha-1 antagonist (FDA approved for hypertension) that has become popular as a treatment for PTSD-associated insomnia/nightmares. More recent studies have cast doubt on its efficacy for nightmares, but many clinicians still believe it is useful.

FDA Indications:
Hypertension.

Off-Label Uses:
PTSD; alcohol use disorder.

Dosage Forms:
Capsules (G): 1 mg, 2 mg, 5 mg.

Dosage Guidance:
- PTSD (off-label): Titrate dose slowly to minimize possibility of "first-dose" orthostatic hypotension. Start 1 mg QHS ×3 days, then 2 mg QHS ×4 days. If tolerating but still symptomatic, increase to 3 mg QHS ×7 days. Dose can be increased further, based on response, to 4 mg QHS ×7 days. Target 1–5 mg/day.
- May dose-divide BID to target daytime PTSD-associated arousal symptoms.

Monitoring: Periodic blood pressure.

Cost: $

Side Effects:
- Most common: Somnolence, dizziness, headache, weakness.
- Serious but rare: Orthostasis and syncope; prolonged erections and priapism have been reported.

Mechanism, Pharmacokinetics, and Drug Interactions:
- Alpha-1 adrenergic receptor antagonist.
- Metabolism primarily hepatic (non-CYP450); t ½: 2–3 hours.
- Caution with other antihypertensive agents, diuretics, and PDE5 inhibitors (eg, Viagra) that may have additive hypotensive effects.

Clinical Pearls:
- Initial studies showed improvement in trauma-related nightmares and sleep quality when dosed at bedtime, as well as positive effects on daytime PTSD symptoms when dosed BID.
- Prazosin failed to work in a more recent controlled trial of military veterans with chronic PTSD. This was the largest study to date on this drug, but it had some flaws: The placebo rate was unusually high, and the investigators may have enriched their sample with patients who were less likely to respond to prazosin (Raskind MA et al, *N Engl J Med* 2018;378:507–517).
- Increasing data on efficacy in alcohol use disorder are promising, making prazosin a reasonable second-line option particularly for patients with any combination of anxiety, insomnia, nightmares, PTSD, or hypertension.

Fun Fact:
Prazosin is an older drug that is now rarely used for its original indication (hypertension). Aside from its uses in psychiatry, it is used most often as a second-line agent for urinary hesitancy in benign prostatic hyperplasia.

Anxiolytic and Hypnotic Medications

PROPRANOLOL (Inderal) Fact Sheet [G]

Bottom Line:

Propranolol has several uses in psychiatry, including performance anxiety, drug-induced tremor, and akathisia. Some clinicians favor it as an "as needed" drug for a variety of anxiety issues, especially when benzos are contraindicated.

FDA Indications:

Hypertension; angina; post-MI cardioprotection; atrial fibrillation; migraine prophylaxis; essential tremor.

Off-Label Uses:

Performance anxiety; tremor due to medication side effects (especially lithium); akathisia.

Dosage Forms:

Tablets (G): 10 mg (scored), 20 mg (scored), 40 mg (scored), 60 mg (scored), 80 mg (scored).

Dosage Guidance:

- Performance anxiety (off-label): Give 10 mg about 60 minutes prior to performance; usual effective dose is 10–40 mg.
- Medication-induced tremor (off-label): Start 10 mg BID as needed; can go up to 30–120 mg daily in two or three divided doses. Can also use Inderal LA, long-acting version of propranolol, 60–80 mg once a day.
- Akathisia (off-label): Start 10 mg BID; can go up to 30–90 mg daily in two or three divided doses.

Monitoring: Periodic blood pressure/pulse.

Cost: $

Side Effects:

Most common: Dizziness, fatigue, bradycardia, and hypotension.

Mechanism, Pharmacokinetics, and Drug Interactions:

- Non-selective beta-1 and beta-2 adrenergic receptor antagonist.
- Metabolized primarily through CYP2D6, also CYP1A2 and CYP2C19; t ½: 3–6 hours.
- Caution with other antihypertensives (additive effects). CYP2D6 inhibitors, as well as inhibitors or inducers of CYP1A2 and CYP2C19, may affect propranolol levels.

Clinical Pearl:

With beta blockade, propranolol reduces some of the somatic symptoms of anxiety (tremor, sweating, flushing, tachycardia).

Fun Fact:

The list of notable people who suffer or have suffered from performance anxiety or stage fright is long. It includes Barbra Streisand, Carly Simon, Van Morrison, Frédéric Chopin, Renee Fleming, Jay Mohr, Hugh Grant, Laurence Olivier, Mahatma Gandhi, and Thomas Jefferson, among others.

RAMELTEON (Rozerem) Fact Sheet [G]

Bottom Line:

Ramelteon is a melatonin receptor agonist. Compared to other hypnotics, ramelteon poses a lower risk for respiratory depression and hangover effect (morning grogginess). A good agent to have in your bag of tricks, but consider the possibility of rare hormonal effects. Also consider that over-the-counter melatonin (which ramelteon mimics) may do the same job, possibly at a lower price.

FDA Indications:

Insomnia (sleep onset).

Off-Label Uses:

Jet lag; shift-work sleep disorder.

Dosage Forms:

Tablets (G): 8 mg.

Dosage Guidance:

Start, target, and maximum dose 8 mg QHS, 30 minutes before bedtime. Avoid administering with high-fat meal (delays therapeutic effect by 45 minutes).

Monitoring: No routine monitoring recommended unless clinical picture warrants.

Cost: $$

Side Effects:

- Most common: Headache, somnolence, fatigue, dizziness, nausea.
- Serious but rare: Anaphylaxis, angioedema, complex sleep-related behavior (sleep driving, cooking, eating, phone calls), increased prolactin, abnormal cortisol or testosterone levels.

Mechanism, Pharmacokinetics, and Drug Interactions:

- Melatonin-1 and melatonin-2 receptor agonist.
- Metabolized primarily through CYP1A2 (major), and to a lesser extent CYP2C9 and CYP3A4; t ½: 1–2.6 hours.
- Avoid concomitant use with CNS depressants (additive effects). Exercise caution in patients taking potent CYP1A2 inhibitors (eg, fluvoxamine), which could increase ramelteon's effects.

Clinical Pearls:

- Because ramelteon's mechanism of action relates to melatonin receptors and regulation of circadian rhythms, it does not cause patients to "feel" sedated. Often patients say that it doesn't start working for several days—however, clinical trials have shown efficacy from the first night of use. It's good to warn patients about this ahead of time, or they may conclude it's ineffective after a single night and stop using it.
- No evidence of abuse potential or physical dependence.
- Hormonal alterations occur very rarely and usually with high-dose (16 mg in one study) and longer-term use (six to 12 months). If unexplained amenorrhea, galactorrhea, decreased libido, or fertility problems occur, consider evaluating patient's prolactin or testosterone levels.

Fun Fact:

Another melatonin agonist, agomelatine, has been studied as an antidepressant, partly because circadian rhythms are disrupted in depression. It is approved overseas, but the manufacturer scrapped its development in the US.

SUVOREXANT (Belsomra) Fact Sheet

Bottom Line:

Suvorexant is an orexin receptor antagonist, and as such it treats insomnia differently from existing agents. Other than a new mechanism of action, suvorexant doesn't have any clear advantages. It is no more effective than benzos or Z-drugs, and it has a similar abuse liability. We're concerned that next-day impairment is a potential side effect at the highest approved dose of 20 mg, particularly since sleepless patients may decide on their own to take even higher doses. It's not a first-line hypnotic.

FDA Indications:

Insomnia (sleep onset and sleep maintenance).

Dosage Forms:

Tablets: 5 mg, 10 mg, 15 mg, 20 mg.

Dosage Guidance:

Start 10 mg QHS, 30 minutes before bedtime and with at least seven hours remaining before planned awakening time. If tolerated but not effective, may increase to max 20 mg QHS. For more rapid onset, patients should wait at least an hour after a meal before taking it. Avoid administering within an hour of a high-fat meal (delays therapeutic effect by about 1.5 hours).

Monitoring: No routine monitoring recommended unless clinical picture warrants.

Cost: $$$$

Side Effects:

- Most common: Somnolence, headache, abnormal dreams, dry mouth.
- Serious but rare: Impaired alertness and motor coordination, including impaired driving; dose-related worsening depression or suicidal ideation; sleep paralysis (inability to speak or move for up to a few minutes during the sleep-wake transition), hypnagogic/hypnopompic hallucinations (including vivid and disturbing perceptions), and cataplexy-like symptoms (leg weakness for seconds up to a few minutes both in the nighttime and the daytime) reported, especially at higher doses.

Mechanism, Pharmacokinetics, and Drug Interactions:

- "DORA" or dual orexin (OX1 and OX2) receptor antagonist.
- Metabolized primarily through CYP3A4, with minor contribution from 2C19; t ½: 12 hours.
- Caution with CYP3A4 inhibitors and inducers; suvorexant dose adjustment recommended. Caution with alcohol and other CNS depressants.

Clinical Pearls:

- Schedule IV controlled substance. One study found that drug abusers "liked" suvorexant as much as Ambien.
- Suvorexant is contraindicated in patients with narcolepsy.
- The incidence of suicidal ideation reported with suvorexant seemed to be dose related, unlike lemborexant. However, all patients taking suvorexant should be monitored for suicidality, particularly those with depression.
- Suvorexant has a unique mechanism of action. Unlike other hypnotics, it does not act by stimulating GABA or melatonin receptors or by blocking histamine. Instead, suvorexant blocks orexin receptors (orexins are neurotransmitters that promote wakefulness).
- Risk of next-day impairment increases with dose; caution patients taking 20 mg against next-day driving and other activities requiring mental alertness.
- Suvorexant's package label was updated in 2020 to include findings on its use in 285 patients with mild to moderate Alzheimer's disease and insomnia. Suvorexant improved total sleep time and was well tolerated, with somnolence (4% compared to 1% for placebo), dry mouth (2% compared to 1% for placebo), and falls (2% compared to 0% for placebo) as the most common side effects.

Fun Fact:

Merck expected to gain FDA approval for suvorexant in summer 2013. However, the FDA expressed concerns about safety with the proposed 30–40 mg dosing range and denied approval. It was finally approved in August 2014 at lower doses.

TEMAZEPAM (Restoril) Fact Sheet [G]

Bottom Line:
Temazepam has the advantages of a short half-life and no active metabolites, and is therefore less likely to cause next-day sedation. It's a decent first-line agent for insomnia if a benzodiazepine is appropriate for use.

FDA Indications:
Insomnia (short term).

Off-Label Uses:
Anxiety disorders; acute mania or psychosis; catatonia.

Dosage Forms:
Capsules (G): 7.5 mg, 15 mg, 22.5 mg, 30 mg.

Dosage Guidance:
Start 15 mg QHS. Max 30 mg nightly. Use lower doses in elderly.

Monitoring: No routine monitoring recommended unless clinical picture warrants.

Cost: 15 mg, 30 mg: $; 7.5 mg, 22.5 mg: $$

Side Effects:
- Most common: Somnolence, dizziness, weakness, ataxia.
- Serious but rare: Anterograde amnesia, increased fall risk, paradoxical reaction (irritability, agitation), respiratory depression (avoid in patients with sleep apnea or on opioids).

Mechanism, Pharmacokinetics, and Drug Interactions:
- Binds to benzodiazepine receptors to enhance GABA effects.
- Metabolized primarily through liver but no CYP450 involvement; t ½: 9–18 hours.
- Avoid concomitant use with other CNS depressants, including alcohol and opioids (additive effects). No risk for CYP450 drug interactions.

Clinical Pearls:
- Schedule IV controlled substance.
- Temazepam has long been a favored hypnotic for the elderly because of the lack of active metabolites, its short half-life, and absence of drug interactions.
- If abruptly discontinued, withdrawal symptoms are usually seen on the first day and last for five to seven days in patients taking this type of short-intermediate half-life benzodiazepine.
- Tolerance to sedative effect may develop within two to four weeks of use, and benzodiazepines affect sleep architecture; thus, long-term use is discouraged.

Fun Fact:
The US Air Force uses temazepam as one of the approved "no-go pills" to help aviators and special duty personnel sleep in support of mission readiness; "ground tests" are required prior to authorization being issued to use the medication in an operational situation.

TRIAZOLAM (Halcion) Fact Sheet [G]

Bottom Line:
Triazolam gained notoriety as the benzodiazepine that may have caused President George Bush to faint at a state dinner in 1992. It is rarely used due to the higher likelihood for adverse effects (anterograde amnesia, psychiatric disturbances) compared to other benzos.

FDA Indications:
Insomnia (short term).

Off-Label Uses:
Anxiety disorders; acute mania or psychosis; catatonia.

Dosage Forms:
Tablets (G): 0.125 mg, 0.25 mg (scored).

Dosage Guidance:
Start 0.25 mg QHS; max 0.5 mg QHS. Take immediately before bedtime. Use lower doses in elderly.

Monitoring: No routine monitoring recommended unless clinical picture warrants.

Cost: $

Side Effects:
- Most common: Drowsiness, headache, dizziness, ataxia.
- Serious but rare: Anterograde amnesia, increased fall risk, paradoxical reaction (irritability, agitation); respiratory depression (avoid in patients with sleep apnea or opioid use).

Mechanism, Pharmacokinetics, and Drug Interactions:
- Binds to benzodiazepine receptors to enhance GABA effects.
- Metabolized primarily through CYP3A4; t ½: 1.5–5.5 hours.
- Avoid concomitant use with other CNS depressants, including alcohol and opioids (additive effects). Avoid use with potent CYP3A4 inhibitors (eg, erythromycin, ketoconazole, fluvoxamine) as they may increase triazolam levels significantly, whereas CYP3A4 inducers (eg, carbamazepine) may decrease triazolam levels; adjust triazolam dosing.

Clinical Pearls:
- Schedule IV controlled substance.
- Rapid onset of effect; best to take when already in bed.
- Due to its short half-life, triazolam is not effective for patients who suffer from frequent awakenings or early wakening; mostly useful for sleep onset.
- Rebound insomnia and other withdrawal symptoms are more likely and more severe with a short-acting benzodiazepine such as triazolam.
- Tolerance to sedative effect may develop within two to four weeks of use, and benzodiazepines affect sleep architecture; thus, long-term use is discouraged.
- May induce more anterograde amnesia than other benzodiazepines; concomitant use of alcohol or use of higher dose (0.5 mg) increases risk.
- Due to studies that suggest the frequency of severe psychiatric disturbances is higher with triazolam compared to other benzodiazepines, the United Kingdom and Brazil have banned it.

Not-So-Fun Fact:
Serial killer Jeffrey Dahmer used triazolam to sedate his victims.

ZALEPLON (Sonata) Fact Sheet [G]

Bottom Line:

Zaleplon is the only sleeping pill that can be taken at 3 or 4 a.m. without causing functional impairment when the patient gets out of bed a few hours later. It's great for inducing sleep, but not great for sleep maintenance throughout the night.

FDA Indications:

Insomnia (short term, sleep onset).

Dosage Forms:

Capsules (G): 5 mg, 10 mg.

Dosage Guidance:

Start 10 mg QHS, which is the usual dose for most adults. Max 20 mg QHS in those who tolerate but don't benefit from the usual 10 mg dose. Avoid administering with a high-fat meal (delays onset of effect by two hours). Use lower doses in elderly.

Monitoring: No routine monitoring recommended unless clinical picture warrants.

Cost: $

Side Effects:

- Most common: Somnolence, dizziness, headache.
- Serious but rare: Anaphylaxis, complex sleep-related behavior (sleep driving, cooking, eating, phone calls).

Mechanism, Pharmacokinetics, and Drug Interactions:

- Selective GABA-A alpha-1 subunit agonist.
- Metabolized primarily through aldehyde oxidase and also CYP3A4; t ½: 1 hour.
- Avoid concomitant use with other CNS depressants, including alcohol and opioids (additive effects). Potent CYP3A4 inhibitors (eg, fluvoxamine, erythromycin) may increase effects of zaleplon significantly, whereas CYP3A4 inducers (eg, carbamazepine) may decrease zaleplon levels; adjust zaleplon dosing.

Clinical Pearls:

- Schedule IV controlled substance.
- Patients should take it immediately before going to bed or once they are in bed to minimize amnesic episodes.
- Because of zaleplon's very short half-life, it rarely causes next-day impairment.
- Unlike benzodiazepines, zaleplon does not disrupt normal sleep stages.
- Most useful for sleep initiation disorders; does not substantially increase total sleep time or decrease number of awakenings.
- Classified as a Schedule IV drug, but at therapeutic doses, abuse potential is somewhat less than benzodiazepines. However, abuse potential at high doses (2.5–7.5 times recommended dose) is similar to that of benzodiazepines.
- Fewer withdrawal effects than with benzodiazepines, but abrupt discontinuation, particularly from higher doses, can cause withdrawal symptoms (mostly rebound insomnia).

Fun Fact:

The name "Sonata" calls to mind the classical music composition featuring three or four movements, much like the phases of sleep.

ZOLPIDEM (Ambien, Edluar, Intermezzo, Zolpimist) Fact Sheet [G]

Bottom Line:
Ambien is the original Z-drug, having been initially FDA approved in 1992. It is a good hypnotic that can also help with sleep maintenance, particularly in the ER formulation. The lower-dose sublingual version (Intermezzo) has a shorter duration of action and can be taken in the middle of the night—but we recommend using cheaper generic zaleplon instead for middle-of-the-night awakening.

FDA Indications:
Insomnia (IR: short term, sleep onset; CR: sleep onset and maintenance; Intermezzo: difficulty falling asleep after middle-of-the-night awakening).

Dosage Forms:
- **Tablets (G):** 5 mg, 10 mg.
- **ER tablets (G):** 6.25 mg, 12.5 mg.
- **SL tablets (Edluar):** 5 mg, 10 mg.
- **SL tablets (Intermezzo, [G]):** 1.75 mg, 3.5 mg.
- **Oral spray (Zolpimist):** 5 mg/spray.

Dosage Guidance:
- Start 10 mg QHS (5 mg in women). ER: Start 12.5 mg QHS (6.25 mg in women). Take immediately before bed, with at least seven to eight hours remaining before planned awakening time. Dose may be increased to max 10 mg (or 12.5 mg ER) QHS if no daytime grogginess. Higher doses may lead to greater abuse potential. Use lower doses in elderly.
- Lower doses of 3.5 mg (men), 1.75 mg (women) SL QHS can be used with at least four hours remaining before wake time.

Monitoring: No routine monitoring recommended unless clinical picture warrants.

Cost: $; Intermezzo, Zolpimist: $$; Edluar: $$$$

Side Effects:
- Most common: Headache, somnolence, dizziness, diarrhea.
- Serious but rare: Complex sleep-related behavior (sleep driving, cooking, eating, phone calls).

Mechanism, Pharmacokinetics, and Drug Interactions:
- Selective GABA-A alpha-1 subunit agonist.
- Metabolized primarily through CYP3A4; t ½: 2.5–3 hours.
- Avoid concomitant use with other CNS depressants, including alcohol and opioids (additive effects). Potent CYP3A4 inhibitors may increase effects of zolpidem, whereas CYP3A4 inducers (eg, carbamazepine) may decrease zolpidem levels; adjust zolpidem dosing.

Clinical Pearls:
- Schedule IV controlled substance.
- Unlike benzodiazepines, zolpidem does not disrupt normal sleep stages.
- At therapeutic doses, abuse potential is somewhat less than with benzodiazepines.
- Less withdrawal effects than with benzodiazepines, but abrupt discontinuation, particularly from higher doses, can cause withdrawal symptoms (mostly rebound insomnia).
- The CR formulation's dual layer allows some medication to be released immediately, with the rest released gradually, resulting in higher levels through the night.

Fun Fact:
Bioavail Labs received FDA approval for an orally disintegrating tablet form of zolpidem called Tovalt in 2007. It has since been discontinued due to poor sales.

Dementia Medications

GENERAL PRESCRIBING TIPS

Cognitive Impairment

While cholinesterase inhibitors do not improve patients' memory, they do stop the decline of memory loss for six to 12 months. After that reprieve, the clock starts ticking down again, and a person's memory will decline along the same slope that it did before the medication was started. If the medication is interrupted, the person's memory quickly drops by another six to 12 months of function—usually within a week or two. Unfortunately, the research shows that restarting the cholinesterase inhibitor will not bring the person's memory back to where it was before the treatment interruption.

For mild to moderate dementia, use one of the three approved cholinesterase inhibitors. These include donepezil, galantamine, and rivastigmine. We recommend starting with donepezil (we have the most data and experience with this agent, though the others are equally effective). Start with 5 mg daily for a month, then increase to 10 mg and maintain that dose if the patient is doing well. Later, if the patient is continuing to worsen, try to push the dose up to 15 or 20 mg. The main limiting side effects are gastrointestinal issues and, occasionally, vivid dreams at night.

Some clinicians start with 8 mg of sustained-release galantamine in the morning, increasing after a month to 16 mg, which is equivalent to 10 mg of donepezil. Increase to 24 mg of galantamine if needed. If the patient is bothered by vivid dreams, switch to immediate-release galantamine and start with 4 mg in the morning, increasing to 8 mg if tolerated.

The rivastigmine patch is another option to consider, mainly for patients who are having intolerable GI side effects on one of the pills. While the patch causes fewer GI side effects, it's more expensive than pills, and it's more cumbersome because you need another person to take it off or put it on. The patch comes in 4.6 mg/24 hour, 9.5 mg/24 hour, and 13.3 mg/24 hour doses. In general, start patients on the 4.6 mg patch and then move them up to the 9.5 mg. We rarely use the 13.3 mg dose, because that tends to cause the GI side effects that we are using the patch to avoid.

In patients with moderate to severe Alzheimer's dementia, for an FDA-approved approach, you can start with either memantine IR or high-dose donepezil (either by combining two 10 mg tablets or using the 23 mg version). Reserve the more expensive memantine XR for those rare situations in which IR is poorly tolerated.

An alternative approach is to follow the same protocol for all your patients with dementia, whether or not it is "severe" or "moderate." Start with a combination of donepezil and memantine, and for patients who have trouble taking two pills, consider Namzaric, which is the combination donepezil/memantine.

The FDA's approval of the amyloid beta monoclonal antibody aducanumab (Aduhelm) for treating mild cognitive impairment in Alzheimer's disease has been fraught with controversy. Two pivotal Phase 3 trials showed decreases in amyloid plaque in the brain but showed minimal to no slowing of cognitive decline. In fact, these studies were closed early because the drug didn't seem to be helping patients. Based on this, the FDA Advisory Committee took a pass on the drug in 2020, but it was later given accelerated approval in 2021. We don't recommend it, due to its questionable efficacy, its potential serious side effects, and its high cost ($62,000 per year).

When working with these patients, don't forget to review their medications for agents that may be worsening cognition or causing confusion. These include benzodiazepines, non-benzo Z-drugs, and anticholinergic agents. You'll find a list of medications with a heavy anticholinergic load in Appendix G.

Behavioral and Psychological Symptoms of Dementia (BPSD)

90% of patients with dementia have secondary symptoms, including agitation, aggression, wandering, psychosis, depression, and anxiety. Because of the frailty of this population, you should prioritize nonpharmacological treatments such as recreational therapy, art and music therapy, and habilitation therapy. However, meds are often needed to maintain safety, and here is a brief run-down of your options:

- *Cholinesterase inhibitors.* The medications we discussed above not only delay cognitive decline but also often help with behavioral issues. They may be especially helpful in patients with dementia due to Parkinson's or Lewy body disease.

- *SSRIs.* Several studies have shown that SSRIs help with mild to moderate levels of agitation, including psychomotor restlessness, irritability, hostility, and tearful dysphoria. While the largest study was done with citalopram, it has become less popular due to a recent FDA warning about QT interval prolongation. Thus, many clinicians prefer to use escitalopram (begin with 5 mg and titrate gradually to 20 mg) or sertraline (begin with 12.5 mg and titrate as high as 100 mg). Be wary of the possibility of upper GI bleeding and hyponatremia, both of which are uncommon SSRI side effects but more likely in the elderly.

- *Mirtazapine (Remeron)*. Mirtazapine is helpful for insomnia as well as symptoms of depression. This drug has two other nice features for the elderly: It is less likely than SSRIs to cause hyponatremia, and it does not cause nausea (in fact, mirtazapine is an effective treatment for hyperemesis gravidarum, the severe nausea during pregnancy). Start at 7.5 mg at bedtime and titrate up as needed.

- *Benzodiazepines*. We try to avoid these agents in the elderly because of potential side effects that include loss of balance, impaired cognition, and paradoxical agitation. If you do use benzos, it's best to choose short-acting agents such as lorazepam 0.25 mg as needed, which may be more effective in patients with a history of alcohol use disorder. For patients with REM sleep disorder, use the longer-acting clonazepam at bedtime.

- *Antipsychotics*. In 2005, the FDA required a black box warning on the use of antipsychotics in dementia because of a 1.7-fold increase in mortality and an increased risk of stroke. It's important to put this statistic into perspective. This is a proportional increase; in the long-term care setting, it would represent a change in the 180-day cumulative mortality rate from 15.1% to 16.6% (Gill SS, *Ann Intern Med* 2007;146(11):775–786). In both Canada and the United Kingdom, risperidone is approved for short-term treatment of BPSD. The bottom line is that you should consider antipsychotics in the elderly when they display psychotic symptoms or severe aggression. Start with low-dose risperidone (0.125 mg to 0.25 mg) at bedtime and slowly titrate upwards. Switch to twice-daily dosing if there are breakthrough symptoms during the day. Avoid risperidone in patients with Parkinson's disease—in these patients, use quetiapine or clozapine, or try the newly approved (but currently prohibitively expensive) pimavanserin (Nuplazid) if the others are not tolerated or effective.

- *Mood stabilizers and anticonvulsants*. Gabapentin appears to be the most commonly used of the anticonvulsants, because it is well tolerated and effective for agitation. The usual dose is 100 mg timed to symptoms. Other lower side effect medications to consider are lamotrigine and oxcarbazepine. Depakote is used for impulsivity and disinhibition, though it can cause hyperammonemia leading to confusion. Lithium, though effective, is less commonly prescribed because of a range of side effects, risk for toxicity, and the need for blood level monitoring.

- *Other agents:*

  - Acetaminophen, oddly enough, is often helpful to prescribe to dementia patients, probably because it eases pain syndromes that are so common and underdiagnosed in the elderly. Prescribe 500 mg BID or TID, generally on a standing basis, since patients' impaired cognition makes it unlikely that they will be able to communicate their needs for medication.

  - Opiates. While on the subject of pain relief, we should mention low-dose opiates, which are highly effective for agitation related to pain. Use Roxanol liquid (morphine sulfate), beginning with 2.5 mg daily. Monitor for increased confusion or fall risk, especially early in therapy.

  - Trazodone, at a starting dose of 12.5 mg, is helpful both for agitation and insomnia, and can be given either at bedtime or at midday.

  - Prazosin is well tolerated. Start with 1 mg at bedtime and titrate as needed up to 4 mg or more, divided BID, watching for blood pressure changes.

  - Clonidine patch, 0.1 mg, is often effective for anxiety and agitation, and has the added benefit of ensuring compliance for patients who resist oral meds (as long as the patient can't take it off).

  - Dronabinol (Marinol) is a preparation of cannabinoids that is FDA approved for weight loss in AIDS and nausea in chemotherapy, but it is often used off-label for agitation in dementia. Start at 2.5 mg daily, increasing to 5 mg as needed.

*We gratefully acknowledge the contributions of Dr. Andrew Budson and Dr. Alexis Freedberg for their practical advice regarding treatment of dementia and BPSD.

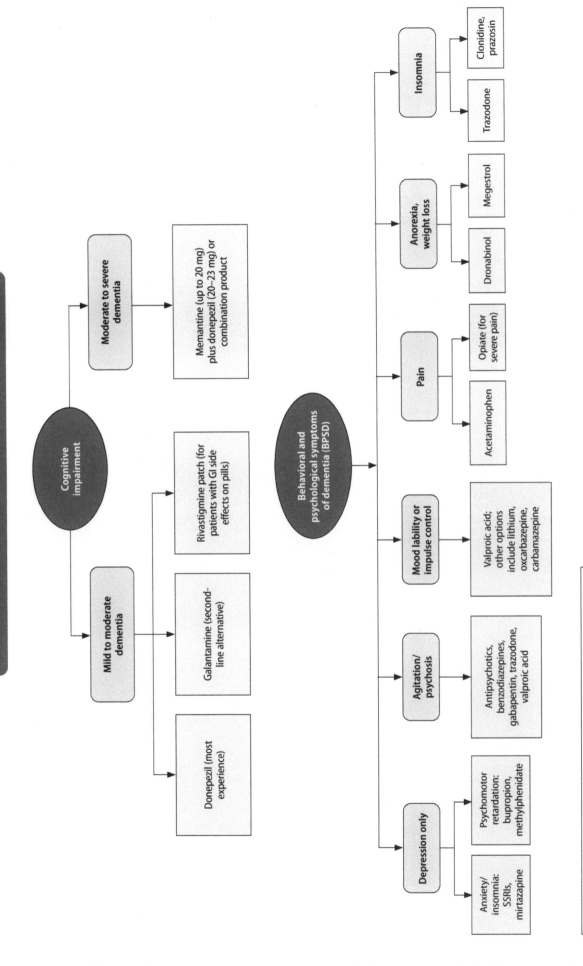

Dementia Treatment Algorithm

Cognitive impairment

- **Mild to moderate dementia**
  - Donepezil (most experience)
  - Galantamine (second-line alternative)
  - Rivastigmine patch (for patients with GI side effects on pills)

- **Moderate to severe dementia**
  - Memantine (up to 20 mg) plus donepezil (20–23 mg) or combination product

Behavioral and psychological symptoms of dementia (BPSD)

- **Depression only**
  - Anxiety/insomnia: SSRIs, mirtazapine
  - Psychomotor retardation: bupropion, methylphenidate

- **Agitation/psychosis**
  - Antipsychotics, benzodiazepines, gabapentin, trazodone, valproic acid

- **Mood lability or impulse control**
  - Valproic acid; other options include lithium, oxcarbazepine, carbamazepine

- **Pain**
  - Acetaminophen
  - Opiate (for severe pain)

- **Anorexia, weight loss**
  - Dronabinol
  - Megestrol

- **Insomnia**
  - Trazodone
  - Clonidine, prazosin

Supportive and environmental measures (eg, music therapy, structured activity, supportive staff, walking) should be tried before medications.

Table 14: **Dementia Medications**

Generic Name (Brand Name) Year FDA Approved *[G] denotes generic availability*	Relevant FDA Indication(s)	Available Strengths (mg except where noted)	Usual Dosage Range (starting–max) (mg)
Aducanumab (Aduhelm) 2021	Mild Alzheimer's dementia	Injection: 170 mg/1.7 mL, 300 mg/3 mL	10 mg/kg IV Q4 weeks
Donepezil [G] (Aricept, Aricept ODT) 1996	Mild to moderate Alzheimer's dementia (5, 10 mg) Moderate to severe Alzheimer's dementia (10, 23 mg)	Tablet: 5, 10, 23 ODT: 5, 10	5–23 QAM
Galantamine [G] (Razadyne) 2001	Mild to moderate Alzheimer's dementia	Tablet: 4, 8, 12 Liquid: 4 mg/mL	4–12 BID
Galantamine ER [G] (Razadyne ER) 2004	Mild to moderate Alzheimer's dementia	ER capsule: 8, 16, 24	8–24 ER QAM
Memantine [G] (Namenda) 2003	Moderate to severe Alzheimer's dementia	Tablet: 5, 10 Liquid: 2 mg/mL	5 QAM–10 BID
Memantine ER [G] (Namenda XR) 2010	Moderate to severe Alzheimer's dementia	ER capsule: 7, 14, 21, 28	7–28 QD
Memantine ER/donepezil [G] (Namzaric) 2014	Moderate to severe Alzheimer's dementia (in patients already stabilized on both medications)	ER capsule: 7/10, 14/10, 21/10, 28/10	Patients on memantine (10 mg BID or 28 mg XR QD) and donepezil 10 mg QD can be switched to Namzaric 28/10 mg QPM
Rivastigmine [G] (Exelon) 2000	Mild to moderate Alzheimer's dementia Mild to moderate dementia associated with Parkinson's disease	Capsule: 1.5, 3, 4.5, 6	1.5–6 BID
Rivastigmine [G] (Exelon Patch) 2007	Mild to moderate and severe Alzheimer's dementia Mild to moderate dementia associated with Parkinson's disease	ER patch: 4.6, 9.5, 13.3/24 hr	4.6–13.3/24 hr QD

ADUCANUMAB (Aduhelm) Fact Sheet

Bottom Line:

Aducanumab is an antibody that attacks and dissolves the amyloid protein that is thought to contribute to Alzheimer's dementia. It is the first new drug approved for Alzheimer's since 2003. Unfortunately, it is marginally effective at best, requires monthly IV infusion, has cumbersome monitoring requirements, and carries potentially significant side effects, all at very high cost. We don't recommend it.

FDA Indications:

Mild Alzheimer's dementia.

Dosage Forms:

Injection: 170 mg/1.7 mL, 300 mg/3 mL.

Dosage Guidance:

Start 1 mg/kg IV infused over one hour Q4 weeks for the first two infusions; ↑ to 3 mg/kg IV Q4 weeks for the next two infusions; ↑ to 6 mg/kg IV Q4 weeks for infusions five and six; ↑ and continue recommended dose of 10 mg/kg IV Q4 weeks for infusion seven and beyond.

Monitoring: Baseline brain magnetic resonance imaging (MRI), repeat MRI prior to the seventh and 12th infusions. If there are 10 or more incident microhemorrhages or more than two focal areas of superficial siderosis, continue with caution only if follow-up MRI shows stabilization.

Cost: $$$$$

Side Effects:

- Most common: Amyloid-related imaging abnormalities in 41% of patients including edema, headache, microhemorrhage, superficial siderosis; confusion; dizziness; nausea; falls.
- Serious but rare: Angioedema, urticarial; discontinue if hypersensitivity reaction occurs.

Mechanism, Pharmacokinetics, and Drug Interactions:

- Recombinant human immunoglobulin gamma-1 (IgG1) anti-amyloid beta monoclonal antibody.
- Degraded into small peptides and amino acids through catabolic pathways, similar to endogenous IgG; t ½: 25 days.
- No drug interactions known.

Clinical Pearls:

- Aducanumab was granted accelerated approval based on reduction in amyloid beta plaques; continued approval may be contingent on verification of clinical benefit in further studies.
- Aducanumab, if used, should only be used in patients with mild cognitive impairment. There are no data on its effects in earlier or later stages.
- Amyloid-related imaging abnormalities are very common. Associated clinical symptoms, most commonly headache, confusion, dizziness, visual disturbance, and nausea, were present in 24% of patients treated with aducanumab.

Fun Fact:

Allegations about improper collaboration between the FDA and aducanumab's manufacturer Biogen have led to calls for an investigation by the inspector general. A number of health systems have publically stated they will not use the drug until more convincing data are available.

Dementia Medications

DONEPEZIL (Aricept) Fact Sheet [G]

Bottom Line:

Donepezil is the cholinesterase inhibitor with the longest track record and with which we have the most experience. It is generally considered the first-line agent for dementia. Though not a cure, it delays dementia progression by six to 12 months.

FDA Indications:

Mild to moderate Alzheimer's dementia (5 mg, 10 mg); **moderate to severe Alzheimer's dementia** (10 mg, 23 mg).

Off-Label Uses:

Other memory disorders; mild cognitive impairment.

Dosage Forms:

- **Tablets (G):** 5 mg, 10 mg, 23 mg.
- **Orally disintegrating tablets (Aricept ODT, [G]):** 5 mg, 10 mg.

Dosage Guidance:

- Mild to moderate dementia: Start 5 mg QAM and ↑ to 10 mg QAM after four to six weeks.
- Moderate to severe dementia: May ↑ further to 23 mg QAM after at least three months (range 10–23 mg/day).

Monitoring: No routine monitoring recommended unless clinical picture warrants.

Cost: $

Side Effects:

- Most common: Dose-related diarrhea, nausea, vomiting, weight loss (especially 23 mg/day dose), anorexia, insomnia, abnormal dreams.
- Serious but rare: Cholinesterase inhibitors may have vagotonic effects that may cause bradycardia and/or heart block with or without a history of cardiac disease; syncope reported.

Mechanism, Pharmacokinetics, and Drug Interactions:

- Acetylcholinesterase (AChE) inhibitor.
- Metabolized primarily through CYP2D6 and CYP3A4; t ½: 70 hours.
- Avoid use with anticholinergic agents as they will diminish therapeutic effects; avoid beta blockers due to risk of bradycardia. P450 interactions not usually clinically important.

Clinical Pearls:

- Donepezil is our first-line AChE inhibitor because of its good track record and tolerability.
- Donepezil is the second drug to be approved for dementia after tacrine, which was pulled from the market due to liver toxicity; donepezil is also the most prescribed of the three cholinesterase inhibitors. It received additional FDA approval for use in severe dementia (in addition to its initial approval for mild to moderate dementia).
- Although the manufacturer recommends bedtime dosing, we recommend starting it in the morning to minimize insomnia and vivid dreams.
- GI side effects usually resolve in one to two weeks.
- Based on a Cochrane review, donepezil causes fewer side effects than rivastigmine.

Fun Fact:

Donepezil has been studied in children for autism, pervasive developmental disorders, ADHD, and tic disorders; however, the minimal data do not support such use.

GALANTAMINE (Razadyne, Razadyne ER) Fact Sheet [G]

Bottom Line:
Galantamine has no appreciable benefit over donepezil; however, its availability in a liquid formulation is helpful for patients who have difficulty swallowing pills.

FDA Indications:
Mild to moderate Alzheimer's dementia.

Off-Label Uses:
Other memory disorders; mild cognitive impairment.

Dosage Forms:
- **Tablets (G):** 4 mg, 8 mg, 12 mg.
- **ER capsules (Razadyne ER, [G]):** 8 mg, 16 mg, 24 mg.
- **Oral solution (G):** 4 mg/mL.

Dosage Guidance:
- IR: Start 4 mg BID (breakfast and dinner), ↑ by 4 mg BID increments every four weeks.
- ER: Start 8 mg QAM (breakfast), ↑ by 8 mg/day every four weeks.
- For both, max 24 mg/day (target dose: 16–24 mg/day).
- If using oral solution, mix dose with three to four ounces of any nonalcoholic beverage; mix well and drink immediately.
- If therapy is interrupted for three or more days, restart at the lowest dose and increase to current dose.

Monitoring: No routine monitoring recommended unless clinical picture warrants.

Cost: $$; liquid: $$$

Side Effects:
- Most common: Diarrhea, nausea, vomiting, weight loss, anorexia, insomnia, abnormal dreams.
- Serious but rare: Cholinesterase inhibitors may have vagotonic effects that may cause bradycardia and/or heart block with or without a history of cardiac disease; syncope reported.

Mechanism, Pharmacokinetics, and Drug Interactions:
- Acetylcholinesterase (AChE) inhibitor and cholinergic nicotinic receptor modulator.
- Metabolized primarily through CYP2D6 and CYP3A4; t ½: 7 hours.
- Avoid use with anticholinergic agents as they will diminish therapeutic effects; avoid beta blockers due to risk of bradycardia. CYP450 interactions not usually clinically important.

Clinical Pearls:
- Galantamine's claim to fame is that it has a "dual" mechanism of action, modulating cholinergic nicotinic receptors in addition to inhibiting AChE. The manufacturer may use this factoid to argue that galantamine is more effective than the other cholinesterase inhibitors. However, accumulating evidence seems to show no difference in efficacy (Birks J, *Cochrane Database Syst Rev* 2006;(1):CD005593).
- ER formulation seems to be used more often due to ease of once-daily dosing.

Fun Fact:
Razadyne was approved in 2001 with its original name, Reminyl. However, pharmacists sometimes confused written scripts for Reminyl with Amaryl, a diabetes medication. In April 2005, the trade name was changed to Razadyne to avoid future dispensing errors.

MEMANTINE (Namenda, Namenda XR) Fact Sheet [G]

Bottom Line:

Memantine's indication (moderate to severe dementia only) may limit its use, but it does boast a unique mechanism of action and has some data to support its usefulness as an augmenter of donepezil. Many prescribers put the majority of their dementia patients on a combination of one of the cholinesterase inhibitors and memantine; we recommend adding memantine when dementia has progressed to the moderate or severe level, possibly earlier. There's no clinical benefit to using the more expensive XR version.

FDA Indications:

Moderate to severe Alzheimer's dementia.

Off-Label Uses:

Mild to moderate Alzheimer's dementia; other memory disorders; mild cognitive impairment; chronic pain.

Dosage Forms:

- **Tablets (G):** 5 mg, 10 mg.
- **Oral solution (G):** 2 mg/1 mL.
- **ER capsules (Namenda XR, [G]):** 7 mg, 14 mg, 21 mg, 28 mg.

Dosage Guidance:

- IR: 5 mg QD week one; 5 mg BID week two; 10 mg QAM and 5 mg QHS week three; 10 mg BID week four and beyond.
- XR: Start 7 mg QD; ↑ by 7 mg/day in increments of at least one week to max dose 28 mg/day (10 mg BID equivalent to 28 mg XR QD). Can be opened and sprinkled on food.

Monitoring: No routine monitoring recommended unless clinical picture warrants.

Cost: IR: $; ER: $$; liquid: $$$

Side Effects:

Most common: Dizziness (XR), transient confusion (IR), headache (XR), diarrhea (XR), constipation, sedation.

Mechanism, Pharmacokinetics, and Drug Interactions:

- N-methyl-D-aspartate (NMDA) receptor antagonist.
- Metabolism primarily hepatic, but not CYP450; t ½: 60–80 hours.
- Pharmacokinetic interactions unlikely.

Clinical Pearls:

- FDA approved for moderate to severe Alzheimer's dementia only; may also be effective as augmentation added to donepezil in patients with moderate to severe Alzheimer's dementia (see memantine ER/donepezil fact sheet).
- Data comparing 10 mg BID and 20 mg QD of IR formulation, as well as pharmacokinetic profile, support use of once-daily IR dosing; IR is used QD in Europe.

Fun Fact:

Forest Pharmaceuticals had announced it was discontinuing sales of the IR formulation as of August 15, 2014, in order to "focus on" the XR formulation—just ahead of the IR patent expiration. However, the New York attorney general filed an antitrust lawsuit, claiming this was an anticompetitive move, and Forest was forced to continue offering both Namenda IR and Namenda XR.

MEMANTINE ER/DONEPEZIL (Namzaric) Fact Sheet

Bottom Line:
Namzaric combines donepezil and memantine in a single capsule. It is helpful for patients who are already on this combination regimen but who have trouble taking two pills.

FDA Indications:
Moderate to severe Alzheimer's dementia.

Off-Label Uses:
Mild to moderate Alzheimer's dementia; other memory disorders; mild cognitive impairment.

Dosage Forms:
Capsules: 7 mg/10 mg, 14 mg/10 mg, 21 mg/10 mg, 28 mg/10 mg memantine ER and donepezil.

Dosage Guidance:
- Patients should first be stabilized on the individual medications; patients on memantine (10 mg BID or 28 mg XR QD) and donepezil 10 mg QD can be switched to Namzaric 28 mg/10 mg QPM.
- Patients with severe renal impairment on memantine 5 mg BID or 14 mg XR QD and donepezil 10 mg QD can be switched to Namzaric 14 mg/10 mg QPM.

Monitoring: No routine monitoring recommended unless clinical picture warrants.

Cost: $$$$

Side Effects:
- Most common: Headache, diarrhea, dizziness, vomiting, weight loss, anorexia, insomnia, abnormal dreams.
- Serious but rare: Cholinesterase inhibitors may have vagotonic effects that may cause bradycardia and/or heart block with or without a history of cardiac disease; syncope reported.

Mechanism, Pharmacokinetics, and Drug Interactions:
- N-methyl-D-aspartate (NMDA) receptor antagonist and acetylcholinesterase (AChE) inhibitor.
- Metabolism: Memantine hepatic but not CYP450, and donepezil primarily through CYP2D6 and CYP3A4; t ½: 60–80 hours (memantine) and 70 hours (donepezil).
- Avoid use with anticholinergic agents as they will diminish therapeutic effects; avoid beta blockers due to risk of bradycardia. CYP450 interactions not usually clinically important.

Clinical Pearls:
- Many experts now stabilize patients on an AChE inhibitor like donepezil and then add memantine.
- The manufacturer recommends bedtime dosing, but taking it in the morning may prevent the insomnia and vivid dreams some patients report with donepezil.
- Once-a-day dosing makes this agent easiest to use.
- Be mindful of other medications that may have intrinsic anticholinergic activity; these will counteract donepezil's therapeutic effects.

Fun Fact:
In 2014, Actavis Pharmaceuticals acquired Forest Pharmaceuticals, manufacturer of Namzaric. That same year, Actavis also acquired Allergan, manufacturer of Botox, another medication targeting the aging process but in a different way.

RIVASTIGMINE (Exelon, Exelon Patch) Fact Sheet [G]

Bottom Line:

Rivastigmine is the only cholinesterase inhibitor available in patch form, which may be an advantage for patients who refuse or have difficulty swallowing medication. We generally consider rivastigmine a second-line agent due to the need for twice-daily dosing, its high cost, and its high rate of nausea and vomiting.

FDA Indications:

Mild to moderate Alzheimer's dementia (capsules); **mild to moderate and severe Alzheimer's dementia** (patch); **dementia associated with Parkinson's disease** (capsules and patch).

Off-Label Uses:

Other memory disorders; mild cognitive impairment.

Dosage Forms:

- **Capsules (G):** 1.5 mg, 3 mg, 4.5 mg, 6 mg.
- **Transdermal patches (G):** 4.6 mg/24 hour, 9.5 mg/24 hour, 13.3 mg/24 hour, containing rivastigmine 9 mg, 18 mg, and 27 mg, respectively.

Dosage Guidance:

- Start 1.5 mg BID with meals for four weeks, ↑ by 1.5 mg BID increments every four weeks, up to max 6 mg BID with meals.
- Patch: For mild to moderate dementia, start 4.6 mg/24 hours; if tolerated, ↑ after at least four weeks to 9.5 mg/24 hours (target and max dose). For severe dementia, titrate to 13.3 mg/24 hours (effective and max dose).
- Converting oral to patch: <6 mg/day: Use 4.6 mg/24 hour patch; 6–12 mg/day: Use 9.5 mg/24 hour patch; apply patch on next day following last oral dose.

Monitoring: No routine monitoring recommended unless clinical picture warrants.

Cost: Oral: $; patch: $$$

Side Effects:

- Most common: Dizziness, headache, diarrhea, anorexia, nausea, vomiting, skin reactions (patch).
- Serious but rare: Cholinesterase inhibitors may have vagotonic effects that may cause bradycardia and/or heart block with or without a history of cardiac disease; syncope reported.

Mechanism, Pharmacokinetics, and Drug Interactions:

- Acetylcholinesterase (AChE) and butyrylcholinesterase (BuChE) inhibitor.
- Metabolized extensively, although CYP enzymes minimally involved; t ½: 1.5 hours (oral); 3 hours (after patch removal).
- Avoid use with anticholinergic agents as they will diminish therapeutic effects; avoid beta blockers due to risk of bradycardia. P450 interactions not likely.

Clinical Pearls:

- Only cholinesterase inhibitor with additional indication for Parkinson's-related dementia.
- Rivastigmine inhibits both AChE and the nonspecific BuChE (also known as pseudocholinesterase), which is mostly found in the liver and GI tract; this may explain why rivastigmine causes significant GI side effects.
- Rivastigmine transdermal patches may cause less nausea and vomiting.

Fun Fact:

Exelon is also the name of a corporation that provides energy services (electric and natural gas) and is the largest nuclear operator in the United States.

Mood Stabilizers and Anticonvulsants

GENERAL PRESCRIBING TIPS

In this chapter, we focus on the non-antipsychotic mood stabilizers—meaning lithium, valproic acid, lamotrigine, carbamazepine, and oxcarbazepine. The antipsychotics, most of which are effective for bipolar disorder, are covered in their own chapter. This chapter also includes anticonvulsants that may not be particularly useful in treating bipolar but may be used from time to time in psychiatric practice.

Here are some general observations:

- *Manic episodes.* Generally the most effective drugs for rapid control of acute mania are antipsychotics and mood stabilizers, often combined with benzodiazepines. While head-to-head studies are scant, clinical lore has it that olanzapine, quetiapine, and haloperidol are the most rapidly effective antipsychotics in highly agitated and psychotic patients. Unfortunately, all three medications are highly likely to cause side effects.

- *Bipolar depression.* The medications with FDA indications for the treatment of bipolar depression include the combination of fluoxetine and olanzapine (Symbyax), quetiapine (Seroquel), lurasidone (Latuda), and most recently cariprazine (Vraylar) and lumateperone (Caplyta). All five have their drawbacks, related to side effects (Symbyax and Seroquel) or cost (Latuda, Vraylar, and Caplyta). There's good evidence for lithium, lamotrigine, and aripiprazole for bipolar depression, and you can add bupropion to any mood stabilizer—bupropion being the antidepressant least likely to cause a manic switch.

- *Maintenance treatment of bipolar disorder.* Maintenance treatment should include a mood stabilizer with a proven record of reducing cycling and increasing the time period between acute episodes. Only a few meds have such a record. These include lithium (more effective at preventing mania than depression), lamotrigine (more effective at preventing depression than mania), and some second-generation antipsychotics (olanzapine, aripiprazole, quetiapine, and ziprasidone, all more effective at preventing mania than depression). In addition, valproic acid and carbamazepine are commonly used as maintenance treatment.

Class Warnings

Several mood stabilizers are also classified as anticonvulsants, and you should note that the FDA issued a black box warning regarding suicide for anticonvulsants as a class. The warning is based on pooled analysis of 199 trials involving various antiepileptics (regardless of indication) that showed an increased risk of suicidal thoughts/behavior (incidence rate: 0.43% of treated patients compared to 0.24% of patients receiving placebo). The risk was observed as early as one week after initiation and continued through duration of trials (most of which were ≤24 weeks). The risk was higher for patients with seizure disorders compared to those receiving anticonvulsants for other indications.

Another class warning for the anticonvulsants regards a potentially serious, sometimes fatal multi-organ hypersensitivity reaction syndrome (drug rash with eosinophilia and systemic symptoms, or DRESS), which has rarely been reported with some antiepileptic drugs. Symptoms may include fever, rash, and/or lymphadenopathy; monitor for signs and symptoms of possible disparate manifestations associated with lymphatic, hepatic, renal, and/or hematologic organ systems. Early symptoms of hypersensitivity reaction (eg, lymphadenopathy, fever) may occur without rash. If this occurs, discontinuation and conversion to alternate therapy may be required.

Switching or Discontinuing Mood Stabilizers

Patients with bipolar disorder are at relatively high risk for relapsing to either manic or depressive episodes. For this reason, switching or discontinuing mood stabilizers requires special caution. For instance, patients who discontinue maintenance lithium have a 60%–90% risk of recurrence of a mood episode within a year. And this risk is greater the more abruptly the lithium is stopped: Discontinuing lithium over two to four weeks is significantly less likely to lead to relapse than discontinuing in two weeks or less (Baldessarini RJ et al, *Am J Psychiatry* 1997;154(4):551).

While we don't have as much data on how to discontinue mood stabilizers other than lithium, it's reasonable to assume that relapse risks are higher with more rapid tapering. When switching among lithium, valproate, carbamazepine, or lamotrigine, you should cross-taper as gradually as is feasible—typically over at least a two-week period.

Here's an example of how you might take two weeks to gradually transition a patient from lithium 1500 mg daily to a therapeutic dose of valproate:

- Days one to three: Continue lithium at 1500 mg daily as you start valproate at 250–500 mg QHS.

- Days four to six: Decrease lithium to 1200 mg daily. Increase valproate to 750–1000 mg QHS.

- Days seven to nine: Decrease lithium to 900 mg daily. Increase valproate to 1000–1250 mg daily QHS or in divided doses.

- Days 10–12: Decrease lithium to 600 mg daily. Increase valproate or hold depending on side effects/blood level.

- Days 13–15: Decrease lithium to 300 mg daily. Maintain valproate dose.

- Day 16: Discontinue lithium. Maintain valproate dose.

This guideline is applicable to most switches, with the exception of switching from any mood stabilizer to lamotrigine, which requires a very slow dosing schedule to lower the risk of a serious rash. In switching to lamotrigine, you will typically maintain the first mood stabilizer at a nearly full therapeutic dose while titrating lamotrigine in small increments (see lamotrigine fact sheet for details) up to 100 mg daily, which requires about four weeks. You can then start tapering the first medication as you continue to increase lamotrigine. In the special case of switching from valproate to lamotrigine, you must slow down the titration even more.

Anticonvulsants

There's a great tradition in psychiatry of adopting antiepileptic drugs for use in psychiatric syndromes. In some cases, as above, this strategy has yielded effective treatments. But for gabapentin, pregabalin, and topiramate, the payoff has been fairly scant. All three were initially touted as having efficacy in bipolar disorder, based on uncontrolled trials. However, subsequent data from randomized controlled trials did not support this indication.

Nonetheless, these drugs have found their places in other spheres, especially disorders related to anxiety or substance use. For example, pregabalin is approved for generalized anxiety disorder in parts of Europe. It also has pretty convincing data for effectiveness in helping patients discontinue benzodiazepines. Topiramate seems to have a niche for patients with alcohol dependence and for any patient who wants to lose weight. Gabapentin is a non-addictive alternative to benzodiazepines for anxiety and alcohol dependence.

Side Effects

The newer anticonvulsants are appealing because they are generally less toxic than the older agents, do not require serum level monitoring, and in most cases have a lower risk of drug interactions. However, the antiepileptics have a class warning for increased risk of suicidal thoughts and behavior; this warning stems from pooled analysis of trials (for seizure disorders as well as other indications) that showed a nearly doubled incidence of suicidal thought and behavior (0.43% for anticonvulsants vs 0.24% for placebo).

You'll note that the DEA has deemed pregabalin a controlled substance (Schedule V). Some states are reclassifying gabapentin as a controlled substance or mandating reporting to prescription drug monitoring programs (PDMPs). Reports of diversion and misuse of both pregabalin and gabapentin have been accumulating. Recreational use seems to be higher among individuals with opioid use disorder, and this may be related to the potentiation of euphoria described when the two are used together. Similar to combining benzos with opioids, the combination of gabapentinoids and opioids also increases the risk of opioid-related death. When using these in patients, be sure to monitor for misuse or diversion.

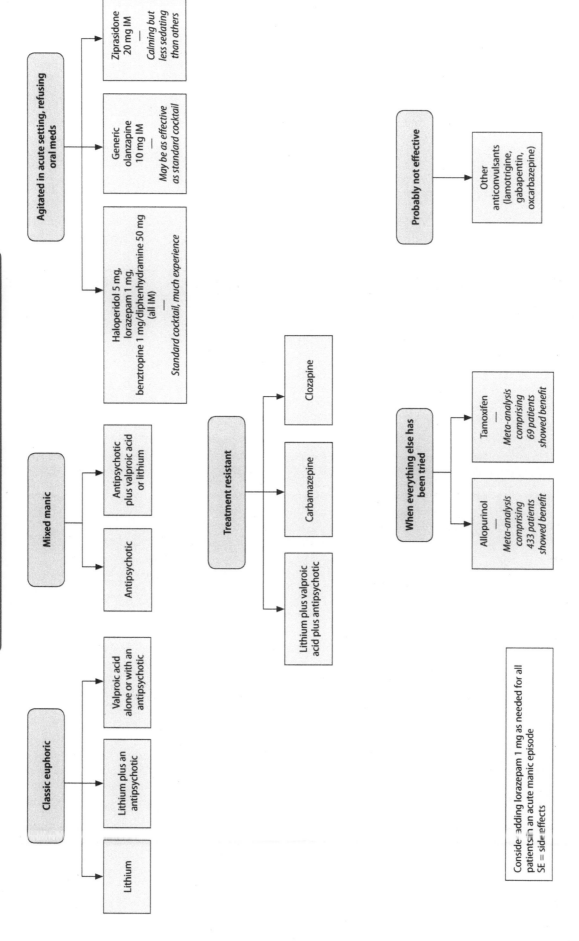

Bipolar Mania Treatment Algorithm

Classic euphoric
- Lithium
- Lithium plus an antipsychotic
- Valproic acid alone or with an antipsychotic

Mixed manic
- Antipsychotic
- Antipsychotic plus valproic acid or lithium

Agitated in acute setting, refusing oral meds
- Haloperidol 5 mg, lorazepam 1 mg, benztropine 1 mg/diphenhydramine 50 mg (all IM)
  —
  Standard cocktail, much experience
- Generic olanzapine 10 mg IM
  —
  May be as effective as standard cocktail
- Ziprasidone 20 mg IM
  —
  Calming but less sedating than others

Treatment resistant
- Lithium plus valproic acid plus antipsychotic
- Carbamazepine
- Clozapine

When everything else has been tried
- Allopurinol
  —
  Meta-analysis comprising 433 patients showed benefit
- Tamoxifen
  —
  Meta-analysis comprising 69 patients showed benefit

Probably not effective
- Other anticonvulsants (lamotrigine, gabapentin, oxcarbazepine)

Consider adding lorazepam 1 mg as needed for all patients in an acute manic episode
SE = side effects

Table 15: **Mood Stabilizers**

Generic Name (Brand Name) Year FDA Approved for Bipolar Disorder or Mania [G] denotes generic availability	Relevant FDA Indication(s)	Available Strengths (mg)	Usual Dosage Range (starting–max) (mg)
Carbamazepine [G] (Carbatrol, Epitol, Equetro, Tegretol, Tegretol XR, Teril) 2004	Bipolar disorder (Equetro: Acute mania)	CH: 100, 200 IR: 100, 200, 300, 400 ER: 100, 200, 300, 400 Oral solution: 100 mg/5 mL	200–800 BID
Lamotrigine [G] (Lamictal, Lamictal CD, Lamictal ODT, Lamictal XR, Subvenite) 2003	Bipolar disorder (maintenance)	IR: 25, 50, 100, 150, 200 CH: 2, 5, 25 ODT: 25, 50, 100, 200 ER: 25, 50, 100, 200, 250, 300	25 QD–100 BID 25 QD–50 BID if on VPA
Lithium [G] (Eskalith, Lithobid) 1970	Acute mania Bipolar maintenance	IR: 150, 300, 600 ER: 300, 450 Oral solution: 300 mg/5 mL	300–600 QHS–1200 BID
Oxcarbazepine [G] (Oxtellar XR, Trileptal) 2000	Not approved for any bipolar indication	IR: 150, 300, 600 ER: 150, 300, 600 Oral suspension: 300 mg/5 mL	300–1200 BID
Valproic acid [G] (Depakene, Depakote, Depakote ER, Depakote Sprinkles) 1995	Bipolar disorder (acute mania)	IR: 250 Liquid: 250 mg/5 mL DR: 125, 250, 500 ER: 250, 500	250–500 QHS–2000 BID

CH = chewable, IR = immediate release, ER = extended release, ODT = orally disintegrating tablet, DR = delayed release

Table 16: **Anticonvulsants**

Generic Name (Brand Name) Year FDA Approved [G] denotes generic availability	Off-Label Psychiatric Uses	Available Strengths (mg)	Usual Dosage Range (starting–max) (mg)
Gabapentin [G] (Gralise, Horizant, Neurontin) 1993	Anxiety disorders Withdrawal from alcohol or benzodiazepines Alcohol dependence	Capsule: 100, 300, 400 Tablet: 600, 800 Oral solution: 50 mg/mL ER tablet: 300, 600	100 QHS–300 TID
Pregabalin [G] (Lyrica, Lyrica CR) 2004	Generalized anxiety disorder Withdrawal from alcohol or benzodiazepines Alcohol dependence	Capsule: 25, 50, 75, 100, 150, 200, 225, 300 Oral solution: 20 mg/mL ER tablet: 82.5, 165, 330	75–300 BID
Topiramate [G] (Eprontia, Qudexy XR, Topamax, Trokendi XR) 1996	Alcohol dependence Bipolar disorder PTSD Binge-eating disorder Obesity	Tablet: 25, 50, 100, 200 Capsule: 15, 25 ER capsule: 25, 50, 100, 150, 200 Oral solution: 25 mg/mL	25–150 BID

CARBAMAZEPINE (Epitol, Equetro, Tegretol, others) Fact Sheet [G]

Bottom Line:
Equetro is the only FDA-approved formulation of carbamazepine for bipolar disorder, but use of other formulations would result in the same effects at a lower price. Generally, carbamazepine is not considered a first-line treatment for bipolar disorder due to its side effect profile and high likelihood of significant drug interactions.

FDA Indications:
Bipolar disorder (Equetro: acute mania); seizures; trigeminal neuralgia.

Off-Label Uses:
Bipolar maintenance; impulse control disorders; violence and aggression.

Dosage Forms:
- **Chewable tablets (G):** 100 mg, 200 mg (scored).
- **Tablets (Tegretol, Epitol, [G]):** 100 mg, 200 mg, 300 mg, 400 mg (scored).
- **ER tablets (Tegretol XR, [G]):** 100 mg, 200 mg, 400 mg.
- **ER capsules (Equetro, Carbatrol, [G]):** 100 mg, 200 mg, 300 mg.
- **Oral solution (Tegretol, Teril, [G]):** 100 mg/5 mL.

Dosage Guidance:
- Bipolar disorder: Start at 200 mg BID and gradually ↑ by 200 mg/day every three to four days, to target 400–600 mg BID (guided by clinical response). Max 800 mg BID. Dosing is the same for IR and ER versions of carbamazepine; both are BID.
- Extended-release formulations of carbamazepine are better tolerated than immediate release.

Monitoring: Carbamazepine level, complete blood count, sodium, LFT, pregnancy test, HLA-B*1502 in Asians.

Cost: $

Side Effects:
- Most common: Dizziness, somnolence, nausea, headache.
- Serious but rare: Hematologic abnormalities including agranulocytosis, aplastic anemia, neutropenia, leukopenia, thrombocytopenia, and pancytopenia reported; hepatic complications including slight increases in hepatic enzymes, cholestatic and hepatocellular jaundice, hepatitis and (rarely) hepatic failure, hyponatremia, SIADH; rash (5%–10%), including exfoliation, reported. Severe reactions including toxic epidermal necrolysis and Stevens-Johnson syndrome are rare, but can be fatal.

Mechanism, Pharmacokinetics, and Drug Interactions:
- Sodium channel blocker.
- Metabolized primarily through CYP3A4; t ½: 15 hours (initially 25–65 hours, but induces its own metabolism within two to four weeks and then stabilizes).
- High potential for significant interactions: Potent inducer of CYP1A2, CYP2B6, CYP2C19, CYP2C8, CYP2C9, CYP3A4, P-glycoprotein; use caution with medications significantly metabolized through these pathways as their levels may become subtherapeutic; caution in patients taking strong CYP3A4 inducers or inhibitors that can affect carbamazepine levels.
- Avoid concomitant use with oral contraceptives (can lower serum levels of these contraceptives and cause unplanned pregnancies) and with clozapine (additive risk of agranulocytosis).

Clinical Pearls:
- ER capsules such as Carbatrol have been shown to cause less fluctuation in serum CBZ level and fewer side effects, so start with this formulation when possible (some insurance companies might require pre-authorization).
- Therapeutic levels: 4–12 mcg/mL in seizure disorders. Studies in bipolar haven't shown correlation between levels and clinical response, so it's best dosed clinically.
- Lab monitoring: Baseline and periodic (at six weeks and every three months) CBC and LFTs.
- Patients of Asian descent should be screened for the variant HLA-B*1502 allele prior to starting carbamazepine; this variant is associated with significantly increased risk of developing Stevens-Johnson syndrome and/or toxic epidermal necrolysis. Avoid use in such patients.

Fun Fact:
Carbamazepine may cause a false-positive serum TCA screen—indeed, its chemical structure contains the familiar tricyclic nucleus common to all TCAs.

GABAPENTIN (Gralise, Horizant, Neurontin) Fact Sheet [G]

Bottom Line:
Gabapentin used to be considered a non-addictive medication for anxiety and for alcohol dependence, but we now know it may be misused and diverted for its euphoriant effect. If monitored closely, it can still be helpful for anxiety and insomnia, especially if your patient also suffers from one of the approved indications—such as neuropathic pain and restless legs syndrome.

FDA Indications:
Partial seizures (Neurontin); post-herpetic neuralgia (Gralise, Neurontin); restless legs syndrome (Horizant).

Off-Label Uses:
Anxiety disorders; withdrawal from alcohol or benzodiazepines; alcohol dependence.

Dosage Forms:
- **Capsules (G):** 100 mg, 300 mg, 400 mg.
- **Tablets (G):** 600 mg, 800 mg.
- **Oral solution (G):** 50 mg/mL.
- **Tablets, ER (Gralise):** 300 mg, 600 mg.
- **Tablets, ER (Horizant):** 300 mg, 600 mg (gabapentin enacarbil, a prodrug with better bioavailability).

Dosage Guidance:
- Anxiety (off-label): Start 100 mg QHS and ↑ by 100 mg/day increments every few days as tolerated to 300 mg TID. Max 3600 mg/day (highest doses often used for pain indications). Use lower doses in patients with renal impairment.
- Restless legs syndrome: Use gabapentin enacarbil (Horizant) 600 mg QD at 5 p.m.

Monitoring: No routine monitoring recommended unless clinical picture warrants.

Cost: IR: $; ER: $$$$$

Side Effects:
- Most common: Dizziness, somnolence, ataxia, weight gain.
- Serious but rare: Potentially serious, sometimes fatal multiorgan hypersensitivity (also known as drug reaction with eosinophilia and systemic symptoms, or DRESS); respiratory depression.

Mechanism, Pharmacokinetics, and Drug Interactions:
- Blocks voltage-dependent calcium channels and modulates excitatory neurotransmitter release.
- Not metabolized; excreted unchanged by kidneys; t ½: 5–7 hours.
- Few significant drug interactions, although you may see additive sedative effects with other sedating drugs. Analgesic control may be affected when gabapentin is added to opiates, including decreased levels of hydrocodone (Vicodin) or increased levels of morphine.

Clinical Pearls:
- Gabapentin is structurally related to GABA. However, it does not bind to GABA-A or GABA-B receptors, and it does not appear to influence synthesis or uptake of GABA.
- Controlled trials have shown no effect as monotherapy or adjunctive therapy for bipolar disorder.
- Data with acute alcohol or benzodiazepine withdrawal (both inpatient and outpatient) are limited but promising.
- There have been reports of recreational use of gabapentin in correctional facilities, some of which have restricted its use.
- Recreational use and abuse in the general population is also increasing and seems to occur more often with pregabalin than gabapentin, often at supratherapeutic dosing for the euphoric effects. Those with opioid use disorders have much higher gabapentin and pregabalin abuse rates.
- FDA added a warning regarding potential for respiratory depression particularly in combination with other CNS depressants (especially opioids) or in patients at risk (eg, elderly, those with COPD).

Fun Fact:
Gabapentin recently was reclassified as a controlled substance in Kentucky (Schedule V). Prescribers must have a DEA license, and prescriptions will be logged in the state's PDMP database. More states and the federal government likely will follow.

LAMOTRIGINE (Lamictal, Lamictal XR, Subvenite) Fact Sheet [G]

Bottom Line:
Lamotrigine is a good choice for maintenance treatment of bipolar disorder, especially to prevent depressive episodes. It has a good side effect profile. Its main disadvantage is the very slow titration schedule recommended to decrease the risk of Stevens-Johnson syndrome—as well as its ineffectiveness in the treatment of manic episodes.

FDA Indications:
Bipolar disorder (maintenance) in adults; seizures in adults and children.

Off-Label Uses:
Bipolar depression; neuropathic pain; major depression.

Dosage Forms:
- **Tablets (Lamictal, Subvenite, [G]):** 25 mg, 50 mg, 100 mg, 150 mg, 200 mg (scored).
- **Chewable tablets (Lamictal CD, [G]):** 2 mg, 5 mg, 25 mg.
- **Orally disintegrating tablets (Lamictal ODT, [G]):** 25 mg, 50 mg, 100 mg, 200 mg.
- **ER tablets (Lamictal XR, [G]):** 25 mg, 50 mg, 100 mg, 200 mg, 250 mg, 300 mg.

Dosage Guidance:
- Bipolar disorder: Start 25 mg QD for two weeks, ↑ to 50 mg QD for two weeks, then 100 mg QD; max 200 mg/day; can increase up to 400 mg/day if needed.
- Patients on valproic acid: Start 25 mg QOD (every other day) for two weeks, ↑ to 25 mg QD for two weeks, then 50 mg QD; max 100 mg/day (VPA doubles lamotrigine levels).
- Dosing is the same with all versions of lamotrigine. However, patients taking more than 200 mg should either split the dose or take the Lamictal XR formulation.
- Dose timing: Can be taken either in the morning or night; it rarely causes drowsiness.

Monitoring: No routine monitoring recommended unless clinical picture warrants.

Cost: IR: $; ER: $$

Side Effects:
- Most common: Dizziness, headache, nausea, sedation, benign rash (7%).
- Serious but rare: Skin reactions (black box warning): Severe, potentially life-threatening skin rashes requiring hospitalization reported; incidence is higher in pediatric patients; risk increased by co-administration with valproic acid, higher than recommended starting doses, and exceeding recommended dose titration. The majority of cases occur in the first eight weeks, but isolated cases may occur beyond eight weeks or even in patients without risk factors. Discontinue at first sign of rash and do not reinitiate unless rash is clearly not drug-related; rare cases of Stevens-Johnson syndrome, toxic epidermal necrolysis, and angioedema reported. Cardiac arrhythmias (slowed ventricular conduction and widening of the QRS) in susceptible patients.

Mechanism, Pharmacokinetics, and Drug Interactions:
- Sodium channel blocker.
- Metabolism primarily hepatic (non-P450); t ½: 25–33 hours (with VPA 48–70 hours; with carbamazepine 13–14 hours).
- Caution with enzyme-inducing medications (eg, carbamazepine), which may decrease lamotrigine levels. Caution with hormonal contraceptives, which may decrease lamotrigine levels; lamotrigine maintenance dose may need to be increased (two-fold). Gradual increases of lamotrigine levels may occur during the inactive "pill-free" week. Lamotrigine may decrease levels of some hormonal contraceptives (greater effect with estrogens than progestins); alternative birth control methods should be considered. Valproic acid may double lamotrigine levels, necessitating dosage adjustments (as above).

Clinical Pearls:
- Lamotrigine is useful for the maintenance treatment of bipolar disorder, with best efficacy in the prophylaxis of depressive episodes. Not useful in acute episodes.
- If lamotrigine has been stopped/missed for more than five half-lives (see above), consider restarting according to initial dosing recommendations to minimize rash risk.
- Routine baseline ECG is not necessary, but similar to use of other mood stabilizers that can affect heart rhythm (lithium, carbamazepine, oxcarbazepine), monitor or get consultation in patients with cardiac conduction delay or significant ischemic or structural heart disease.

Fun Fact:
The first FDA-approved drug for bipolar disorder (not just acute mania) since lithium, a drug approved more than 30 years earlier (2003 for lamotrigine; 1970 for lithium).

LITHIUM (Eskalith, Lithobid) Fact Sheet [G]

Bottom Line:

Lithium is the gold standard for bipolar disorder. It is more useful for euphoric mania than for mixed and rapid-cycling types of bipolar disorder, but it is effective for depressive episodes and maintenance treatment of bipolar disorder. It is also known for its antisuicide effects in bipolar and unipolar mood disorders. It is likely underprescribed due to side effect concerns—though most patients tolerate lithium quite well.

FDA Indications:

Acute mania; bipolar disorder (maintenance) in children and adults.

Off-Label Uses:

Bipolar depression; treatment-resistant depression; neutropenia; vascular headache.

Dosage Forms:

- **Capsules (lithium carbonate, [G]):** 150 mg, 300 mg, 600 mg.
- **Tablets (lithium carbonate, [G]):** 300 mg.
- **ER tablets (Lithobid, [G]):** 300 mg.
- **ER tablets (Eskalith CR, [G]):** 450 mg (scored).
- **Oral solution (lithium citrate, [G]):** 300 mg/5 mL.

Dosage Guidance:

- Start 300–600 mg QHS; gradually ↑ by 300–600 mg/day every two to three days to target serum lithium level of 0.8 mEq/L (usually 900–1200 mg/day). Can be dosed BID–TID or all QHS. Max 2400 mg/day.
- Extended-release formulations of lithium are better tolerated than immediate release.

Monitoring: Lithium level, TSH, BUN/creatinine, pregnancy test, ECG if cardiac disease.

Cost: $

Side Effects:

- Most common: Nausea/diarrhea (take with meals, split dosing, switch to ER), fine tremor (lower dose or use propranolol), polyuria/excessive thirst (dose all at bedtime), memory problems, weight gain, hypothyroidism (7%–8%; nine times more common in women), acne or worsening psoriasis, benign increase in WBC.
- Serious but rare: Chronic use may result in diminished renal concentrating ability (nephrogenic diabetes insipidus); usually reverses when discontinued, or treat with hydrochlorothiazide 25–50 mg/day or amiloride 5–10 mg twice daily. Cardiac: Bradycardia, cardiac arrhythmia, flattened or inverted T waves, sinus node dysfunction may occur rarely.

Mechanism, Pharmacokinetics, and Drug Interactions:

- Alters neuronal sodium transport.
- Eliminated by kidneys; t ½: 18–24 hours.
- Drugs that ↑ lithium levels: "**No ACE** in the **H**ole" (**N**SAIDs, **ACE** inhibitors, and **H**CTZ); excess sweating can ↑ levels; low-sodium diet may ↑ lithium levels. Caffeine may ↓ levels.

Clinical Pearls:

- Check lithium level, TSH/T4, BUN/Cr, electrolytes after one week of treatment, at one to two months, then every six to 12 months. Target levels for acute mania: 0.8–1.2 mEq/L; maintenance: 0.6–1.0 mEq/L; toxicity >1.5 mEq/L but may see signs at lower levels, especially in elderly.
- An increase or decrease of 300 mg/day will change serum level by roughly 0.25±0.1 mEq/L.
- Dehydration: Use with caution in patients with significant fluid loss (protracted sweating, diarrhea, or prolonged fever); temporary reduction or discontinuation may be necessary.
- Some evidence suggests that patients with bipolar disorder who are treated with lithium have better concentration and memory over the long term. Lithium has also been associated with reduced rate of dementia. In some patients, though, it can cause cognitive side effects like mental slowing.

Fun Fact:

The soft drink 7-Up was originally called "Bib-Label Lithiated Lemon-Lime Soda" and contained lithium until 1950.

OXCARBAZEPINE (Oxtellar XR, Trileptal) Fact Sheet [G]

Bottom Line:
Oxcarbazepine, an analog of carbamazepine, is popular because of its reputation as a kinder, gentler carbamazepine, which it's gained due to its more favorable side effect and drug interaction profile. However, due to the paucity of efficacy data in bipolar disorder, it is reserved for second-line use after lithium and valproic acid, and even after carbamazepine.

FDA Indications:
Seizure disorders in adults and children.

Off-Label Uses:
Bipolar disorder.

Dosage Forms:
- **Tablets (G):** 150 mg, 300 mg, 600 mg (scored).
- **Oral suspension (G):** 300 mg/5 mL.
- **ER tablets (Oxtellar XR):** 150 mg, 300 mg, 600 mg.

Dosage Guidance:
- Bipolar disorder (off-label): Start 300 mg BID; ↑ by 300 mg/day every three days or 600 mg/day weekly to target dose 600–1200 mg BID. Max 2400 mg/day. No data on use of XR for bipolar disorder; caution as higher doses of XR likely needed when converting from IR to XR (not interchangeable on dose-for-dose basis).
- Dose timing: It can cause sedation; the entire dose can be taken at bedtime if needed.

Monitoring: Sodium, HLA-B*1502 in Asians.

Cost: IR: $; ER: $$$$

Side Effects:
- Most common: Dizziness, somnolence, headache, ataxia, nausea, vomiting.
- Serious but rare: Potentially serious, sometimes fatal, dermatologic reactions (eg, Stevens-Johnson, toxic epidermal necrolysis) reported; monitor for skin reactions. Rare cases of anaphylaxis and angioedema reported, even after initial dosing; permanently discontinue should symptoms occur.
- Use caution in patients with previous hypersensitivity to carbamazepine (cross-sensitivity occurs in 25%–30%). Clinically significant hyponatremia (serum sodium <125 mmol/L) may develop (1%–3%; higher rate than with carbamazepine); monitor serum sodium, particularly during first three months of therapy, especially in patients at risk for hyponatremia.

Mechanism, Pharmacokinetics, and Drug Interactions:
- Sodium channel blocker and neuronal membrane stabilizer.
- Metabolized primarily through CYP450; potent inducer of CYP3A4 and inhibitor of CYP2C19; t ½: 2 hours (9 hours for active metabolite).
- No auto-induction of metabolism and fewer interactions than with carbamazepine. However, there is still potential for interactions. Avoid concomitant use with medications metabolized by CYP3A4 since oxcarbazepine may reduce their levels. Oxcarbazepine may reduce efficacy of oral contraceptives; nonhormonal measures recommended.

Clinical Pearls:
- Oxcarbazepine is the 10-keto analog of carbamazepine (its "chemical cousin").
- Not bioequivalent to carbamazepine. Increase total daily dose by 20%–30% if switching from carbamazepine to oxcarbazepine.
- Patients of Asian descent should be screened for the variant HLA-B*1502 allele prior to starting oxcarbazepine; this variant may increase risk of developing Stevens-Johnson syndrome and/or toxic epidermal necrolysis. Avoid use in such patients.
- Oxcarbazepine failed to work in patients with bipolar disorder in two small and flawed placebo-controlled studies. Some limited data suggest it may fare better when used as augmentation with other mood stabilizers.

Fun Fact:
While first synthesized in 1965, oxcarbazepine first appeared on the US market in 2000. In 2010, Novartis pleaded guilty to marketing oxcarbazepine for non-FDA-approved uses, including neuropathic pain and bipolar disorder, in 2000 and 2001.

PREGABALIN (Lyrica, Lyrica CR) Fact Sheet [G]

Bottom Line:

Pregabalin is structurally related to gabapentin and is likely more effective for psychiatric disorders, especially generalized anxiety disorder and social anxiety disorder. It can also be helpful for patients struggling to discontinue benzodiazepines. Now that the generic is available, it's no longer more expensive than gabapentin and preferable in most cases.

FDA Indications:

Diabetic peripheral neuropathy; spinal cord injury–associated neuropathic pain; post-herpetic neuralgia; partial seizures; fibromyalgia.

Off-Label Uses:

Generalized anxiety disorder; withdrawal from alcohol or benzodiazepines; alcohol dependence.

Dosage Forms:

- **Capsules (G):** 25 mg, 50 mg, 75 mg, 100 mg, 150 mg, 200 mg, 225 mg, 300 mg.
- **Oral solution:** 20 mg/mL.
- **ER tablets (G):** 82.5 mg, 165 mg, 330 mg.

Dosage Guidance:

- Start 75 mg BID and ↑ by 75–150 mg/day every week as tolerated to max 300 mg BID (based on trials for generalized anxiety disorder, an off-label use). Use lower doses in renal impairment.
- Dose timing: Although the package insert recommends BID dosing, it can cause sedation, so consider starting it at bedtime.

Monitoring: No routine monitoring recommended unless clinical picture warrants.

Cost: IR: $; liquid, ER: $$$

Side Effects:

- Most common: Peripheral edema, dizziness, somnolence, ataxia, weight gain.
- Serious but rare: Hypersensitivity reactions, including skin redness, blistering, hives, rash, dyspnea, and wheezing. Angioedema, possibly life threatening, reported; use with caution in patients with a history of angioedema or patients on ACE inhibitors. Increases in CPK and rare cases of rhabdomyolysis reported.

Mechanism, Pharmacokinetics, and Drug Interactions:

- Binds alpha-2 delta subunit of calcium channels and reduces neurotransmitter release.
- Negligible metabolism; mostly excreted unchanged by kidneys; t ½: 6 hours.
- No significant drug interactions, although you may see additive sedative effects with other sedating drugs.

Clinical Pearls:

- Schedule V controlled substance (same category as cough suppressants containing codeine). Following abrupt withdrawal, patients may experience insomnia, nausea, headache, or diarrhea; this may be suggestive of physical dependence.
- Recreational use and abuse seems to occur more often with pregabalin than gabapentin, often at supratherapeutic dosing for the euphoric effects. Those with opioid use disorders have much higher gabapentin and pregabalin abuse rates.
- Pregabalin is related in structure to gabapentin, which is (so far, according to the DEA) not a controlled substance but is more potent, with faster absorption and greater bioavailability.
- For generalized anxiety disorder, pregabalin appears more effective than placebo, but data comparing it to benzodiazepines are inconsistent.
- FDA added a warning regarding potential for respiratory depression particularly in combination with other CNS depressants (especially opioids) or in patients at risk (eg, elderly, those with COPD).

Fun Fact:

Other drugs related to gabapentin and pregabalin are being studied; Pfizer was developing atagabalin for use in insomnia, but it discontinued development due to disappointing trial results.

TOPIRAMATE (Eprontia, Qudexy XR, Topamax, Trokendi XR) Fact Sheet [G]

Bottom Line:

Topiramate is a reasonable off-label choice for alcohol use disorder and antipsychotic-induced weight gain. Otherwise, relegate it to the "try when out of other ideas" category.

FDA Indications:

Seizure disorders for patients ≥2 years; migraine prophylaxis.

Off-Label Uses:

Alcohol dependence; bipolar disorder; PTSD; binge-eating disorder; obesity.

Dosage Forms:

- **Tablets (G):** 25 mg, 50 mg, 100 mg, 200 mg.
- **Capsules (G):** 15 mg, 25 mg.
- **Capsules, ER (Trokendi XR, Qudexy XR, [G]):** 25 mg, 50 mg, 100 mg, 150 mg, 200 mg.
- **Oral solution (Eprontia):** 25 mg/mL.

Dosage Guidance:

Seizures/migraine: Start 25–50 mg QHS and ↑ by 50 mg/day in weekly increments. Doses used in psychiatry have typically been 50–300 mg/day, divided BID (ER can be given QHS).

Monitoring: Baseline and periodic serum bicarbonate.

Cost: IR: $; ER: $$$

Side Effects:

- Most common: Somnolence, dizziness, nervousness, ataxia, speech problems, memory difficulties, confusion, anorexia.
- Serious but rare: Decreases in serum bicarbonate (metabolic acidosis) relatively common but usually mild to moderate; more severe cases, including marked reductions to <17 mEq/L, may occur more rarely. Watch for kidney stones, osteomalacia.

Mechanism, Pharmacokinetics, and Drug Interactions:

- Sodium channel blocker.
- Not metabolized, excreted primarily unchanged; t ½: 21 hours (56 hours for XR); mild CYP3A4 inducer.
- Avoid concomitant use with hydrochlorothiazide, which can increase risk for hypokalemia; monitor potassium. Avoid in patients with metabolic acidosis taking concomitant metformin. Additive effects with sedatives or alcohol. Concurrent use with valproic acid may increase risk of hyperammonemia and associated encephalopathy. Higher doses (>200 mg/day) may decrease levels of some drugs, including contraceptives (P450 induction).

Clinical Pearls:

- Many published articles have shown some efficacy in a wide range of disorders, including bipolar disorder, PTSD, alcohol dependence, binge-eating disorder, and obesity.
- Most compelling data are for preventing relapse in alcoholism.
- Some patients may lose weight, but this is not common; greatest decrease in weight seems to occur in heaviest patients (>100 kg). When weight loss occurs, it is often not a large effect (mean of 6 kg) nor is it a sustained effect (patients return to pretreatment weight after 12–18 months).
- A combination of extended-release topiramate and phentermine was FDA approved in 2012 for the long-term treatment of obesity as Qsymia (Vivus Pharmaceuticals).

Fun Fact:

Dose-related cognitive effects of topiramate have led some to refer to Topamax as "Dopamax."

VALPROIC ACID (Depakene, Depakote, others) Fact Sheet [G]

Bottom Line:

Valproic acid is the go-to antimanic agent for acute manic episodes, featuring faster onset of response and better adverse effect profile compared to lithium, fewer drug interactions than carbamazepine, and efficacy for rapid cycling and relapse prevention.

FDA Indications:

Bipolar disorder (acute mania); migraine prophylaxis; seizures.

Off-Label Uses:

Bipolar maintenance; impulse control disorders; violence and aggression.

Dosage Forms:

- **Capsules (valproic acid, [G]):** 250 mg.
- **Oral liquid (Depakene, [G]):** 250 mg/5 mL.
- **Delayed-release tablets (Depakote, [G]):** 125 mg, 250 mg, 500 mg.
- **Delayed-release capsules (Depakote Sprinkles, [G]):** 125 mg.
- **ER tablets (Depakote ER, [G]):** 250 mg, 500 mg.

Dosage Guidance:

- Acute mania: Start 250–500 mg QHS; ↑ rapidly to effective dose (serum level 50–125 mcg/mL, target 1000–1500 mg/day); max 4000 mg/day, or 60 mg/kg.
- Depakote ER is generally better tolerated in terms of side effects. When converting from regular Depakote to Depakote ER, be aware that patients will get about 20% less valproic acid with the ER formulation.

Monitoring: Valproic acid level, LFTs, CBC for platelets, pregnancy test, ammonia if confusion.

Cost: $

Side Effects:

- Most common: Somnolence, nausea, fatigue, dizziness, hair loss, tremor, thrombocytopenia (up to 24% of patients; dose-related; reversible).
- Serious but rare: Hepatotoxicity—rare idiosyncratic reaction, not dose related; most cases occur within three months; risk factors: age <2 years, multiple anticonvulsants, and presence of neurologic disease in addition to epilepsy. Asymptomatic elevations of liver enzymes may occur, not necessarily associated with hepatic dysfunction. Pancreatitis (rare but potentially fatal). Polycystic ovary syndrome (PCOS) in about 10% of women. Hyperammonemia, encephalopathy (sometimes fatal) reported and may present with normal liver enzymes.

Mechanism, Pharmacokinetics, and Drug Interactions:

- Sodium channel blocker.
- Metabolized primarily by liver with only minimal (10%) role of CYP450 enzymes (2A6, 2B6, 2C9); t ½: 9–16 hours.
- VPA causes ↑ levels of lamotrigine and risk for rash. Taking with topiramate can lead to encephalopathy.

Clinical Pearls:

- ER tablets have 10%–20% less fluctuation in serum concentration than delayed-release (DR) tablets. Divalproex sodium ER and DR tablets are *not* bioequivalent; increase total daily dose by 10%–20% if switching from DR to ER.
- ER formulation should be dosed QAM so that peak levels and sedation occur in the evening.
- Elevations of ammonia can often occur at normal doses and serum levels of VPA. Reducing dose when clinically appropriate typically reverses ammonia elevation. Treating with L-carnitine is also effective.
- Once steady state levels reached (within two to four days of initiation or dose adjustment), trough serum levels should be drawn just before once daily ER dose in the morning (21–24 hours post administration) and 12-post dose with IR formulation. Target levels between 50–125 mcg/mL.
- Several major malformations, most notably neural tube defects, have been clearly associated with first-trimester exposure to valproic acid. Educate and exercise caution in women of childbearing age.

Fun Fact:

Valproic acid was first synthesized in 1882 by B.S. Burton as an analogue of valeric acid, found naturally in valerian.

Natural Treatments

GENERAL PRESCRIBING TIPS

If you're interested in natural treatments (also known as complementary and alternative medicine, or CAM), you will likely recommend various strategies other than the nine medications we cover in this chapter. These would include exercise (helpful for depression and for preventing cognitive impairment), light therapy (for seasonal affective disorder), massage, meditation, and other modalities.

We have included fact sheets on those natural products that have been shown to be effective via standard randomized controlled trials. Some natural products not included here might be effective but have not been adequately tested vs placebo (eg, adaptogens such as ashwagandha and rhodiola).

Because most of these products are not regulated by the FDA, there are quality control issues. The amount of active constituents can vary not only from brand to brand, but also from batch to batch, and some products may be adulterated with other herbs, chemicals, drugs, or toxins. We recommend that patients stick to well-known brands sold by trusted retailers.

For additional information, you may also find these resources helpful:

- NIH National Center for Complementary and Integrative Health: https://www.nccih.nih.gov/health/herbsataglance

- National Library of Medicine: www.medlineplus.gov/druginfo/herb_All.html

- Natural Medicines Comprehensive Database (requires subscription): http://naturaldatabase.therapeuticresearch.com

- ConsumerLab (requires subscription): www.consumerlab.com

Table 17: **Natural Treatments**

Name (Brand name, if applicable)	Commonly Available Strengths (mg)	Reported Uses in Psychiatry	Usual Dosage Range (starting–max) (mg)
Lavender essential oil (Silexan, CalmAid)	80	Generalized anxiety disorder	80–160 QHS
L-methylfolate (Deplin and others)	0.4, 0.8, 1, 3, 5, 7.5, 15	Depression (adjunct)	15 QD
L-tryptophan	500	Depression	500–2000 divided BID or TID
Melatonin	0.5, 1, 2.5, 3, 5, 10	Insomnia	1–20 QHS
N-acetylcysteine	500, 600, 750, 1000	OCD, trichotillomania, nail biting, skin picking	1200–2400 divided BID
Omega-3 fatty acids (fish oil)	500, 1000, 1200	Depression (unipolar, bipolar)	500–2000 QD or divided BID–TID
S-adenosyl-L-methionine (SAMe)	100, 200, 400	Depression	800 BID
St. John's wort	100, 300, 450	Depression	300 TID
Vitamin D	1000 IU, 2000 IU, 5000 IU, 10,000 IU (as D3)	Depression	1000–5000 IU QD

LAVENDER ESSENTIAL OIL (CalmAid, Silexan) Fact Sheet [G]

Bottom Line:

Lavender essential oil is a reasonable option in patients who have not responded to FDA-approved treatments for generalized anxiety disorder (GAD) or in patients who request a natural alternative.

FDA Indications:

None.

Off-Label Uses:

GAD.

Dosage Forms:

Softgels (CalmAid): 80 mg.

Dosage Guidance:

Start 80 mg QHS; ↑ to 160 mg QHS after one week if needed.

Monitoring: No routine monitoring recommended unless clinical picture warrants.

Cost: $

Side Effects:

- Most common: Lavender-flavored burping; well tolerated in most.
- Serious but rare: Weak estrogenic properties may contribute to rare cases of breast development in adolescents (avoid in those under 18).

Mechanism, Pharmacokinetics, and Drug Interactions:

- Several mechanisms proposed, but most relevant may be serotonin-1A agonism.
- Drug metabolism pathway unclear; t ½: 9 hours.
- Drug interactions: Limited information, though studies thus far show no inhibition or induction of P450 enzymes by Silexan.

Clinical Pearls:

- Silexan is a proprietary blend of linalool and linalyl acetate, along with over 100 compounds from the lavender plant.
- In a large randomized, double-blind controlled study, Silexan 80 mg and 160 mg both beat out paroxetine 20 mg/day and placebo on the Hamilton Anxiety Rating Scale with a large effect size of 0.87. Silexan also performed best on secondary outcome measures such as depression, sleep quality, and quality of life.
- One smaller study found Silexan 80 mg/day was comparable to lorazepam 0.5 mg/day in patients with GAD.
- Benefits are typically seen after two weeks and continue to build over three months.
- While Silexan is not sedating, patients report improved sleep quality, likely secondary to its anxiolytic effect.

Fun Fact:

Silexan is regulated as a prescription and licensed for anxiety in 14 countries. In the US, it is available over the counter as CalmAid, through Schwabe's "Nature's Way" line.

L-METHYLFOLATE (Deplin) Fact Sheet [G]

Bottom Line:
L-methylfolate is a metabolite of dietary folic acid, and is necessary for the synthesis of the main neurotransmitters relevant to psychiatric disorders. Though the data are not robust, folate supplementation *might* be effective for some patients with depression, but we recommend that patients try the cheap stuff (folic acid) before springing for Deplin (L-methylfolate).

FDA Indications:
None.

Off-Label Uses:
Adjunctive treatment for depression (considered a "medical food product" by the FDA, not an FDA-approved drug product, although available as prescription only).

Dosage Forms:
- **Capsules (Deplin):** 7.5 mg, 15 mg.
- **Tablets and capsules (various other L-methylfolate products, [G]):** 0.4 mg, 0.8 mg, 1 mg, 3 mg, 5 mg.

Dosage Guidance:
Depression (Deplin only): Start 7.5 mg QD; target and max dose 15 mg/day.

Monitoring: No routine monitoring recommended unless clinical picture warrants.

Cost: [G]: $$; Deplin: $$$

Side Effects:
- Most common: Not well known; likely well tolerated.
- Serious but rare: Folic acid supplementation may mask symptoms of vitamin B12 deficiency (administration of folic acid may reverse the hematological signs of B12 deficiency, including megaloblastic anemia, while not addressing neurological manifestations). L-methylfolate may be less likely than folic acid to mask B12 deficiency, though the possibility should be considered.

Mechanism, Pharmacokinetics, and Drug Interactions:
- May enhance synthesis of monoamine neurotransmitters.
- No typical drug metabolism pathway as it is naturally stored and used by body; t ½: 3 hours.
- Drug interactions generally unlikely, although L-methylfolate may decrease anticonvulsant levels (including carbamazepine and valproic acid). Drugs that lower folate, such as anticonvulsants (including carbamazepine, valproic acid, and lamotrigine), may necessitate higher doses of L-methylfolate.

Clinical Pearls:
- Dietary folic acid is normally transformed to L-methylfolate by the enzyme MTHFR, and L-methylfolate is necessary for the synthesis of monoamines (serotonin, norepinephrine, dopamine). The marketing pitch for prescribing Deplin is that in about 50% of the population, genetic variations impair the function of MTHFR, leading to low levels of methylfolate. A recent review of the data on one of these genetic polymorphisms (called C677T) found that overall, it did not put people at any higher risk of depression (in fact, schizophrenia was more common).
- A few small studies over the years have shown that both folate (over the counter) and L-methylfolate may be somewhat helpful as adjunctive agents in the treatment of depression, particularly in those with low baseline folate levels.

Fun Fact:
"Medical foods" are foods that are specially formulated and intended for the dietary management of a disease with distinctive nutritional needs that cannot be met by normal diet alone. These include total parenteral nutrition as well as nasogastric tube feeds and oral rehydration products. Depression has no accepted distinctive nutritional needs.

L-TRYPTOPHAN Fact Sheet [G]

Bottom Line:

L-tryptophan is an amino acid that is eventually converted to serotonin. The evidence base to support using L-tryptophan in depression is extremely limited, but more and more patients are turning to it, especially in combination "serotonin boost" products being marketed today. We recommend sticking to the serotonergic agents we know to be safe and effective: SSRIs and SNRIs.

FDA Indications:

None.

Off-Label Uses:

Depression; premenstrual dysphoric disorder (PMDD); smoking cessation.

Dosage Forms:

Capsules: 500 mg.

Dosage Guidance:

For depression, doses as low as 300 mg/day in combination with antidepressants have been used. For other uses, dose is typically 500–1000 mg BID or 500 mg TID. PMDD dosing studied is 6 g/day.

Monitoring: No routine monitoring recommended unless clinical picture warrants.

Cost: $$

Side Effects:

- Most common: Abdominal pain, nausea, vomiting, diarrhea, flatulence, headache.
- Serious but rare: Over 1,500 reports of eosinophilia-myalgia syndrome (EMS) and 37 deaths were reported in the US, leading to it being pulled from the market in 1990; nearly all cases were tied to contaminated batches out of Japan. Symptoms of EMS include eosinophilia, fatigue, myalgia, neuropathy, rash, and inflammation. There have been no reported recurrences of these reactions since that outbreak.

Mechanism, Pharmacokinetics, and Drug Interactions:

- Essential amino acid found in plant and animal proteins. Absorbed from dietary protein sources and converted to 5-hydroxytryptophan (5-HTP) and then to serotonin (5-hydroxytryptamine).
- Metabolized by non-P450 liver pathway; t ½: 3–4 hours.
- Combining with serotonergic antidepressants may increase risk of serotonin syndrome. Avoid use with MAOIs.

Clinical Pearls:

- Best efficacy in PMDD and smoking cessation. Evidence for use in depression is limited but suggestive.
- L-tryptophan has also been studied in ADHD, anxiety, depression, fibromyalgia, insomnia, and migraines, but there is insufficient evidence to support these uses.
- While both L-tryptophan and 5-HTP can cross the blood-brain barrier, L-tryptophan more readily does so.
- Combination formulations are sold as "serotonin boosters" and include amino acids (tryptophan, 5-HTP, SAMe), vitamins (B6, B9, B12, C, D), minerals (magnesium, zinc), and herbs (theanine, curcumin, garcinia, rhodiola). These formulations all have extremely limited evidence to support efficacy in depression.

Fun Fact:

Especially around Thanksgiving, many will talk about "turkey coma" as a result of ingesting too much tryptophan contained in turkey. Actually, the drowsiness is more likely due to all the carbs eaten with the turkey. Turkey has no more tryptophan than other meats.

MELATONIN Fact Sheet [G]

Bottom Line:

Melatonin is secreted by the pineal gland, and its rise in serum levels correlates with the time course of natural sleep. Short-term melatonin treatment appears to only modestly reduce the time it takes to fall asleep (about 12 minutes, which might not be considered clinically relevant) and does not appear to significantly improve overall sleep time. However, some patients report minor improvement in subjective feelings of sleep quality. It is cheaper than the melatonin agonist ramelteon (Rozerem); however, like ramelteon, it lacks good long-term safety data, especially with regard to effects on hormones.

FDA Indications:

None.

Off-Label Uses:

Insomnia; jet lag; shift-work sleep disorder.

Dosage Forms:

Supplied over the counter (OTC) in various forms including liquid, tablet, capsule, sublingual, and time-release formulations; usually in 0.5 mg, 1 mg, 2.5 mg, 3 mg, 5 mg, and 10 mg.

Dosage Guidance:

- Insomnia (adults): 0.5–20 mg in early evening. Emerging data suggest lower doses are effective; start low (0.5–1 mg) and gradually increase to desired effect ("normal" melatonin levels vary widely among individuals, and the same dose can induce different levels depending on age or health).
- Jet lag: 1–3 mg on day of departure at a time that corresponds to the anticipated bedtime at arrival destination, followed by 1–3 mg at bedtime for next three to five days.

Monitoring: No routine monitoring recommended unless clinical picture warrants.

Cost: $

Side Effects:

- Most common: Generally well tolerated in the short term. Drowsiness, headaches, and dizziness most common but at similar rates to placebo; next-day grogginess or irritability (higher doses); vivid dreams or nightmares (higher doses).
- Serious but rare: No serious side effects reported; however, long-term human studies have not been conducted. Theoretically, melatonin may alter other hormones (inhibiting ovulation in women and gonadal development in children and adolescents); avoid use in women who are pregnant or are attempting to become pregnant, and use caution in children.

Mechanism, Pharmacokinetics, and Drug Interactions:

- Melatonin receptor agonist.
- Metabolized primarily through CYP1A2, may inhibit CYP1A2; t ½: 35–50 minutes.
- Some suggest melatonin may reduce glucose tolerance and insulin sensitivity and may increase efficacy of calcium channel blockers for blood pressure.

Clinical Pearls:

- Melatonin is secreted from the pineal gland in a 24-hour circadian rhythm. It rises at sunset and peaks in the middle of the night, regulating the normal sleep/wake cycle.
- Melatonin should only be taken in its synthetic form; the "natural" form comes from ground-up cow pineal glands and may spread disease (eg, mad cow disease).
- Melatonin taken at bedtime doesn't seem to affect nocturnal sleep. Taken in the early evening, it appears to be similar to temazepam in hypnotic effect.
- Although melatonin products have been available OTC in the US since the mid-1990s, many countries require a prescription, and some do not permit its sale.

Fun Fact:

Foods containing melatonin include cherries, bananas, grapes, rice, cereals, herbs, olive oil, wine, and beer.

N-ACETYLCYSTEINE (NAC) Fact Sheet [G]

Bottom Line:

NAC is a glutamate modulator and is derived from the amino acid cysteine. It has been tested for many psychiatric conditions, but is most likely effective as an add-on treatment to SSRIs in OCD, trichotillomania, nail biting, and skin picking.

FDA Indications:

None.

Off-Label Uses:

OCD; trichotillomania; nail biting; skin picking.

Dosage Forms:

Capsules: 500 mg, 600 mg, 750 mg, 1000 mg.

Dosage Guidance:

NAC doses studied have ranged from 600 mg to 6000 mg/day, with the majority of the studies using 1200–2400 mg/day. Divide dose BID to minimize GI side effects.

Monitoring: No routine monitoring recommended unless clinical picture warrants.

Cost: $

Side Effects:

• Most common: Usually well tolerated with nausea/vomiting, diarrhea, cramping, flatulence being most common.
• Serious but rare: May exacerbate asthma.

Mechanism, Pharmacokinetics, and Drug Interactions:

• NAC is derived from the amino acid cysteine, a precursor of a key brain antioxidant, glutathione. It works as a glutamate modulator, which may have effects on oxidative stress, mitochondrial dysfunction, inflammatory mediators, neurotransmission, and neural plasticity.
• Metabolized extensively by liver with minimal P450 involvement; t ½: 6 hours.
• No known drug interactions; not likely an issue for the majority of patients.

Clinical Pearls:

• Amino acid derivate with antioxidant properties.
• NAC is most recognized for its use as a treatment for acetaminophen overdose.
• Although NAC has been studied in autism, Alzheimer's, cocaine and cannabis addiction, bipolar disorder, depression, trichotillomania, nail biting, skin picking, OCD, and schizophrenia, the results are generally mixed. Best data are in patients with OCD, trichotillomania, nail biting, and skin picking (including Prader-Willi syndrome).
• Most patients develop tolerance to GI symptoms, and they go away after a few weeks.
• No long-term data; most studies were eight weeks long, and a few followed patients for three to six months.

Fun Fact:

Many of the published studies have come from an individual Australian researcher who holds a patent on a particular formulation of NAC, raising the issue of bias or a potential conflict of interest.

OMEGA-3 FATTY ACIDS (Fish Oil) Fact Sheet [G]

Bottom Line:
Omega-3 fatty acids form the lipid bilayers of cell membranes, and supplementing our natural dietary supply may have psychological and cardiological benefits. Based on the limited data available, the best use of omega-3 fatty acids (particularly 1–2 g with at least 60% EPA) is as an adjunct in the treatment of unipolar and bipolar depression. There is not enough evidence to recommend omega-3 fatty acids in other psychiatric disorders at this time.

FDA Indications:
High triglycerides (as Lovaza).

Off-Label Uses:
Unipolar and bipolar depression.

Dosage Forms:
- Supplied over the counter in various dosages and formulations; 500 mg, 1000 mg, and 1200 mg softgel capsules most common.
- By prescription only: Lovaza: 1000 mg softgel capsules (GSK). Dosage on label usually reflects fish oil dosage, which is not the same as omega-3 fatty acid dosage (eg, 1000 mg fish oil in some brands may provide 300 mg of omega-3 fatty acids, including EPA and DHA). Dosing recommendations are based on mg of fish oil.

Dosage Guidance:
Effective dose unclear, but studies have used 300 mg–6 g QD. For depression, start 500 mg/day, increase as tolerated (target dose 1–2 g/day); doses >3 g/day should be used cautiously. Dividing dose BID–TID helps with side effect tolerability.

Monitoring: No routine monitoring recommended unless clinical picture warrants.

Cost: $

Side Effects:
- Most common: Well tolerated up to 4 g/day. Nausea, loose stools, fishy aftertaste.
- Serious but rare: Caution in those who are allergic to seafood. Increased risk of bleeding, particularly at higher doses.

Mechanism, Pharmacokinetics, and Drug Interactions:
- Exact mechanism unknown, but may improve cell membrane fluidity and membrane function, change neurotransmitter binding, and promote anti-inflammatory effects.
- Metabolism is hepatic, primarily through CYP450; t ½: Unknown.
- For most patients, drug interactions not likely an issue; however, may prolong bleeding time. Fish oils may lower blood pressure and have additive effects when used with antihypertensives.

Clinical Pearls:
- Fish oils contain eicosapentaenoic acid (EPA) and docosahexaenoic acid (DHA); both are omega-3 fatty acids. Although the body can synthesize these fats from alpha-linolenic acid (ALA), this is believed to be inefficient in many people.
- EPA and DHA are derived from fish; ALA is derived from flax seed and other vegetable matter. Mercury accumulates in fish meat more than in fish oil, which might explain the lack of detectable mercury in most fish oil supplements. Also, the manufacturing process that is used to deodorize fish oil supplements seems to lower the levels of PCBs and other contaminants.
- Omega-3 fatty acids have been tested in the treatment of schizophrenia, bipolar disorder, depression, anxiety, OCD, ADHD, autism, aggression, borderline personality disorder, substance use disorder, anorexia nervosa, and dementia. With the exception of depressive disorders, overall consensus is still lacking for the majority of these uses due to limited sample sizes, selection of patients, doses and formulations used, and study durations.
- Omega-3 fatty acids appear helpful as augmentation in unipolar depression in some individual studies, but several meta-analyses have not been able to show robust benefit. In positive studies, most benefit seen at 1 g/day, with EPA more effective than DHA and more severely ill patients showing greater improvement.

Fun Fact:
Inuit people have been reported to ingest up to 16 g/day (via fish) with no dangerous side effects.

S-ADENOSYL-L-METHIONINE (SAMe) Fact Sheet [G]

Bottom Line:

SAMe is a natural methyl donor important in neurotransmitter synthesis and function. Several clinical studies (lasting up to 42 days) have shown that taking SAMe is more effective than placebo and appears to be as effective as tricyclic antidepressants, though the studies were limited in various ways. Consider using it for those patients with mild to moderate depression who are interested in using alternative therapies, or as an augmentation strategy in partial responders.

FDA Indications:

None.

Off-Label Uses:

Depression; osteoarthritis; cirrhosis and fatty liver disease.

Dosage Forms:

Supplied over the counter most often as 100 mg, 200 mg, 400 mg tablets, usually enteric coated.

Dosage Guidance:

Effective dose is variable, but most antidepressant studies have used doses of about 400–1600 mg/day (1600 mg most common), usually divided BID.

Monitoring: No routine monitoring recommended unless clinical picture warrants.

Cost: $

Side Effects:

- Most common: Well tolerated. Higher doses may result in flatulence, nausea, vomiting, diarrhea, constipation, dry mouth, headache, mild insomnia, anorexia, sweating, dizziness, and nervousness. Anxiety and tiredness have occurred in people with depression, and hypomania has occurred in people with bipolar disorder.
- Serious but rare: Theoretical concern of elevated homocysteine since SAMe is converted to this during normal metabolism. No reports to date, but some recommend taking folate and vitamin B supplements anyway.

Mechanism, Pharmacokinetics, and Drug Interactions:

- Methyl group donor that may increase synthesis of neurotransmitters, increase responsiveness of neurotransmitter receptors, and increase fluidity of cell membranes through the production of phospholipids.
- Metabolism similar to endogenous SAMe (transmethylation, trans-sulphuration, and aminopropylation); t ½: 100 minutes.
- No drug interactions reported. Theoretically, serotonin syndrome possible but risk likely minimal.

Clinical Pearls:

- SAMe is produced by our bodies as a derivative of the amino acid methionine. It is necessary for the production of serotonin and norepinephrine (and in more than 100 other biochemical reactions) throughout virtually all body tissues and fluids. Concentrations are highest in childhood and decrease with age.
- SAMe is difficult to formulate as a stable oral salt, and the FDA halted trials of an investigational prescription product in 1993 due to concerns about tablet dissolution; concerns have been raised that some supplements may also have these problems.

Fun Facts:

SAMe has been available as a dietary supplement in the US since 1999, but it has been used as a prescription drug in Italy since 1979, in Spain since 1985, and in Germany since 1989. Patients in trials of SAMe for depression noted improvement in their arthritis symptoms, suggesting another possible use.

ST. JOHN'S WORT Fact Sheet [G]

Bottom Line:

St. John's wort can be considered an option along with conventional antidepressants for short-term treatment of mild depression; however, be wary of its many drug interactions.

FDA Indications:

None.

Off-Label Uses:

Depression.

Dosage Forms:

Supplied over the counter most commonly as 100 mg, 300 mg, 450 mg tablets and capsules.

Dosage Guidance:

For mild to moderate depression, most clinical trials have used St. John's wort extract containing 0.3% hypericin and/or 3% hyperforin; most common dose is 300 mg TID. Doses of 1200 mg QD have also been used. Some studies have also used a 0.2% hypericin extract dosed at 250 mg BID. A St. John's wort extract standardized to 5% hyperforin and dosed at 300 mg TID has also been used.

Monitoring: No routine monitoring recommended unless clinical picture warrants.

Cost: $

Side Effects:

- Most common: Well tolerated at recommended doses. Insomnia (decrease dose or take in morning), vivid dreams, restlessness, anxiety, agitation, irritability, gastrointestinal discomfort, diarrhea, fatigue, dry mouth, dizziness, and headache reported. Sexual dysfunction may occur, but less often than with SSRIs.
- Serious but rare: Risk of severe phototoxic skin reactions and photosensitivity at high doses (2–4 g/day).

Mechanism, Pharmacokinetics, and Drug Interactions:

- Thought to exert antidepressant effects by modulating effects of monoamines, and may inhibit reuptake of these neurotransmitters.
- Metabolized primarily through the liver; t ½: 24–48 hours.
- Avoid concomitant use with serotonergic agents: Rare cases of serotonin syndrome reported. Potent inducer of many CYP450 enzymes (3A4, 2C9, 1A2) and P-glycoprotein transporter, which results in increased metabolism and reduced plasma concentrations of a large number of drugs. St. John's wort can decrease oral contraceptive levels by 13%–15%, resulting in bleeding or unplanned pregnancy; women should use an additional or nonhormonal form of birth control.

Clinical Pearls:

- Also known as *Hypericum perforatum*; active constituents (predominantly hypericin and hyperforin) are derived from the flowering buds.
- St. John's wort is more effective than placebo, likely as effective as low-dose tricyclic antidepressants and SSRIs in milder forms of depression; however, a study in *JAMA* found it no more effective than placebo or sertraline for moderate to severe depression.
- Avoid abrupt discontinuation due to the risk of withdrawal effects.

Fun Facts:

Although not indigenous to Australia and long considered a weed, St. John's wort is now grown as a cash crop, and Australia produces 20% of the world's supply. The use of St. John's wort dates back to the ancient Greeks; Hippocrates documented the medical use of St. John's wort flowers. St. John's wort is so named because it blooms near June 24th, which is the birthday of John the Baptist. "Wort" is an old English word for plant.

VITAMIN D Fact Sheet [G]

Bottom Line:
Vitamin D supplementation may be beneficial in depression, but reserve its use for those who have low vitamin D levels, and make sure patients take adequate doses, in the range of 1000–5000 IU daily.

FDA Indications:
None.

Off-Label Uses:
Depression.

Dosage Forms:
Supplied over the counter as vitamin D2 and D3, as tablets, capsules, and softgels in "international units" (IU) dosing. We recommend D3: 1000 IU, 2000 IU, 5000 IU, 10,000 IU.

Dosage Guidance:
Dosing guidelines vary. For depression, use 1000–5000 IU per day.

Monitoring: Periodic vitamin D [25(OH)D] levels.

Cost: $

Side Effects:
- Most common: Well tolerated.
- Serious but rare: Vitamin D toxicity possible but very rare.

Mechanism, Pharmacokinetics, and Drug Interactions:
- Thought to play a role in brain plasticity, neuroimmunomodulation, and inflammation.
- Metabolized by liver and kidneys; t ½: 12–50 days (varies based on level, source, dose, obesity, and race).
- No known significant interactions.

Clinical Pearls:
- Sources of vitamin D include exposure to sunlight, dietary intake, and supplements.
- It's difficult to obtain sufficient daily needs from dietary intake alone. Two types of vitamin D are obtained from dietary sources: D2 (ergocalciferol) from plant sources such as mushrooms and soy milk and D3 (cholecalciferol) from animal sources such as raw fish, mackerel, smoked salmon). D3 is approximately three times stronger than D2.
- Majority of vitamin D is produced through conversion of 7-dehydrocholesterol via ultraviolet B, after penetration of sunlight on the skin, to vitamin D3.
- Vitamin D is metabolized in the liver to 25-hydroxyvitamin D or 25(OH)D and then in the kidneys to its active form calcitriol, or 1,25-dihydroxyvitamin D. There is no consensus about the optimal total 25(OH)D level, which may vary with the assay used. Many labs report 25(OH)D level of 30–60 ng/mL as normal range, 21–29 ng/mL as insufficiency, and ≤20 ng/mL as deficiency.
- Several meta-analyses have found no beneficial effects of vitamin D supplementation on depression. When studies were limited to depressed patients with both vitamin D insufficiency at baseline and adequate dosing of supplementation (>800 mg/day), statistically significant benefits were seen.
- Studies in anxiety, psychosis, and dementia have not shown positive results of supplementation.

Fun Fact:
A number of things affect your vitamin D status, including how far away you live from the equator, the air quality in your community, your skin color, and your use of sunscreen.

Sexual Dysfunction Medications

GENERAL PRESCRIBING TIPS

Many psychiatric medications cause sexual dysfunction. Most antidepressants (the main exceptions being bupropion and mirtazapine) cause sexual problems, which can include low libido, anorgasmia, and erectile dysfunction. Antipsychotics often lower libido, whether due to increased prolactin or other unknown factors.

Before jumping to treat the side effect of one medication with another medication, try other potential solutions: decreasing the dose of the offending medication, switching medications, adding an "antidote" such as bupropion or mirtazapine in the case of antidepressant-induced effects, or prescribing two- or three-day drug holidays. If none of these strategies work, you might want to prescribe one of the medications in this chapter.

For men with erectile dysfunction, prescribe one of the four PDE-5 inhibitors. Sildenafil (Viagra) has the benefit of being well known, which might enhance the placebo effect. Tadalafil (Cialis) has the advantage of a long duration of action (up to 36 hours). Avanafil (Stendra) works a little more quickly than Viagra: 15 minutes as opposed to 30 minutes. Vardenafil (Levitra) is available as a peppermint-flavored orally disintegrating pill—though it has no therapeutic advantages beyond whatever aphrodisiac power peppermint might provide, as its onset of action is no faster than the regular Levitra tablet.

For women with low sexual desire (hypoactive sexual desire disorder), there are two approved medications—flibanserin (Addyi) and bremelanotide (Vyleesi). Low sexual desire can stem from a number of psychological, physiological, or other factors such as stress, and there's controversy around how to diagnose, whether to treat with medication, and how well the medications work. When medication is used, there are differences between the two: Flibanserin must be taken by mouth daily and alcohol must be avoided within two hours of taking it, whereas bremelanotide can be taken as needed but must be injected. For both men and women who suffer sexual dysfunction from serotonergic antidepressants, you can try off-label cyproheptadine. It works pretty well sometimes, but other times it doesn't work at all. As above, adjunctive bupropion or mirtazapine sometimes helps as well.

For men with low testosterone, prescribe... testosterone. It will add zip to patients who suffer low libido as a result of low T. However, don't get roped into prescribing this for anyone who asks for it, since there's no evidence it helps men with normal T levels.

Class Warning for PDE-5 Inhibitors

Avoid concomitant use with nitrates in any form—eg, nitroglycerin, isosorbide dinitrate, amyl nitrite ("poppers").

Table 18: **Sexual Dysfunction Medications**

Generic Name (Brand Name) Year FDA Approved [G] denotes generic availability	Relevant FDA Indication(s)	Available Strengths (mg)	Starting Dose (mg)	Usual Dosage Range (starting–max) (mg)	Special Features
Avanafil (Stendra) 2012	Erectile dysfunction	50, 100, 200	100	50–200	More rapid onset (15 minutes); food doesn't affect absorption
Bremelanotide (Vyleesi) 2019	Hypoactive sexual desire disorder in premenopausal women	1.75 mg/0.3 mL	1.75	1.75	Subcutaneous autoinjector; no more than 1 dose per 24 hours or 8 doses per month
Cyproheptadine [G] 1961 Brand name Periactin discontinued; generic only	None	4; 2/5 mL	4	4–12	Sedating; most effective for anorgasmia
Flibanserin (Addyi) 2015	Hypoactive sexual desire disorder in premenopausal women	100	100	100	Can't be combined with alcohol
Sildenafil [G] (Viagra) 1998 Generic only available as 20 mg tablet	Erectile dysfunction	25, 50, 100	25	25–100	Takes 30 minutes; fatty meals decrease absorption
Tadalafil [G] (Cialis) 2003	Erectile dysfunction	2.5, 5, 10, 20	5	5–20	Takes one hour, lasts 36 hours; no meal effect
Testosterone	Hypogonadism	Various formulations and dosages; see fact sheet for details			No evidence of beneficial effect in the absence of low T
Vardenafil [G] (Levitra) 2003	Erectile dysfunction	2.5, 5, 10, 20	10	10–20	Works in 30 minutes; fatty meals decrease absorption
Vardenafil ODT (Staxyn) 2010	Erectile dysfunction	10 ODT	10	10	Peppermint flavored

AVANAFIL (Stendra) Fact Sheet

Bottom Line:
Avanafil is the newest PDE-5 inhibitor to come to market. Its potential advantage is a somewhat faster onset than any of the other ED drugs.

FDA Indications:
Erectile dysfunction.

Dosage Forms:
Tablets: 50 mg, 100 mg, 200 mg.

Dosage Guidance:
- Start 100 mg ×1 taken 15 minutes before sexual activity. Max dose 200 mg/dose, up to one dose/24 hours.
- May be taken with or without food.

Monitoring: No routine monitoring recommended unless clinical picture warrants.

Cost: $$$$

Side Effects:
- Most common: Headache, nasal congestion, flushing.
- Serious but rare: May cause dose-related impairment of color discrimination. Sudden decrease or loss of hearing has been reported rarely; hearing changes may be accompanied by tinnitus and dizziness. Decreases in blood pressure may occur due to vasodilator effects; concurrent use with alpha-adrenergic antagonists or substantial alcohol consumption may cause symptomatic hypotension. Avoid use with nitrates (see below). Painful erection greater than six hours in duration (priapism) may occur rarely.

Mechanism, Pharmacokinetics, and Drug Interactions:
- Phosphodiesterase type 5 (PDE-5) inhibitor.
- Metabolized primarily through CYP3A4, also 2C9/19 to a lesser degree; t ½: 5 hours.
- Avoid concomitant use with nitrates in any form (eg, nitroglycerin, isosorbide dinitrate, amyl nitrite "poppers"). Use with caution in patients taking alpha-adrenergic blockers; may cause symptomatic hypotension (maximum of 50 mg in 24 hours). Use with caution in patients taking strong CYP3A4 inhibitors, which may increase or extend effects of avanafil (maximum of 50 mg in 24 hours).

Clinical Pearls:
Onset of effect is usually 15–30 minutes after a dose (and not affected by meals). About two-thirds of men will have therapeutic effect within 15 minutes. Usual duration is approximately two hours.

Fun Fact:
Avanafil was initially approved with the recommendation to take it 30 minutes before sexual activity. Its manufacturer decided it was tough to compete with blockbusters like Viagra and Cialis without some sort of competitive edge, so it presented some data to the FDA and had the dosing changed to "as early as approximately 15 minutes before sexual activity." Spontaneity became the hallmark of the drug's marketing campaign, with taglines like "This time, he was ready before dessert."

BREMELANOTIDE (Vyleesi) Fact Sheet

Bottom Line:

Bremelanotide (marketed as the "female Viagra") is a melanocortin receptor agonist that is modestly effective in increasing sexual desire in women, though it doesn't affect sexual functioning. Disadvantages include the fact that it requires self-injection and carries a 40% rate of nausea as a side effect. It's worth trying in some patients, but don't expect miracles.

FDA Indications:

Hypoactive sexual desire disorder in premenopausal women.

Dosage Forms:

Subcutaneous self-injection: 1.75 mg/0.3 mL.

Dosage Guidance:

Patient to self-inject 1.75 mg subcutaneously via the autoinjector to the abdomen or thigh, as needed, at least 45 minutes before anticipated sexual activity. Do not use more than one dose within 24 hours or eight doses per month.

Monitoring: No routine monitoring recommended unless clinical picture warrants.

Cost: $$$$

Side Effects:

- Most common: Nausea (seen in 40% of women in clinical trials), flushing, injection site reactions, headache, and vomiting.
- Serious but rare: Transient increase in blood pressure and decrease in heart rate may occur after each dose; usually resolves within 12 hours. Focal hyperpigmentation has been reported by 1% of patients, including involvement of the face, gingiva, and breasts; higher risk in patients with darker skin. Hyperpigmentation may resolve in about half of patients; discontinue if it develops.

Mechanism, Pharmacokinetics, and Drug Interactions:

- Melanocortin receptor agonist.
- As a peptide with seven amino acids, metabolism primarily involves hydrolysis (non-P450); t ½: 2.7 hours.
- Avoid concomitant use with naltrexone; bremelanotide significantly decreases systemic exposure of oral naltrexone.

Clinical Pearls:

- Bremelanotide has not been studied in postmenopausal women or in men.
- Bremelanotide does not enhance sexual performance; rather, it increases interest.
- In the two preclinical trials, nearly 40% dropped out of the trial and only 4%–8% benefited over placebo.

Fun Fact:

Even before the FDA approved Vyleesi, its manufacturer was sponsoring a campaign called "unblush" to spread the word on hypoactive sexual desire disorder (www.unblush.com).

CYPROHEPTADINE (Periactin) Fact Sheet [G]

Bottom Line:
Cyproheptadine is sometimes effective in reversing SSRI-induced anorgasmia, but with continued use it could interfere with antidepressant efficacy. As-needed occasional use is the best strategy.

FDA Indications:
Allergic rhinitis; urticaria.

Off-Label Uses:
Antidepressant-induced sexual dysfunction; anorexia and bulimia nervosa; appetite stimulant; acute management of serotonin syndrome.

Dosage Forms:
- **Tablets (G):** 4 mg (scored).
- **Syrup (G):** 2 mg/5 mL syrup.

Dosage Guidance:
Take 4–12 mg one to two hours before sexual activity.

Monitoring: No routine monitoring recommended unless clinical picture warrants.

Cost: $

Side Effects:
Most common: Sedation, confusion, weight gain, anticholinergic effects, potential reversal of antidepressant therapeutic effect.

Mechanism, Pharmacokinetics, and Drug Interactions:
- Histamine H1 receptor antagonist with mild antiserotonergic effects.
- Metabolized primarily through hepatic glucuronidation via UGT1A; t ½: 16 hours.
- Avoid concomitant use with MAOIs. Additive effects with other sedating agents.

Clinical Pearls:
- Appears to work best for anorgasmia. Average effective dose in one study was 8.6 mg.
- Excessive sedation may impede therapeutic efficacy in some patients.

Fun Facts:
Cyproheptadine's antagonistic effects at serotonin receptors have been shown to be useful as part of the management of serotonin syndrome. It's been used to counteract the more rarely occurring serotonergic side effects of serotonergic antidepressants, such as sweating and vivid dreams. It is also the most commonly used appetite stimulant for cats.

Sexual Dysfunction Medications

FLIBANSERIN (Addyi) Fact Sheet

Bottom Line:

Flibanserin, marketed as the "pink Viagra," is mildly effective for enhancing sexual desire, but with potentially significant side effects and precautions regarding alcohol use around the time of administration.

FDA Indications:

Hypoactive sexual desire disorder in premenopausal women.

Dosage Forms:

Tablets: 100 mg.

Dosage Guidance:

Start and continue 100 mg QHS; taking during the daytime may increase risk of hypotension, syncope, and CNS depression. Discontinue after eight weeks if no improvement.

Monitoring: No routine monitoring recommended unless clinical picture warrants.

Cost: $$$$

Side Effects:

- Most common: Dizziness, somnolence, nausea, fatigue, insomnia, dry mouth.
- Serious but rare: May have potential to cause severe hypotension or syncope.

Mechanism, Pharmacokinetics, and Drug Interactions:

- Mixed agonist-antagonist on postsynaptic serotonergic receptors with 5-HT1A agonist and 5-HT2A antagonist effects.
- Metabolized primarily through CYP3A4 and to a lesser extent, 2C19; t ½: 11 hours.
- Avoid concomitant use with alcohol, with CYP3A4 inhibitors, or in patients with hepatic impairment as there may be an increased risk for hypotension and syncope.

Clinical Pearls:

- Flibanserin has not been studied in postmenopausal women or in men.
- Flibanserin does not enhance sexual performance; rather, it increases interest.
- While studies of Viagra show around 80% of men improving (50%–60% more than placebo), only 8%–13% more women on flibanserin had benefits over placebo.
- The manufacturer wanted the black box warning and contraindication about alcohol removed, so the FDA reviewed postmarketing studies. The FDA decided to modify rather than remove the warning. They determined that there is still cause for concern about drinking alcohol close in time to taking flibanserin but that it doesn't have to be avoided completely. Now the warning specifies that women shouldn't drink two hours before or at least until the morning after taking flibanserin at bedtime.

Fun Fact:

Based on mediocre efficacy data, Dr. Carlat has made the analogy that "if Viagra is a Starbucks triple espresso, flibanserin is a Dixie cup of cafeteria coffee."

SILDENAFIL (Viagra) Fact Sheet [G]

Bottom Line:

Sildenafil is the original PDE-5 inhibitor, and as such it has the best evidence and longest track record.

FDA Indications:

Erectile dysfunction; pulmonary arterial hypertension (Revatio brand name).

Dosage Forms:

Tablets (G): 25 mg, 50 mg, 100 mg.

Dosage Guidance:

Start 50 mg ×1 (25 mg if >65 years old or with CYP3A4 inhibitors) from 30 minutes to four hours before sexual activity. Max 100 mg/dose and one dose/day. Avoid taking with a high-fat meal.

Monitoring: No routine monitoring recommended unless clinical picture warrants.

Cost: $

Side Effects:

- Most common: Headache, dyspepsia/heartburn, flushing.
- Serious but rare: May cause dose-related impairment of color discrimination. Sudden decrease or loss of hearing has been reported rarely; hearing changes may be accompanied by tinnitus and dizziness. Decreases in blood pressure may occur due to vasodilator effects; concurrent use with alpha-adrenergic antagonists or substantial alcohol consumption may cause symptomatic hypotension. Avoid use with nitrates (see below). Painful erection greater than six hours in duration (priapism) may occur rarely.

Mechanism, Pharmacokinetics, and Drug Interactions:

- Phosphodiesterase type 5 (PDE-5) inhibitor.
- Metabolized primarily through CYP3A4 and to a lesser extent, 2C9; t ½: 4 hours.
- Avoid concomitant use with nitrates in any form (eg, nitroglycerin, isosorbide dinitrate, amyl nitrite "poppers"). Use with caution in patients taking alpha-adrenergic blockers; may cause symptomatic hypotension (use 25 mg dose). Use with caution in patients taking strong CYP3A4 inhibitors, which may increase or extend effects of sildenafil (maximum of 25 mg in 48 hours).

Clinical Pearl:

Onset of effect is usually 15–20 minutes after a dose (but may be delayed 60 minutes by a high-fat meal), and usual duration is approximately two hours.

Fun Fact:

Sildenafil has been used recreationally. Some users mix it with MDMA (ecstasy) to counteract the erectile dysfunction MDMA can cause; this combination is known as "sextasy."

TADALAFIL (Cialis) Fact Sheet [G]

Bottom Line:

We have fewer data for tadalafil in the psychiatric setting; however, compared to other agents in the class, its long duration of action may improve spontaneity, and the lack of interaction with meals may offer advantages. Tadalafil is an especially good choice for men who have both prostatic hypertrophy and erectile dysfunction.

FDA Indications:

Erectile dysfunction; benign prostatic hyperplasia; pulmonary arterial hypertension (Adcirca brand name).

Dosage Forms:

Tablets (G): 2.5 mg, 5 mg, 10 mg, 20 mg.

Dosage Guidance:

- PRN dosing: Start 10 mg ×1, 30–60 minutes prior to sexual activity; adjust dose to 5–20 mg based on response. Max 20 mg/dose and one dose/24 hours.
- Daily dosing: Start 2.5 mg QD; may increase to max of 5 mg QD based on response.

Monitoring: No routine monitoring recommended unless clinical picture warrants.

Cost: $

Side Effects:

- Most common: Headache, dyspepsia/nausea, flushing, back pain, muscle aches.
- Serious but rare: May cause dose-related impairment of color discrimination. Sudden decrease or loss of hearing has been reported rarely; hearing changes may be accompanied by tinnitus and dizziness. Decreases in blood pressure may occur due to vasodilator effects; concurrent use with alpha-adrenergic antagonists or substantial alcohol consumption may cause symptomatic hypotension. Avoid use with nitrates (see below). Painful erection greater than six hours in duration (priapism) may occur rarely.

Mechanism, Pharmacokinetics, and Drug Interactions:

- Phosphodiesterase type 5 (PDE-5) inhibitor.
- Metabolized primarily through CYP3A4; t ½: 15–17.5 hours.
- Avoid concomitant use with nitrates in any form (eg, nitroglycerin, isosorbide dinitrate, amyl nitrite "poppers"). Use with caution in patients taking alpha-adrenergic blockers; may cause symptomatic hypotension (use lower tadalafil dose). Use with caution in patients taking strong CYP3A4 inhibitors, which may increase or extend effects of tadalafil (maximum of 10 mg/dose and one dose/72 hours with PRN dosing or 2.5 mg/day with daily dosing).

Clinical Pearls:

- Onset of effect of tadalafil is usually within one hour, and its effects may last 36 hours.
- Daily tadalafil has the advantage of allowing users to always be "ready," but it can also cause daily side effects.

Fun Fact:

Cialis' 36-hour effectiveness earned it the nickname "the weekend pill."

TESTOSTERONE (various) Fact Sheet [G]

Bottom Line:
Successful marketing has convinced the public that "low T" is a public health scourge, leading to over-prescribing of testosterone for patients who don't need it. Prescribe it only for men with demonstrably low testosterone levels and accompanying symptoms.

FDA Indications:
Hypogonadism.

Dosage Forms:
- **Capsules (Android):** 10 mg methyltestosterone.
- **Buccal ER tablet (Striant):** 30 mg.
- **Topical gel (AndroGel, Androderm, others):** 1%, 2%.
- **Long-acting depot injection (Depo-Testosterone, [G]):** 100 mg/mL, 200 mg/mL.

Dosage Guidance:
- Dosing varies from daily dosing of oral, buccal, and topical agents to Q2–4 week or Q3–6 month dosing of injectable formulations.
- Schedule III controlled substance.

Monitoring: Hematocrit, bone density, LFTs.

Cost: Capsule: $$$$$; buccal: $$$$$; gel: $$$$; depot injectable: $

Side Effects:
- Most common: Nausea, headache, insomnia, anxiety, acne, water and electrolyte retention, local effects (eg, gum irritation with buccal formulation, application site irritation with gel, injection site pain with injectables).
- Serious but rare: Thromboembolic events (DVT, PE), myocardial infarction, stroke, worsening BPH, risk of prostate cancer.

Mechanism, Pharmacokinetics, and Drug Interactions:
- Anabolic and andronergic testosterone receptor agonist.
- Metabolized primarily through liver (non-CYP450); t ½: Varies.

Clinical Pearls:
- Hypogonadism may play a significant role in erectile dysfunction, and a threshold level of testosterone may be necessary for normal erectile function. However, testosterone levels needed for normal sexual function vary widely; some men may have normal function even with age-adjusted lower normal range levels. Testosterone replacement may be appropriate when both clinical symptoms and biochemical evidence of hypogonadism exist.
- Available data indicate that all testosterone products may be equally effective and associated with similar side effect profiles.

Fun Fact:
Stephen Braun, a medical writer, described how he was funded by Abbott Pharmaceuticals to help write a "consensus panel" statement for a physician's organization. Two of his paragraphs casting doubt on the dangers of low testosterone were deleted from the final document (Braun S, *JAMA Internal Medicine* 2013;173(15):1458–1460).

VARDENAFIL (Levitra) Fact Sheet [G]

Bottom Line:

Vardenafil doesn't offer any benefits compared to sildenafil, which has more data in the psychiatric setting, more clinical experience, and lower cost.

FDA Indications:

Erectile dysfunction.

Dosage Forms:

* **Tablets (Levitra, [G]):** 2.5 mg, 5 mg, 10 mg, 20 mg.
* **Orally disintegrating tablets (Staxyn):** 10 mg.

Dosage Guidance:

* Start 10 mg ×1 one hour prior to sexual activity (5 mg if >65 years old). Max 20 mg/dose and one dose/day.
* Orally disintegrating tablets (Staxyn): Start 10 mg ×1 one hour prior to sexual activity. Max 10 mg/day.
* Taking with a high-fat meal may decrease serum vardenafil levels by as much as 50%.

Monitoring: No routine monitoring recommended unless clinical picture warrants.

Cost: $$$

Side Effects:

* Most common: Flushing, headache, nasal congestion, heartburn.
* Serious but rare: May cause dose-related impairment of color discrimination. Sudden decrease or loss of hearing has been reported rarely; hearing changes may be accompanied by tinnitus and dizziness. Decreases in blood pressure may occur due to vasodilator effects; concurrent use with alpha-adrenergic antagonists or substantial alcohol consumption may cause symptomatic hypotension. Avoid use with nitrates (see below). Painful erection greater than six hours in duration (priapism) may occur rarely.

Mechanism, Pharmacokinetics, and Drug Interactions:

* Phosphodiesterase type 5 (PDE-5) inhibitor.
* Metabolized primarily through CYP3A4 and to a lesser extent, 2C9; t ½: 4–5 hours.
* Avoid concomitant use with nitrates in any form (eg, nitroglycerin, isosorbide dinitrate, amyl nitrite "poppers"). Use with caution in patients taking alpha blockers; may cause symptomatic hypotension (use 5 mg dose). Use with caution in patients taking strong CYP3A4 inhibitors, which may increase or extend effects of vardenafil (maximum of 2.5 mg/day).

Clinical Pearl:

Usual onset of effect of vardenafil is within one hour of a dose; effects usually last two hours.

Fun Fact:

Staxyn, the orally disintegrating tablet form of vardenafil, is peppermint flavored.

Side Effect Management

GENERAL MANAGEMENT TIPS

If you're like most psychiatrists, you probably severely underestimate the number of side effects your patients are experiencing. According to one survey, patients on antidepressants reported *20 times* more side effects than were actually recorded by their psychiatrists (Zimmerman M et al, *J Clin Psychiatry* 2010;71(4):484–490).

Sometimes we don't ask about side effects because we're not sure what to do about them. In order to help you expand your side effect battling arsenal, we have provided this side effect management chapter. We've included 20 fact sheets, including three new ones (diarrhea, neuroleptic malignant syndrome, and serotonin syndrome), covering some of the most common side effects you are likely to encounter in your patients. We had to pick and choose which ones to include, so if there are important symptoms that are missing, please let us know so we can add them to the next edition.

In addition to the side effect management sheets, we've included seven regular medication fact sheets on agents that we use primarily to treat side effects. These include amantadine, benztropine, and trihexyphenidyl for extrapyramidal symptoms of antipsychotics; deutetrabenazine, tetrabenazine, and valbenazine for tardive dyskinesia; and metformin for weight gain caused by psychotropic drugs.

Here's a quick orientation to the side effect fact sheet format:

- *Characteristics:* We describe what the side effect feels like for patients and how you can recognize it.

- *Meds That Cause It:* These are the medications that are most likely to cause the side effect in question. We include only psychotropics in this list.

- *Mechanism:* Although we usually don't know exactly how psychotropics cause most side effects, we posit mechanisms that seem to be most popular with experts.

- *General Management:* This refers to everything other than prescribing specific antidotes. Included here are things like watchful waiting, reducing the dose, switching to a different medication, shifting the timing of the dose (usually to bedtime), taking with food, and so on. Mostly these are commonsense interventions, which you should try before prescribing a new anti–side effect medication.

- *First-Line Medications:* In some cases, most experts agree on a few medications that are most likely to be effective for managing specific side effects. That said, since there are very few clinical trials testing meds for side effects, judgments about what qualifies as a first-line vs a second-line medication are fallible, and we won't be offended if you disagree.

- *Second-Line Medications:* This section is reserved for the various nostrums—drugs that have been tried by various people and might work. You would likely resort to these only out of desperation.

- *Clinical Pearls:* Hard-won wisdom from the trenches.

- *Fun Fact:* Sometimes entertaining, sometimes intriguing... and sometimes just present.

A note on information sources: It's not easy to find reliable information on side effect management. There are very few well-designed clinical trials on such uses, meaning that we must rely on uncontrolled trials, small case series, anecdotes, or simply expert opinion. In doing research for the symptom fact sheets in this chapter, we relied primarily on the following three sources, supplemented by various articles and our own clinical experiences:

- Annamalai A. *Medical Management of Psychotropic Side Effects*. New York, NY: Springer Publishing; 2017.

- Goldberg JF and Ernst CL. *Managing the Side Effects of Psychotropic Medications*. 2nd ed. Arlington, VA: American Psychiatric Association; 2019.

- Mago R. *Side Effects of Psychiatric Medications*. Createspace Independent Pub; 2014.

Side Effect Management:
MEDICATIONS

AMANTADINE (Gocovri, Symmetrel) Fact Sheet [G]

Bottom Line:
Amantadine is a dopaminergic medication used primarily in Parkinson's disease, but it is also helpful in drug-induced Parkinsonism and has fewer anticholinergic side effects (eg, cognitive impairment, dry mouth, constipation) than other anti-EPS meds like benztropine.

FDA Indications:
Drug-induced extrapyramidal symptoms (EPS); Parkinson's disease; influenza A.

Off-Label Uses:
Tardive dyskinesia; ADHD; enuresis; treatment-resistant depression; OCD.

Dosage Forms:
- **Capsules (G):** 100 mg.
- **Tablets (G):** 100 mg.
- **Oral solution (G):** 50 mg/5 mL.
- **ER capsules (Gocovri):** 68.5 mg, 137 mg.

Dosage Guidance:
- IR: Start 100 mg HS or BID. Max 300 mg/day.
- ER: Start 137 mg QHS; increase after one week to usual and max dose of 274 mg QHS.

Monitoring: No routine monitoring recommended unless clinical picture warrants.

Cost: $; ER: $$$$$

Side Effects:
- Most common: Nausea, dizziness, orthostatic hypotension, insomnia, blurred vision, constipation, dry mouth.
- Serious but rare: Rare cases of intense urges to gamble, spend money, or have sex reported.

Mechanism, Pharmacokinetics, and Drug Interactions:
- Weak NMDA antagonist and potentiates dopaminergic neurons. Antiviral (inhibits replication of influenza A virus).
- Not metabolized; excreted primarily through kidneys; t ½: 17 hours.
- Minimal clinically significant drug interactions.

Clinical Pearls:
- Because of dopaminergic effects, theoretically amantadine could worsen psychosis. At doses typically used to manage EPS, though, this doesn't generally happen.
- Typically used when anticholinergic side effects of other anti-EPS medications (benztropine, trihexyphenidyl) are intolerable.
- Adjust dose in elderly patients or those with impaired renal function.
- Gocovri is an extended-release once-daily version of amantadine, approved for treatment of dyskinesia in Parkinson's patients taking levodopa. It costs patients an estimated $45 per capsule, ringing in at over $30,000 per year.

Fun Fact:
Memantine (Namenda), an NMDA antagonist used in dementia, is an analogue of amantadine.

Side Effect Management: Medications

BENZTROPINE (Cogentin) Fact Sheet [G]

Bottom Line:

Benztropine is an anticholinergic medication that is the go-to agent for treating and preventing antipsychotic-induced EPS.

FDA Indications:

Drug-induced extrapyramidal symptoms (EPS); Parkinson's disease.

Off-Label Uses:

Sialorrhea (excessive salivation); hyperhidrosis (excessive sweating).

Dosage Forms:

- **Tablets (G):** 0.5 mg, 1 mg, 2 mg.
- **Injectable:** 1 mg/mL.

Dosage Guidance:

- Start 1 mg BID; ↑ by 1–2 mg/day every three to seven days as needed; max 3 mg BID. May be taken once daily at bedtime.
- For acute dystonic reactions, use 1–2 mg IM ×1 and continue with oral, as above, to prevent recurrence.

Monitoring: No routine monitoring recommended unless clinical picture warrants.

Cost: $

Side Effects:

- Most common: Dry mouth, blurred vision, constipation, urinary retention, sedation.
- Serious but rare: In those at risk (elderly patients), may cause confusion or delirium; may worsen angle-closure glaucoma.

Mechanism, Pharmacokinetics, and Drug Interactions:

- Anticholinergic, antihistaminergic.
- Metabolized primarily through liver via unknown P450; t ½: 12–24 hours.
- Minimal clinically significant drug interactions; avoid combining with other anticholinergic agents due to additive effects.

Clinical Pearl:

If starting a patient on a high-potency antipsychotic such as haloperidol or risperidone, some clinicians will start benztropine prophylactically to prevent EPS. If you do so, consider taper and withdrawal of benztropine after one or two weeks to see if it's really needed.

Fun Fact:

Veterinarians use benztropine to treat priapism in stallions.

DEUTETRABENAZINE (Austedo) Fact Sheet

Bottom Line:

Deutetrabenazine was the second of the VMAT inhibitors to be approved for the treatment of tardive dyskinesia (TD) in 2017. Its advantage over off-label tetrabenazine is less frequent dosing and less likelihood of causing depression. However, it is extremely expensive—about $6,000/month as opposed to $400/month for tetrabenazine.

FDA Indications:

TD; Huntington's chorea.

Off-Label Uses:

Tourette's and other tic disorders.

Dosage Forms:

Tablets: 6 mg, 9 mg, 12 mg.

Dosage Guidance:

Start 6 mg BID with food. Titrate at weekly intervals by 6 mg/day increments; increase to maximum dose of 48 mg/day with food (doses ≥12 mg/day should be divided BID).

Monitoring: ECG if cardiac disease.

Cost: $$$$$

Side Effects:

- Most common: Sedation, somnolence, fatigue, diarrhea.
- Serious but rare: QT interval prolongation; caution in those with increased risk (congenital long QT syndrome, electrolyte disturbances, poor 2D6 metabolizers, concomitant 2D6 inhibitors).

Mechanism, Pharmacokinetics, and Drug Interactions:

- Reversible inhibitor of vesicular monoamine transporter 2 (VMAT2). This prevents VMAT2 from transporting monoamines including dopamine back into presynaptic vesicles, resulting in metabolism of monoamines, ultimately leading to depletion of monoamine stores and less dopamine being around. This treats TD symptoms, which are likely caused by hypersensitivity to dopamine.
- Metabolized primarily by CYP450 2D6; t ½: 9–10 hours.
- Avoid MAOIs. Decrease deutetrabenazine dose in presence of 2D6 inhibitors or poor metabolizers.

Clinical Pearls:

- Deutetrabenazine is a deuterated form of tetrabenazine (Xenazine), a similar VMAT2 inhibitor, which is approved for treatment of Huntington's chorea.
- Increased depression and suicidality have been reported with tetrabenazine. Paucity of long-term data with deutetrabenazine makes it difficult to determine whether it will pose these concerns as well.
- A one-year course costs over $70,000.

Fun Fact:

Chemistry course refresher! Deuterated drugs are created by replacing one or more of the hydrogen atoms of the drug molecule with deuterium. This may significantly slow drug metabolism, resulting in a longer half-life of the drug.

METFORMIN (Glucophage, Glumetza, Riomet) Fact Sheet [G]

Bottom Line:

Metformin is a medication for type 2 diabetes that increases insulin sensitivity and decreases appetite. It's somewhat effective for antipsychotic-induced weight gain (average of 3 kg weight loss) and might work better if started prophylactically as a way to prevent excessive weight gain in the first place. It's quite safe and well tolerated (with some GI side effects) and is becoming a standard add-on treatment in patients taking clozapine or olanzapine.

FDA Indications:

Diabetes mellitus, type 2.

Off-Label Uses:

Antipsychotic-induced weight gain; polycystic ovary syndrome; prediabetes; female infertility.

Dosage Forms:

- **Tablets (G):** 500 mg, 850 mg, 1000 mg.
- **ER tablets (Glucophage XR, Glumetza, [G]):** 500 mg, 750 mg, 1000 mg.
- **Oral solution (Riomet, [G]):** 500 mg/5 mL.

Dosage Guidance:

- IR: Start 500 mg BID; ↑ by 500 mg/day increments weekly; max 2250 mg/day.
- ER: Start 500 mg QPM; ↑ by 500 mg/day increments weekly; max 2000 mg/day.
- ER formulation is preferred because it minimizes GI side effects. Better tolerated with taken with meals.

Monitoring: No routine monitoring recommended unless clinical picture warrants.

Cost: $; liquid: $$$

Side Effects:

- Most common: Diarrhea; nausea; abdominal bloating, flatulence, and discomfort.
- Serious but rare: Rare cases of lactic acidosis reported.

Mechanism, Pharmacokinetics, and Drug Interactions:

- Decreases glucose production by liver and increases insulin sensitivity.
- Not metabolized; excreted primarily through kidneys; t ½: 4–9 hours.
- Minimal clinically significant drug interactions.

Clinical Pearls:

- In psychiatry, metformin is used primarily to prevent or reverse weight gain in patients taking certain antipsychotic medications. The best-studied and most widely used dose is 500–1000 mg BID, which typically produces an average of 3 kg of weight loss in patients.
- A recent meta-analysis of 12 studies, representing a total of 743 patients, found metformin use resulted in more weight loss (an average of about 7 lbs) and BMI reduction than placebo in patients taking antipsychotics (de Silva VA et al, *BMC Psychiatry* 2016;16:341).
- Another review of patients with schizophrenia who were treated with antipsychotics found metformin also improved insulin resistance and decreased lipids (Mizuno Y et al, *Schiz Bull* 2014;40(6):1385–1403).
- Taking with food or using XR formulation helps to minimize the nausea and diarrhea that occurs in up to 50% of patients.
- Adjust dose in patients with eGFR less than 60 mL/minute (see Appendix H for guidance).

Fun Fact:

Metformin was introduced in the US in 1995, but it's been used in France since 1957.

TETRABENAZINE (Xenazine) Fact Sheet

Bottom Line:
Tetrabenazine was the original VMAT inhibitor brought to market and approved for the treatment of Huntington's disease. It's an off-label alternative to deutetrabenazine and valbenazine for treating tardive dyskinesia (TD). Although it's much less expensive, it requires more frequent dosing and may have a higher likelihood of causing depression.

FDA Indications:
Huntington's chorea.

Off-Label Uses:
TD; Tourette's and other tic disorders.

Dosage Forms:
Tablets: 12.5 mg, 25 mg.

Dosage Guidance:
Start 12.5 mg QAM for one week. Titrate at weekly intervals by 12.5 mg/day increments; increase to maximum dose of 100 mg/day. Should be given in divided doses of BID to QID with no more than 25 mg/dose.

Monitoring: ECG if cardiac disease.

Cost: $$

Side Effects:
- Most common: Sedation, somnolence, fatigue, diarrhea.
- Serious but rare: Risk of depression and suicidality; QT interval prolongation; caution in those with increased risk (congenital long QT syndrome, electrolyte disturbances, poor 2D6 metabolizers, concomitant 2D6 inhibitors).

Mechanism, Pharmacokinetics, and Drug Interactions:
- Reversible inhibitor of vesicular monoamine transporter 2 (VMAT2). This prevents VMAT2 from transporting monoamines including dopamine back into presynaptic vesicles, resulting in metabolism of monoamines, ultimately leading to depletion of monoamine stores and less dopamine being around. This treats TD symptoms, which are likely caused by hypersensitivity to dopamine.
- Metabolized primarily by CYP450 2D6; t ½: 5–7 hours.
- Avoid MAOIs. Decrease tetrabenazine dose in presence of 2D6 inhibitors or poor metabolizers.

Clinical Pearls:
- One double-blind study and seven open-label studies support the efficacy of tetrabenazine for TD.
- Increased depression and suicidality have been reported with tetrabenazine; use caution in patients with a history of depression and monitor all patients for symptoms.
- Genotyping for 2D6 metabolism is recommended for doses >50 mg/day.

Fun Fact:
Tetrabenazine was initially developed in the 1950s as an antipsychotic to replace reserpine because it had less severe depressive and hypotensive effects.

TRIHEXYPHENIDYL (Artane) Fact Sheet [G]

Bottom Line:

Trihexyphenidyl is an anticholinergic medication that is less favored than benztropine because it must be dosed TID and is only available in oral formulations. Use as a second-line option.

FDA Indications:

Drug-induced extrapyramidal symptoms (EPS); Parkinson's disease.

Off-Label Uses:

Sialorrhea (excessive salivation); hyperhidrosis (excessive sweating).

Dosage Forms:

• **Tablets (G):** 2 mg, 5 mg.
• **Oral solution:** 2 mg/5 mL.

Dosage Guidance:

Start 2 mg QD; ↑ by 2 mg/day increments every three to five days as needed, up to maximum 5 mg TID.

Monitoring: No routine monitoring recommended unless clinical picture warrants.

Cost: $

Side Effects:

• Most common: Dry mouth, blurred vision, constipation, urinary retention, sedation.
• Serious but rare: In those at risk (elderly patients), may cause confusion or delirium; may worsen angle-closure glaucoma.

Mechanism, Pharmacokinetics, and Drug Interactions:

• Anticholinergic, antihistaminergic.
• Metabolized primarily through liver via unknown P450; t ½: 3–4 hours.
• Minimal clinically significant drug interactions; avoid combining with other anticholinergic agents due to additive effects.

Clinical Pearl:

If starting a patient on a high-potency antipsychotic such as haloperidol or risperidone, some clinicians will start trihexyphenidyl prophylactically to prevent EPS. If you do so, consider taper and withdrawal of trihexyphenidyl after one or two weeks to see if it's really needed.

Fun Fact:

There have been many reports of recreational use of trihexyphenidyl over the years: by Iraqi soldiers and police to relieve combat stress, as a more intense substitute for LSD in the 1960s, and by the late Oliver Sacks, who reportedly took 20 trihexyphenidyl pills and hallucinated an entire conversation with friends (check out his book, *Hallucinations*, to read about his experimentation with a range of drugs).

VALBENAZINE (Ingrezza) Fact Sheet

Bottom Line:
Valbenazine was the first of the VMAT inhibitors to be approved for the treatment of tardive dyskinesia (TD) in 2017. Its advantage over off-label tetrabenazine is less frequent dosing (once daily) and less likelihood of causing depression. However, it is extremely expensive—about $6,000/month as opposed to $400/month for tetrabenazine.

FDA Indications:
TD.

Off-Label Uses:
Tourette's and other tic disorders; Huntington's chorea.

Dosage Forms:
Capsules: 40 mg, 60 mg, 80 mg.

Dosage Guidance:
Start 40 mg once daily. After one week, ↑ to usual dose of 80 mg once daily.

Monitoring: ECG if cardiac disease.

Cost: $$$$$

Side Effects:
- Most common: Sedation, somnolence, akathisia, restlessness.
- Serious but rare: QT interval prolongation; caution in those with increased risk (congenital long QT syndrome, electrolyte disturbances, poor 2D6 metabolizers, concomitant 2D6 or 3A4 inhibitors).

Mechanism, Pharmacokinetics, and Drug Interactions:
- Reversible inhibitor of vesicular monoamine transporter 2 (VMAT2). This prevents VMAT2 from transporting monoamines including dopamine back into presynaptic vesicles, resulting in metabolism of monoamines, ultimately leading to depletion of monoamine stores and less dopamine being around. This treats TD symptoms, which are likely caused by hypersensitivity to dopamine.
- Metabolized by CYP450 2D6 and 3A4 (primary); t ½: 15–22 hours.
- Avoid MAOIs. Decrease valbenazine dose in presence of 2D6 or 3A4 inhibitors.

Clinical Pearls:
- Clinical trials of valbenazine for TD found an impressive 40% response rate (meaning a 50% improvement in TD symptoms) vs a 9% response rate for patients taking placebo.
- Increased depression and suicidality have been reported with use of a similar VMAT2 inhibitor, tetrabenazine (Xenazine, used for Huntington's chorea). Paucity of long-term data with valbenazine makes it difficult to determine whether this will be of concern with valbenazine as well.
- A one-year course costs over $72,000.

Fun Fact:
Reserpine, an antihypertensive and antipsychotic used in the 1950s, was a VMAT1/VMAT2 inhibitor. Cases of depression reported with its use led to the monoamine hypothesis of depression.

Side Effect Management:

SYMPTOMS

Akathisia

Characteristics: A sense of restlessness, causing the patient to appear fidgety, to have difficulty sitting still, and to rock from one leg to the other while standing. It can present as an inner sense of restlessness without obvious movement. Can lead to agitation and even suicidal ideation.

Meds That Cause It: Antipsychotics, especially high-potency first-generation antipsychotics (such as haloperidol), but second-generation agents may also cause it (especially aripiprazole, brexpiprazole, paliperidone, risperidone). Occasionally SSRIs and buspirone.

Mechanism: D2 blockade.

General Management:
- Reduce dose.
- Switch to lower-potency first-generation or second-generation agent with lower potential for akathisia (see Table 10).

First-Line Medications:
- Propranolol (Inderal). Start 10 mg BID; ↑ by 10–20 mg/day increments; can go up to 30–90 mg daily in two or three divided doses. SE: Dizziness, fatigue, syncope, low BP.
- Inderal LA. Long-acting version of propranolol that can be dosed once a day. 60–80 mg daily.
- Benzodiazepines. Any of them will work (eg, lorazepam [Ativan] 0.5–1 mg BID). Dosed at the equivalent of diazepam (Valium) 10 mg BID or more frequently as needed.

Second-Line Medications:
- Benztropine (Cogentin) 1 mg BID.
- Cyproheptadine (Periactin) 8–16 mg/day.
- Amantadine (Symmetrel) 100–200 mg BID.
- Clonidine (Klonopin) 0.2–0.8 mg/day.
- Gabapentin (Neurontin) 1200 mg/day.
- Trazodone (Desyrel) 100 mg/day.
- Mirtazapine (Remeron) 15 mg/day.

Clinical Pearls:
- May manifest in a number of ways, such as pacing, inability to sit still, crossing and uncrossing one's legs, rocking back and forth, or other purposeless repetitive motions; patients may complain of crawling feeling under skin or "shocks."
- Don't confuse akathisia with agitation due to the underlying psychiatric disorder—you might make the mistake of increasing the antipsychotic, thus worsening the akathisia.
- Risk factors include high dose, high-potency antipsychotics, and rapid dose escalation; use of caffeine, other stimulants, or illicit drugs may also exacerbate akathisia.
- May appear within first few hours of antipsychotic exposure, but usually takes days to weeks to appear.
- Can occur in a tardive form, with symptoms lasting for greater than six months after discontinuation of the offending agent.
- Clozapine and quetiapine cause no more akathisia than placebo.

Fun Fact:
Akathisia is from the Greek *a-kathisis*, "no sitting." The English word "cathedral" is from the same root: *Kathedra* is a bishop's seat or throne, while a cathedral is a church in which the bishop's seat is placed.

Bruxism

Characteristics: Involuntary grinding of teeth, which especially occurs during sleep but can also occur in the daytime. In 5% of cases this can cause severe health problems, such as destruction of tooth structure, temporomandibular joint dysfunction, myofascial pain, and sleep disturbances.

Meds That Cause It: A variety of medications, including antidepressants (especially SSRIs and the SNRI venlafaxine), psychostimulants, and antipsychotics; drugs of abuse such as methamphetamine, cocaine, and ecstasy.

Mechanism: Unclear, but likely involves central dopaminergic and serotonergic systems.

General Management:

- Reduce dose or switch medication.
- Wear dental guards at night.
- Treat anxiety, which worsens bruxism.
- Decrease or stop using tobacco, caffeine, and alcohol.

First-Line Medications:

Buspirone (BuSpar) 10 mg BID or TID.

Second-Line Medications:

- Benzodiazepines, such as clonazepam (Klonopin) 0.5–1 mg at bedtime.
- Gabapentin (Neurontin) 300 mg QHS.

Clinical Pearls:

- Frequency of bruxism varies from day to day, but symptoms are usually induced or worsened by anxiety and stress.
- Watching and waiting may be indicated as spontaneous remission can occur after one month.
- Botulinum toxin (Botox) injections into the masseter muscle are effective for persistent bruxism.
- Risk factors include obstructive sleep apnea and parasomnias, anxiety, heavy alcohol use, loud snoring, caffeine intake, smoking, and other psychiatric and neurologic disorders.

Fun Fact:

People with bruxism are referred to as "bruxists" or "bruxers."

Constipation

Characteristics: Straining to have bowel movements, often with hard stools, and a sensation of incomplete evacuation. Not necessarily infrequent stools—patients may have a bowel movement every day, but if they strain, they are constipated.

Meds That Cause It: Antipsychotics (especially clozapine and olanzapine, but all can cause it); antidepressants, including SSRIs (particularly paroxetine); SNRIs; mirtazapine; tricyclics; benztropine; antihistamines (eg, diphenhydramine, hydroxyzine); opiates.

Mechanism: Usually due to anticholinergic effects, which lead to decrease in bowel motility.

General Management:
- Decrease dose or switch agents.
- Increase fluid intake.
- Increase dietary fiber (cereals, fruits, bran) and eat prunes.
- Increase physical activity.

First-Line Medications:
- Bulk-forming laxative (SE: Gas, bloating):
  - Psyllium (Metamucil) or methylcellulose (Citrucel) one tablespoon three times daily.
  - Avoid in patients taking clozapine as it may increase risk of perforation in slow-transit constipation.
- Stool softener (SE: Diarrhea):
  - Docusate sodium (Colace) 100–250 mg twice daily. Must be taken with full glass of water.

Second-Line Medications:
- Osmotic laxatives (SE: Bloating, gas, watery stools):
  - Lactulose (Kristalose) 15–30 mL daily or every other day.
  - Polyethylene glycol solution (MiraLax) 8–34 g in eight ounces of fluid.
  - Magnesium citrate 150–300 mL daily.
- Stimulant laxatives (SE: Diarrhea, cramps):
  - Sennosides (Ex-Lax, Senokot), available in different formulations (usual dose is one to two 8.6 mg tablets QD to BID as needed).
  - Bisacodyl (Dulcolax), available as suppository (usual dose is 5–15 mg daily, max 30 mg/day).
  - Magnesium hydroxide (milk of magnesia) 30–60 mL QD as needed (available also in chewable tablet form).

Clinical Pearl:
Constipation can be caused by various illnesses, including irritable bowel syndrome (usually diarrhea interspersed with constipation), hypothyroidism, and colon cancer (red flags include blood in stool and weight loss).

Fun Fact:
According to a crossover trial of 40 patients, prunes worked better than psyllium, producing more spontaneous bowel movements (3.5 vs 2.8 per week) and better stool consistency (Attaluri A, *Aliment Pharmacol Ther* 2011;33(7):822).

Diarrhea

Characteristics: Passing of loose or watery stools, at least three times in a 24-hour period. Often due to infectious etiology (eg, rotovirus, norovirus, adenoviruses, *E. coli*) but can occur as a side effect to medications. Most cases resolve with routine over-the-counter treatment.

Meds That Cause It: Antibiotics, proton pump inhibitors, donepezil, galantamine, memantine, rivastigmine, sertraline, acamprosate, lithium, stool softeners and other laxatives, rapid discontinuation of anticholinergic agents (cholinergic rebound).

Mechanism: Increased water content of stool, usually due to impaired water absorption and/or active water secretion by the bowel.

General Management:

• Push fluids and suggest dietary adjustments like the BRAT diet (bananas, rice, applesauce, and toast). Avoid high-fat foods.

• Get a travel and food history.

• Ask about recent antibiotic use.

• Assess for serotonin syndrome (presence of mental status changes, hyperthermia, hyperreflexia, autonomic instability).

• If on lithium, check serum lithium level for toxicity.

First-Line Medications:

• Antimotility agents: Loperamide (Imodium) two tablets (4 mg) initially, then 2 mg after each loose stool for no more than two days with a max dose of 16 mg/day. Avoid if fever or blood in stool.

• Bismuth salicylate (Pepto-Bismol) 30 mL or two tablets every 30 minutes, up to eight doses.

Second-Line Medications:

• Diphenoxylate/atropine (Lomotil) is an alternative antimotility agent that binds to opioid receptors in the gut. Start two tablets QID for no more than two days.

Clinical Pearls:

• Loperamide is also an agonist at opioid receptors in the gut; misuse and abuse of this over-the-counter drug has increased in recent years. Those using opioids know it can help with withdrawal-related diarrhea. Some have discovered that in high doses (100–200 mg/day), it can produce euphoria. In rare cases, high dose use has resulted in hospitalization for arrhythmias and death.

• If persistent, bloody, or accompanied by severe pain or volume depletion (dry mucous membranes, low BP), refer for further evaluation including need for stool testing.

Fun Fact:

Clear liquids like water, ginger ale, and electrolyte-rich sports drinks (eg, Gatorade) are often recommended for fluid repletion during bouts of diarrhea. Probiotic drinks may help too.

Dry Mouth (Xerostomia)

Characteristics: An uncomfortable sensation of dryness due to diminished saliva; can lead to dental caries, because saliva has an antibacterial effect. Can also cause decreased taste and inflammation of gums.

Meds That Cause It: Most psychotropic meds, especially antipsychotics, antidepressants (including SSRIs), lithium, psychostimulants, and medications used to treat or prevent extrapyramidal symptoms (benztropine, diphenhydramine, trihexyphenidyl).

Mechanism: Anticholinergic and other effects.

General Management:
- Encourage aggressive oral hygiene, including more frequent dental cleanings.
- Chew sugarless gum to stimulate saliva production (especially gum containing xylitol, which can also reduce dental caries).
- Sip water frequently.
- Suck on ice chips.

First-Line Medications:
- Biotene line of products, over the counter (most contain lubricants and humectants to "seal in" moisture):
  - Biotene gum, use as needed.
  - Biotene toothpaste, use as with any toothpaste.
  - Biotene oral rinse (mouthwash), rinse up to five times per day.
  - Biotene Oralbalance Gel, use one inch on tongue as needed (comes out of a tube).
  - Biotene moisturizing mouth spray, spray on tongue as needed.
- Many saliva substitutes are available, such as Oralube saliva substitute, Oasis mouth spray, and others. No studies have demonstrated superiority of any single brand.

Second-Line Medications:
- Procholinergic drugs:
  - Pilocarpine (Salagen) 5–10 mg two or three times daily (SE: Sweating, congestion, diarrhea; start with 2.5 mg test dose to ensure tolerability).
  - Cevimeline (Evoxac) 30 mg up to three times daily.

Clinical Pearls:
- Caffeine can worsen dry mouth, so recommend decreasing caffeine use.
- Don't shy away from trying procholinergic drugs—some patients prefer them over having to constantly use saliva substitute products.

Fun Fact:
Medications are often blamed, particularly in older patients, but aging itself is a common cause of dry mouth.

Dystonia

Characteristics: Involuntary contractions of muscles due to some antipsychotics. Can include torticollis (twisting neck), opisthotonos (arching spine or neck), oculogyric crisis (eyes rolling back), and trismus (jaw clenching). Rare but serious is tongue swelling, which can block the airway or cause choking when eating.

Meds That Cause It: Antipsychotics, especially high-potency first-generation antipsychotics. May rarely occur with second-generation antipsychotics.

Mechanism: D2 blockade.

First-Line Medications (give these IM or IV if dystonia is severe):
- Benztropine (Cogentin) 1–2 mg once or twice per day (SE: Dry mouth, blurred vision, constipation, urinary retention, and cognitive changes).
- Diphenhydramine (Benadryl) 50 mg/day.
- If dystonia is severe, stop the offending drug, and give either of the above agents IM or IV once or twice to stop the dystonia. Then prescribe two to three days of the oral version to prevent another episode.

Second-Line Medications:
- Benzodiazepines (especially diazepam [Valium] 5–10 mg).
- Amantadine (Symmetrel) 100–200 mg BID (no injectable available).
- Trihexyphenidyl (Artane) 1–2 mg TID (no injectable available).

Clinical Pearls:
- Earliest of the extrapyramidal symptoms, with an onset of hours to days after antipsychotic is started or dose is increased; 90% of reactions occur within first five days.
- Risk factors include young male patients, high-potency first-generation antipsychotics, or high dose.
- Prophylaxis with anticholinergic agent for first month of treatment in those with high risk or previous history.
- May be very frightening and painful for the patient.
- Can occur in a tardive form, with symptoms lasting for greater than six months after discontinuation of the offending agent.

Fun Fact:

Dystonia has many causes other than antipsychotics, and it is the third most common movement disorder in the United States, following essential tremor and Parkinson's disease. Neurologists use botulinum toxin (Botox) to treat some dystonias, especially cervical dystonias.

Excessive Sweating (Hyperhidrosis)

Characteristics: Excessive sweating, which tends to be more prominent in the face, neck, and chest, and less prominent in the armpits and palms.

Meds That Cause It: Antidepressants, especially SNRIs (venlafaxine, duloxetine, levomilnacipran) and bupropion.

Mechanism: Dysregulation of cholinergically innervated sweat glands.

General Management:
Reduce dose or switch agents.

First-Line Medications:
- Terazosin (Hytrin) alpha-1 blocker; start 1 mg at bedtime, then gradually ↑ by 1 mg/day increments up to 4–6 mg (SE: Dizziness, dry mouth, hypotension, rebound hypertension if stopped abruptly).
- Clonidine (Catapres) 0.1 mg daily.
- Benztropine (Cogentin) 1 mg BID.
- Glycopyrrolate (Robinul); start 1 mg twice daily and ↑ gradually by 1 mg/day increments up to 2 mg three times a day. Can be used PRN.

Second-Line Medications:
- Oxybutynin (Ditropan) 5–10 mg daily or twice daily.
- Mirtazapine (Remeron) up to 60 mg daily as adjunct.
- Cyproheptadine (Periactin) 4 mg daily or twice daily.
- Aripiprazole (Abilify) 10 mg daily (one trial showed it alleviated hyperhidrosis due to fluoxetine or duloxetine).

Clinical Pearls:
- Patients may not need to take medication for sweating in the winter.
- Often occurs in people who tended to sweat a lot before taking the medication.

Fun Fact:
Glycopyrrolate is so effective at reducing sweating that the label warns it can reduce the body's ability to cool off by sweating—which, in very high temperatures, can cause fever and heatstroke.

Fatigue

Characteristics: Sleepiness as a result of medications, usually due to antidepressants. Typically, patients say they sleep more than enough at night, yet they feel like they could fall asleep at any point throughout the day.

Meds That Cause It: Antidepressants (especially paroxetine, mirtazapine, and tricyclics; bupropion is *least* likely to cause fatigue); antipsychotics (especially clozapine, quetiapine, olanzapine, ziprasidone, but all can cause it); mood stabilizers; benztropine; antihistamines (eg, diphenhydramine, hydroxyzine); opiates.

Mechanism: Various mechanisms, often due to antihistamine or anticholinergic effects.

General Management:
- Watchful waiting for spontaneous resolution (not usually effective).
- Change dosing to bedtime.
- Reduce dose.

Medications:
- If not clinically contraindicated, psychostimulants such as methylphenidate or dextroamphetamine. Depending on the response, you may switch to a long-acting stimulant eventually.
- Modafinil (Provigil) 100–300 mg daily in divided doses.
- Armodafinil (Nuvigil) 150–250 mg daily in divided doses.
- If a serotonergic antidepressant is causing fatigue, consider switching to bupropion.

Clinical Pearls:
- Rule out common non-medication causes of fatigue, such as obstructive sleep apnea, hypothyroidism, and anemia.
- Fatigue can be a residual symptom of partially treated depression.
- If patients are taking a benzodiazepine for anxiety or insomnia, this could be causing daytime fatigue. Consider decreasing the dose or switching to a different agent.

Fun Fact:
Some consider the US to be the most overworked developed country. The number of hours Americans work (86% of men and 67% of women work more than 40 hours weekly) and the absence of a national paid parental leave benefit contribute to this distinction, as does the lack of federal laws requiring maximum work week length, paid sick leave, or vacation days. No wonder so many experience fatigue.

Nausea

Characteristics: Nausea or sensation of upset stomach beginning soon after first dose of a new medication.

Meds That Cause It: Serotonergic antidepressants (especially vilazodone and vortioxetine), lithium, valproic acid, naltrexone.

Mechanism: Various; may be related to stimulation of 5-HT3 receptors.

General Management:
- Reduce dose.
- Wait one or two weeks, since nausea is often transient.
- Switch to a nonserotonergic antidepressant.
- Start drug at half the usual dose and go up gradually.
- Take medication just after meals.
- Split the dose into BID or TID dosing.
- Switch to a delayed-release, extended-release, or enteric-coated formulation, if available (eg, valproic acid, lithium).
- Take a spoonful of peanut butter before taking the medication.

Medications (SE: Most well tolerated especially when used PRN; sedation common with many):
- Ginger root capsules two to three times per day, two capsules per dose.
- Trimethobenzamide (Tigan) 300 mg TID PRN.
- Promethazine (Phenergan) 12.5–25 mg BID PRN.
- Ondansetron (Zofran) 4–8 mg Q8 hours PRN (5-HT3 blocker).
- Mirtazapine (Remeron) 15 mg daily (5-HT3 blocker).
- Metoclopramide (Reglan) 10 mg three times a day as needed.
- Prochlorperazine (Compazine) 5–10 mg Q8 hours PRN.

Clinical Pearls:
- Both metoclopramide and prochlorperazine are phenothiazines and, like others in that class, may cause extrapyramidal symptoms if continued for too long.
- Patients with preexisting GERD may be more susceptible to med-induced nausea. Try prescribing a proton pump inhibitor, such as omeprazole (Prilosec), along with the offending agent.

Fun Fact:
Antipsychotics rarely cause nausea—in fact, several are FDA-approved antiemetics.

Neuroleptic Malignant Syndrome (NMS)

Characteristics: A rare but potentially life-threatening drug reaction presenting with muscle rigidity ("lead pipe"), hyperthermia, and altered mental status. May present similarly to serotonin syndrome although may be less acute in onset (within days vs hours).

Meds That Cause It: Antipsychotics. Occasionally other antidopaminergic medications (eg, metoclopramide).

Mechanism: D2 blockade.

General Management:

- Discontinue antidopaminergic agents.
- Monitor vital signs and creatinine kinase levels to assess severity and to guide supportive care, including stabilizing vital signs and intravenous fluids if necessary.

First-Line Medications:

Benzodiazepines. Any of them will work (eg, lorazepam [Ativan] 0.5–1 mg BID or diazepam [Valium] 10 mg BID).

Second-Line Medications:

- Bromocriptine (Parlodel) 2.5–5 mg Q6–8 hours.
- For severe rigidity, dantrolene (Dantrium) 3–5 mg/kg IV divided TID or 100–400 mg/day oral divided QID. Monitor liver function.
- Bromocriptine or dantrolene should be continued for 10 days beyond symptom resolution.

Clinical Pearls:

- Most cases, especially if caught early, will resolve quickly after antipsychotic discontinuation.
- Avoid bromocriptine if serotonin syndrome is not ruled out (eg, patient taking both antipsychotics and serotonergic agents). Bromocriptine has some proserotonergic activity and could worsen serotonin syndrome.
- Up to 50% of patients who have experienced NMS may have another episode. To minimize risk of recurrence in patients who require ongoing antipsychotic therapy, wait until symptoms have completely resolved (at least two weeks). Choose a different agent, ideally a second-generation antipsychotic as they are less likely to cause NMS. Never use a long-acting antipsychotic injection in patients with a history of NMS.

Fun Fact:

Mortality rates from NMS had previously been reported to be as high as 20%–38%. In more recent years, the mortality rate has fallen to below 10%. This has been attributed to earlier recognition and better management.

Orthostatic Hypotension (Postural Hypotension)

Characteristics: Orthostatic hypotension (OH) is caused by blood pooling in the lower extremities when people stand up, causing less blood flow to the brain and consequent dizziness. Usually caused by medications that block the alpha-1 receptors, which are responsible for telling the body to constrict blood vessels (and maintain blood pressure) after standing up. Patients will report feeling faint when they get up, and occasionally a sense of the room spinning (vertigo).

Meds That Cause It: Antipsychotics, especially clozapine, risperidone, quetiapine, and lower-potency first-generation agents. Antidepressants, especially tricyclics, MAOIs, trazodone, sometimes mirtazapine.

Mechanism: Alpha-1 receptor blockade, also anticholinergic effects.

General Management:
- Review all meds, including nonpsychiatric, since many blood pressure and cardiac meds, as well as alpha blockers like prazosin (Minipress) and tamsulosin (Flomax) used for benign prostatic hyperplasia, can cause OH.
- Start at lower dose and titrate more slowly, especially when using higher-risk agents in higher-risk patients.
- Change dosing to minimize peak blood levels (eg, split dosing or switch to an extended-release version).
- Instruct patient to stand up slowly.
- Prevent dehydration by drinking enough fluids.
- Use compression stockings, also known as TED stockings.
- Increase salt intake (if no hypertension).
- Limit alcohol use.

Medications:
- Fludrocortisone (Florinef) 0.1 mg daily; can ↑ by 0.1 mg/day increments weekly to 0.3 mg daily. SE: Hypokalemia. Use only in severe cases where other measures have not worked.
- Midodrine 10 mg three times daily. SE: Goose bumps, paresthesias. Use only in severe cases where other measures have not worked.

Clinical Pearls:
- OH is defined as a 20 mm drop in systolic pressure or a 10 mm drop in diastolic pressure within three minutes of a patient moving from lying to standing position.
- Ask patients when the symptom is worse; if it is worse an hour or two after taking the medication, it is most likely medication induced.
- More common and problematic in elderly; may contribute to fall risk.

Fun Fact:
A recent epidemiologic observational study out of Johns Hopkins, following nearly 12,000 individuals over 20 years, recently suggested that OH in middle age increases risk of cognitive decline and later dementia.

Parkinsonism

Characteristics: Also known as pseudoparkinsonism, these drug-induced symptoms mimic those of Parkinson's disease:

- Tremor (especially apparent in the hands as a resting, "pill rolling" tremor).
- Rigidity (cog-wheel rigidity).
- Bradykinesia (slow movement), decreased arm swing.
- Shuffling gait.
- Slurred speech.
- Mask-like facies, stooped posture, drooling.
- Psychological side effects, such as cognitive dulling (bradyphrenia), worse negative symptoms (neuroleptic-induced deficit syndrome), worse depression (neuroleptic dysphoria).

Meds That Cause It: Antipsychotics, especially first-generation agents, but second-generation antipsychotics may also cause it. Least likely to cause it are clozapine, olanzapine, quetiapine, and ziprasidone.

Mechanism: D2 blockade, disruption of the balance between dopaminergic vs cholinergic neurons.

General Management:

Decrease dose or switch to a different antipsychotic.

First-Line Medications:

- Benztropine (Cogentin) 1–2 mg once or twice per day.
- Trihexyphenidyl (Artane) 2–5 mg once or twice per day.
- Diphenhydramine (Benadryl) 50 mg/day.

Second-Line Medications:

Amantadine (Symmetrel) 100–200 mg twice per day (enhances dopamine release).

Clinical Pearls:

- May occur at any time, but typically seen within one to two months after antipsychotic is initiated.
- Highest-risk patients: Female, older, those taking higher-potency agents or higher doses.
- In patients at high risk of parkinsonism, start benztropine (or one of the other first-line agents) at the same time as starting the antipsychotic.
- Try discontinuing the anticholinergic agent after several weeks; many patients will not need to remain on it long term.

Fun Fact:

Parkinson's disease is named after Dr. James Parkinson (1755–1824), the doctor who first identified the condition. It's caused by loss of neurons in the substantia nigra, where most dopamine is produced.

Prolactinemia

Characteristics: Elevated prolactin levels (>29 ng/mL in nonpregnant, nonlactating women, >18 ng/mL in men) that can cause the following symptoms:

- Women: Menstrual irregularity or amenorrhea, infertility, lowered libido, galactorrhea, decreased bone density, increase or thickening of hair in unexpected areas such as face.
- Men: Breast enlargement (gynecomastia), erectile dysfunction, low libido, infertility, galactorrhea.

Meds That Cause It: Antipsychotics, especially risperidone, paliperidone, and haloperidol. Other potential medications that cause it include estrogen, metoclopramide, and verapamil. Other causes: Hypothyroidism, pregnancy, kidney disease, polycystic ovarian syndrome, pituitary adenoma.

Mechanism: D2 blockade.

General Management:

- Reduce dose or discontinue offending medication. Prolactin levels normalize within two to four days after discontinuation.
- Switch to a different agent (eg, aripiprazole, quetiapine).

First-Line Medications (if stopping the causative drug is not feasible):

Add aripiprazole 5–20 mg daily.

Second-Line Medications:

- Add a dopamine agonist, such as cabergoline (Dostinex) 0.25 mg twice a week (*not* twice a day) or bromocriptine (Parlodel) 1.25–2.5 mg daily.
- Add an oral contraceptive agent to prevent bone loss in women and treat testosterone deficiency in men (it does not treat hyperprolactinemia).

Clinical Pearls:

- Risperidone is the drug that causes the highest elevation, up to 300–400 mg/mL, whereas other drugs rarely cause elevations higher than 100 ng/mL.
- If your patient has a mild elevation (such as up to 40 ng/mL), get another level, but this time make sure it's a fasting level. Mild elevation can be caused by stress.
- While galactorrhea is often mentioned in discussions of high prolactin, this is a pretty rare symptom, much less common than amenorrhea, low libido, and infertility.
- Patients with levels >100 ng/mL are generally referred for an MRI to rule out a pituitary adenoma, even if they are taking a drug known to increase prolactin.
- Use lowest effective dose of dopaminergic agent as higher doses may worsen psychosis.

Fun Fact:

While prolactin's main function is to promote breast milk during lactation, it has other functions, such as promoting weight gain and modulating anxiety. Some research shows that men have increased prolactin when they become fathers.

QT Interval Prolongation

Characteristics: The QT interval in the cardiac cycle represents depolarization (contraction) and repolarization (relaxation) of ventricles (these interval times are corrected to account for variations in heart rate, specified as "QTc").

Classification	QTc Adult Women (msec)	QTc Adult Men (msec)
Normal	<450	<430
Borderline	451–470	431–450
Prolonged	>470	>450

QT prolongation can lead to serious arrhythmias, including torsades de pointes (TdP), and sudden death. While the link between QT and TdP is not clear, QTc above 500 msec is a significant risk factor for TdP.

Meds That Cause It: First-generation antipsychotics (especially thioridazine, high doses of chlorpromazine, and intravenous haloperidol). Of second-generation antipsychotics, ziprasidone has greatest risk of prolonging QT, though to a lower degree. Of SSRIs, higher-dose citalopram (>40 mg/day) most likely. Of tricyclic antidepressants, amitriptyline and maprotiline. Methadone. In overdose, a large number of medications can prolong QT. A good resource to keep on hand: www.crediblemeds.org (free but requires registration).

Mechanism: The mechanism depends on the offending drug. For example, TCAs prolong the QT through blockade of sodium and calcium channels, while citalopram and chlorpromazine do so through blockade of potassium channels.

Management:
- Prevent: Identify risk factors (see below), get baseline electrolytes, ECG, and monitor periodically in patients at risk.
- Manage reversible factors such as repleting electrolytes, hydration.
- With prolonged QTc (>500 msec), obtain a cardiologist consult.
- In patients with a borderline QTc, switch to a less risky agent.
  - Lower-risk antipsychotics: Aripiprazole has minimal risk; asenapine, lurasidone, olanzapine, and quetiapine are also good options.
  - Lower-risk antidepressants: All antidepressants at usual therapeutic doses are relatively safe (avoid citalopram >40 mg/day). However, sertraline may be the best choice because it is the most studied in cardiac patients and has few drug interactions.

Clinical Pearls:
- Risk factors: Congenital (long QT syndrome), female gender, older age, electrolyte abnormalities (low potassium, calcium, magnesium), and other conditions such as hepatic dysfunction, diabetes, hypothyroidism, AIDS, and hypertension.
- Heart conditions that increase a patient's risk are bradycardia, left ventricular dysfunction, heart failure, mitral valve prolapse, and myocardial infarction.
- Caution in situations that may affect electrolytes, including eating disorders, diuretic use, hypoglycemia, renal dysfunction, and pituitary insufficiency.
- Other common medications that are not related to psychiatry can also be culprits, including antiarrhythmics such as sotalol, amiodarone, and quinidine; macrolide antibiotics such as azithromycin; quinolone antibiotics such as levofloxacin; some antifungals; antimalarials; and other medications such as tamoxifen.
- Overdose with psychotropic medication, even "low risk" agents, can lead to QT prolongation.

Fun Fact:
Torsades de pointes translates to "twisting of the points," illustrating the chaotic nature of the heart rhythm that can lead to sudden death.

Serotonin Syndrome

Characteristics: A rare but potentially life-threatening drug reaction that can range from mild to severe. Presents with muscle rigidity (typically hypertonicity, hyperreflexia, clonus), hyperthermia, and altered mental status. While very similar to neuroleptic malignant syndrome (NMS) in presentation, serotonin syndrome typically has a much more acute onset (drastic change from baseline within three to four hours).

Meds That Cause It: Any drugs that can increase serotonin activity either with increased serotonin release, inhibition of serotonin metabolism, inhibition of serotonin reuptake, or activation of serotonin receptors. Most common culprits include MAOIs, SSRIs, SNRIs, buspirone, lithium. Consider nonpsychiatric medications that can have serotonergic effects (eg, fentanyl, meperidine, tramadol, linezolid, dextromethorphan).

Mechanism: Excess serotonergic activity.

General Management:
- Discontinue any serotonergic medications.
- Consider differential diagnoses, including NMS.
- Monitor vital signs and creatinine kinase levels to assess severity and guide supportive care, including stabilizing vital signs and providing intravenous fluids if necessary.

First-Line Medications:
Benzodiazepines. Any of them will work (eg, lorazepam [Ativan] 0.5–1 mg BID or diazepam [Valium] 10 mg BID).

Second-Line Medications:
Cyproheptadine (Periactin) 12 mg followed by 2 mg Q2 hours until improvement, then 8 mg Q8 hours until resolution.

Clinical Pearls:
- The combination of triptans (eg, sumatriptan) and other serotonergic medications like SSRIs will often trigger an alert in your EMR or at the pharmacy. While triptans are serotonergic, they are fairly weakly serotonergic and typically taken sporadically. Hence, this combination is less likely to result in serotonin syndrome.
- Caution with CYP450 inhibitors, which can raise levels of serotonergic medications and thereby increase risk of serotonin syndrome.
- The most severe cases of serotonin syndrome often involve MAOIs combined with other serotonergic agents or overdose situations involving serotonergic drugs.
- Clonus is more specific to serotonin syndrome (vs "lead pipe" rigidity seen in NMS) and presents as involuntary, rhythmic muscle contractions. Clonus tends to happen more in the lower rather than upper extremities, so be sure to check the patient's legs (flex the patient's foot upward and look for a rhythmic beating of the foot and ankle).
- Avoid using cyproheptadine if anticholinergic syndrome cannot be ruled out as it may exacerbate.
- Patient may be restarted on serotonergic medication 24–48 hours after complete resolution, but limit number of serotonergic agents and use minimally effective dose.

Not-So-Fun Fact:
MDMA (ecstasy) in combination with SSRI can lead to serotonin syndrome. This has been a factor in a number of deaths, particularly in adolescents and young adults, at popular music festivals.

Sexual Dysfunction

Characteristics: Impairment of some aspect of sexual functioning, including low libido, anorgasmia, decreased sensation, erectile dysfunction, or delayed or retrograde ejaculation (in men).

Meds That Cause It: Antidepressants (paroxetine most likely, but all SSRIs and SNRIs can cause it); antipsychotics (primarily risperidone and paliperidone); some mood stabilizers (valproic acid and carbamazepine).

Mechanism: Various, including activation of 5-HT2 receptors by antidepressants; hyperprolactinemia by antipsychotics such as risperidone; and anticholinergic and antiadrenergic effects in other antipsychotics, especially first-generation.

General Management:
- Watchful waiting—works in 10%–20% of patients.
- Drug holiday—no dose Friday or Saturday, resume Sunday or Monday. (Not a good idea with paroxetine or venlafaxine due to discontinuation syndrome, nor with fluoxetine due to long half-life.)
- Decrease dose.
- Switch to a medication with low sexual side effects (eg, bupropion, mirtazapine, or an antipsychotic that does not affect prolactin).

First-Line Medications:
- Add a PDE-5 inhibitor, such as sildenafil (Viagra) or tadalafil (Cialis). Works best for erectile dysfunction, but may help with low libido as well. Less effective in women.
- Add bupropion (possibly more effective in women than men).

Second-Line Medications:
- Buspirone (BuSpar) 30–60 mg daily.
- Cyproheptadine (Periactin) 8 mg 30 minutes before sex.
- Amantadine (Symmetrel) 100 mg daily.

Clinical Pearl:
It can be hard to know if sexual dysfunction (SD) is caused by a medication, the underlying psychiatric condition, or a separate problem predating the medication. For this reason, you should try to obtain a sexual history in your patients before starting medications that can cause SD.

Fun Fact:
Early estimates of SD incidence from antidepressants were very low (in the range of 2%–16%) because researchers relied on spontaneous self-reporting. By contrast, in a prospective study of 1,022 outpatients, all of whom were asked specifically about sexual functioning, the authors estimated that SSRIs and venlafaxine caused rates of SD ranging from 58% to 73% (Montejo AL, *J Clin Psych* 2001;62 Suppl 3:10–21).

Sialorrhea (Hypersalivation)

Characteristics: Excessive drooling, usually more severe at night.

Meds That Cause It: Clozapine is the most common cause (30%–80% incidence). Can be caused by olanzapine, risperidone, or quetiapine.

Mechanism: Procholinergic effect.

General Management:
- Chew sugarless gum, which encourages more frequent swallowing of saliva.
- Place towel over pillow if main bothersome symptom is nocturnal sialorrhea.

First-Line Medications:

Glycopyrrolate (Robinul): Start 1 mg at bedtime, then ↑ to 1–2 mg twice daily if symptoms are prominent during the day. Unlike other anticholinergics, glycopyrrolate does not cross the blood-brain barrier, so there are fewer central anticholinergic side effects. SE: Constipation, dry mouth, blurred vision, urinary retention.

Second-Line Medications:
- Ipratropium (Atrovent) 0.03% nasal spray; use one to two sprays sublingually (rather than intranasally).
- Oxybutinin (Ditropan) 5 mg twice daily.
- Alpha agonists such as clonidine (Catapres) 0.05–0.1 mg daily or weekly transdermal patch 0.1–0.2 mg or guanfacine (Tenex).
- Benztropine (Cogentin) 1 mg twice daily.
- Trihexyphenidyl (Artane) 5 mg twice daily.
- Atropine 1% ophthalmic drops; use one drop TID PRN sublingually.

Clinical Pearls:
- Dose reduction of clozapine usually is not helpful in diminishing symptoms.
- Clozapine has strong anticholinergic properties, so its procholinergic effect of excessive drooling is puzzling. Theories explaining this include specific stimulation of cholinergic salivary receptors and impairment in the autonomically mediated swallowing mechanism (which may also contribute to clozapine-related dysphagia and pneumonia).

Fun Fact:

Ayurvedic medicine recommends a number of natural treatments for hypersalivation, including chewing cloves, drinking cinnamon tea, and eating a combination of pepper, ginger, and honey.

Side Effect Management: Medications

Tardive Dyskinesia

Characteristics: Involuntary movements, usually occurring after months or years of antipsychotic treatment. The most common symptoms are oro-buccal-lingual, such as chewing, lip smacking, and tongue protrusion. Occasionally causes movements of fingers or toes and rarely, in severe cases, may affect torso and gait.

Meds That Cause It: Antipsychotics, especially first-generation antipsychotics (3%–5% per year); the risk is smaller with second-generation antipsychotics. Among second-generation antipsychotics, risperidone confers the highest risk.

Mechanism: D2 blockade leading to dopamine receptor supersensitivity.

General Management:

- Monitor all patients taking antipsychotics regularly with a test such as the AIMS (Abnormal Involuntary Movement Scale).
- Switch to a different antipsychotic, preferably a second-generation antipsychotic with low dopamine occupancy, such as quetiapine or clozapine.

First-Line Medications:

- Valbenazine (Ingrezza) 40 mg/day; increase to 80 mg/day after a week. SE: Sedation, akathisia. FDA approved for TD.
- Deutetrabenazine (Austedo): Start 6 mg BID; ↑ weekly by 6 mg/day increments to maximum dose of 48 mg/day (divide doses >12 mg/day BID).
- Tetrabenazine (Xenazine): Start 12.5 mg QD for one week, increase by 12.5 mg/day increments weekly to usual dose of 75–150 mg QD (divided doses >37.5 mg TID). SE: Sedation, akathisia, tremor. FDA approved for Huntington's disease.

Second-Line Medications:

- Amantadine (Symmetrel) 100–300 mg/day.
- Gingko biloba extract 240 mg/day.
- Vitamin E 400–600 IU/day.
- Benzodiazepines (eg, clonazepam [Klonopin] or lorazepam [Ativan] 0.5–1 mg daily or BID).

Clinical Pearls:

- Risk factors for TD include first-generation antipsychotics more so than second-generation antipsychotics, higher-potency agents, duration of exposure, higher dose, elderly age, and Black ethnicity.
- Increasing the dose of the antipsychotic will improve symptoms temporarily but probably make them worse in the long run.
- Decreasing or discontinuing antipsychotics may often worsen the symptoms temporarily ("withdrawal dyskinesia") or even unmask TD symptoms that were not apparent.

Fun Fact:

Antipsychotics aren't the only medications that may cause TD. Prolonged use of medications for nausea and reflux like metoclopramide (Reglan) and prochlorperazine (Compazine), which also block dopamine, have also been associated with TD.

The Abnormal Involuntary Movement Scale (AIMS) is the best tool for assessing for and monitoring severity of TD. The test has 12 items to be rated and can be completed in about 10 minutes. The patient should not have anything in their mouth (dentures, gum) and should be seated in a firm, armless chair. See the following page for the full AIMS and instructions on how to use it.

Instructions

There are two parallel procedures, the examination procedure, which tells the patient what to do, and the scoring procedure, which tells the clinician how to rate what he or she observes.

Examination Procedure

Either before or after completing the examination procedure, observe the patient unobtrusively at rest (e.g., in the waiting room).

The chair to be used in this examination should be a hard, firm one without arms.

1. Ask the patient whether there is anything in his or her mouth (such as gum or candy) and, if so, to remove it.
2. Ask about the 'current' condition of the patient's teeth. Ask if he or she wears dentures. Ask whether teeth or dentures bother the patient 'now'.
3. Ask whether the patient notices any movements in his or her mouth, face, hands, or feet. If yes, ask the patient to describe them and to indicate to what extent they 'currently' bother the patient or interfere with activities.
4. Have the patient sit in the chair with hands on knees, legs slightly apart, and feet flat on floor. (Look at the entire body for movements while the patient is in this position.)
5. Ask the patient to sit with hands hanging unsupported – if male, between his legs, if female and wearing a dress, hanging over her knees. (Observe hands and other body areas).
6. Ask the patient to open his or her mouth. (Observe the tongue at rest within the mouth.) Do this twice.
7. Ask the patient to protrude his or her tongue. (Observe abnormalities of tongue movement.) Do this twice.
8. Ask the patient to tap his or her thumb with each finger as rapidly as possible for 10 to 15 seconds, first with right hand, then with left hand. (Observe facial and leg movements.) [±activated]
9. Flex and extend the patient's left and right arms, one at a time.
10. Ask the patient to stand up. (Observe the patient in profile. Observe all body areas again, hips included.)
11. Ask the patient to extend both arms out in front, palms down. (Observe trunk, legs, and mouth.) [activated]
12. Have the patient walk a few paces, turn, and walk back to the chair. (Observe hands and gait.) Do this twice. [activated]

Scoring Procedure

Complete the examination procedure before making ratings.

For the movement ratings (the first three categories below), rate the highest severity observed. 0 = none, 1 = minimal (may be extreme normal), 2 = mild, 3 = moderate, and 4 = severe. According to the original AIMS instructions, one point is subtracted if movements are seen **only on activation**, but not all investigators follow that convention.

Facial and Oral Movements

1. Muscles of facial expression,
   e.g., movements of forehead, eyebrows, periorbital area, cheeks. Include frowning, blinking, grimacing of upper face.
   0 1 2 3 4

2. Lips and perioral area,
   e.g., puckering, pouting, smacking.
   0 1 2 3 4
3. Jaw,
   e.g., biting, clenching, chewing, mouth opening, lateral movement.
   0 1 2 3 4
4. Tongue.
   Rate only increase in movement both in and out of mouth, **not** inability to sustain movement.
   0 1 2 3 4

Extremity Movements

5. Upper (arms, wrists, hands, fingers).
   Include movements that are choreic (rapid, objectively purposeless, irregular, spontaneous) or athetoid (slow, irregular, complex, serpentine). Do **not** include tremor (repetitive, regular, rhythmic movements).
   0 1 2 3 4
6. Lower (legs, knees, ankles, toes),
   e.g., lateral knee movement, foot tapping, heel dropping, foot squirming, inversion and eversion of foot.
   0 1 2 3 4

Trunk Movements

7. Neck, shoulders, hips,
   e.g., rocking, twisting, squirming, pelvic gyrations. Include diaphragmatic movements.
   0 1 2 3 4

Global Judgments

8. Severity of abnormal movements.
   0 1 2 3 4
   based on the highest single score on the above items.
9. Incapacitation due to abnormal movements.
   0 = none, normal
   1 = minimal
   2 = mild
   3 = moderate
   4 = severe
10. Patient's awareness of abnormal movements.
   0 = no awareness
   1 = aware, no distress
   2 = aware, mild distress
   3 = aware, moderate distress
   4 = aware, severe distress

Dental Status

11. Current problems with teeth and/or dentures.
   0 = no
   1 = yes
12. Does patient usually wear dentures?
   0 = no
   1 = yes

Reproduced from Guy W. ECDEU Assessment Manual for Psychopharmacology: Revised (DHEW publication number ADM 76-338). Rockville, MD, US Department of Health, Education and Welfare, Public Health Service, Alcohol, Drug Abuse and Mental Health Administration, NIMH Psychopharmacology Research Branch, Division of Extramural Research Programs, 1976: 534–7

Side Effect Management: Medications

Tremor

Characteristics: Rapid regular movements of body parts, especially hands. Classified as fine vs coarse, and as resting vs postural vs intention.

Meds That Cause It: Lithium (fine intention tremor), valproic acid (fine), lamotrigine, bupropion, antipsychotics (Parkinsonian, resting coarse tremor), especially high-potency first-generation agents, risperidone. Occasionally SSRIs and buspirone.

Mechanism: Multiple mechanisms depending on cause. Medication-induced tremor may be induced by excitability in muscle receptors and neuronal reflexes.

General Management:

- Rule out unrelated causes, such as essential tremor or hyperthyroidism.
- Most drug tremors are fine postural tremor (seen best when patient is holding a fixed posture, such as holding hands up with arms extended).
- Reduce use of caffeine, which can worsen all tremors.
- Change dosing to minimize peak blood levels (eg, split dosing, switch to an extended-release version, or give full dose before sleep).
- Reduce dose or switch agents.

First-Line Medications:

- Propranolol (Inderal) 10 mg BID as needed, ↑ by 10–20 mg/day increments weekly; can go up to 30–120 mg daily in two or three divided doses. SE: Dizziness, fatigue, syncope, low BP.
- Inderal LA. Long-acting propranolol that can be dosed 60–80 mg once a day.
- Benztropine (Cogentin) 1 mg BID for Parkinsonian tremor (due to antipsychotics).

Second-Line Medications:

- Primidone (Mysoline) 100 mg three times a day.
- Vitamin B6 for lithium tremor 900–1200 mg daily.
- Amantadine (Symmetrel) 100–200 mg BID for Parkinsonian tremor (due to antipsychotics).
- Various anticonvulsants such as topiramate (Topamax), gabapentin (Neurontin), oxcarbazepine (Trileptal).

Clinical Pearls:

- Try to systematically track the severity of the tremor over time. Options include taking a quick video at each appointment, having patients copy a design or write their name and address, or having them drink a cup of water. Take notes or include samples during visits.
- Don't forget that tremor can signal alcohol or benzodiazepine withdrawal—something you might want to ask patients about.

Fun Fact:

One in five people over the age of 65 may have essential tremor (not associated with medication).

Weight Gain

Characteristics: Typically, patients will report food craving and binging. Weight gain is rapid in the first three months, more gradual over the following year, then often plateaus. Rapid initial weight gain is correlated with greater eventual cumulative weight gain. FDA definition of weight gain is ≥7% increase in weight from baseline.

Meds That Cause It: Antipsychotics, especially clozapine, olanzapine, and quetiapine. Somewhat less weight gain with risperidone and paliperidone. Least weight gain with aripiprazole, haloperidol, ziprasidone, and lurasidone. Antidepressants: Mirtazapine, tricyclics, paroxetine. Mood stabilizers: Lithium, valproic acid.

Mechanism: Blockade of histamine and serotonin 2A receptors, leading to increased hunger.

General Management:
- Monitoring: Weight, BMI, waist circumference every four weeks for three months, then every three months.
- Lifestyle modification, including exercise and dietary changes, is helpful for patients who are motivated; several studies have shown some benefit, but in actual clinical settings it may be difficult to match their results.
- Switch to a medication that is more weight neutral.

First-Line Medications (some evidence specifically for reducing psychotropic-induced weight gain):
- Topiramate (Topamax) 100–300 mg/day; SE: Cognitive dulling.
- Metformin XR (Glucophage XR, Glumetza) 500–2000 mg: Take with largest meal, split into two doses if needed (based on GI side effects).
- Olanzapine/samidorphan (Lybalvi) as an alternative to olanzapine alone to reduce weight gain.
- Orlistat (Xenical) 120 mg three times daily after meals. Interferes with fat absorption; SE: Diarrhea.
- Aripiprazole (Abilify) 15 mg/day. Antipsychotic. May be useful for olanzapine-induced weight gain as adjunct.

Second-Line Medications (effective for weight loss, but little or no evidence specifically for psychotropic-induced weight gain):
- Bupropion SR (Wellbutrin SR) 300–400 mg daily.
- Any psychostimulant either methylphenidate or amphetamine class.
- Naltrexone/bupropion (Contrave) 8 mg/90 mg up to two tabs twice daily. Anti-obesity drug.
- Phentermine (Suprenza) 15–37.5 mg daily. Anti-obesity drug.
- Phentermine/topiramate (Qsymia) 7.5 mg/46 mg up to two tabs daily. Anti-obesity drug.
- Glucagon-like peptide-1 agonists (GLP1 agonists), such as liraglutide (Saxenda) or semaglutide (Ozempic).
- Nizatidine (Axid) 150–300 mg daily. Antacid, H2 blocker, available over the counter.
- Amantadine (Symmetrel) 100–300 mg/day.

Clinical Pearls:
- Weight gain is most likely in the first six weeks of taking an antipsychotic, and it's difficult for patients to ever lose this weight. As such, you should monitor weekly initially, and switch to a more weight-neutral agent at the first sign of weight gain.
- If patient gains 5% or more of body weight, switch to a different drug.
- Ziprasidone and aripiprazole are probably the most weight-neutral antipsychotics and may even cause weight loss, especially if switching from another agent.
- Weight gain tends to be most severe in patients who are taking an antipsychotic for the first time.
- Ask weight-gaining patients about dry mouth; many psychotropics cause this, and such patients may gain weight from drinking sugary beverages to deal with this side effect.

Fun Fact:
Some researchers have hypothesized that treatment-emergent weight gain is related to and predictive of clinical response, but others argue it may be a marker for medication adherence instead.

Sleep Disorder Medications

GENERAL PRESCRIBING TIPS

There are seven medications plus one medication class in this chapter—armodafinil (Nuvigil), modafinil (Provigil), pitolisant (Wakix), sodium oxybate (Xyrem) plus its mixed-salts close cousin Xywav, solriamfetol (Sunosi), tasimelteon (Hetlioz), and the dopamine agonists used for restless legs syndrome (RLS). In reality, very few of you will ever prescribe Xyrem, Xywav, or Hetlioz. Xyrem and Xywav are approved for narcolepsy with cataplexy, which is a rare illness treated by sleep specialists, and Hetlioz is used for another rare condition seen primarily in the blind: non-24-hour sleep-wake disorder.

The two "vigil" drugs, on the other hand, are heavily prescribed by psychiatrists for all manner of situations, including shift-work sleep disorder, jet lag, and antidepressant-induced sleepiness. These meds, along with the stimulants, are sometimes requested for off-label use as "cognitive enhancers" by overachievers. Sunosi is a newer agent and, like the "vigil" drugs, it's a Schedule IV controlled drug approved to be used in excessive daytime sedation due to narcolepsy or apnea. Wakix is the newest on the scene, approved only for cataplexy and excessive sedation in narcolepsy, and its primary distinction is that it's not a controlled substance.

These "wake promoting" agents are often prescribed when patients complain of excessive fatigue. In these clinical scenarios, we recommend a thorough workup to determine potential alternative strategies (eg, labs to rule out hypothyroidism, anemia, and other conditions; a sleep study to rule out apnea or RLS; a review of medications or other substances potentially contributing to daytime sedation; and education on good sleep habits).

There's no clear guidance on which of the wake-promoting agents to prescribe. Nuvigil lasts a few hours longer than Provigil, which can be a blessing for those who want to stay awake longer or a curse for those who find it causes them insomnia. We have less experience with Sunosi and Wakix, which are newer and more expensive. Clear benefits have not yet been identified; trial and error is the way to go with these agents.

We've added the dopamine agonists fact sheet to this chapter because psychiatrists may at times manage patients with RLS. Dopamine agonists (pramipexole, ropinirole, rotigotine) are considered first-line treatments for RLS. Carbidopa/levodopa is not FDA approved for this condition but is used for intermittent RLS since regular or routine use often leads to worsening of symptoms. Gabapentin enacarbil (Horizant) is a prodrug of gabapentin, which is approved for RLS. We've included this in our table, but you'll find the gabapentin fact sheet in the Mood Stabilizers and Anticonvulsants chapter.

Table 19: **Sleep Disorder Medications**

Generic Name (Brand Name) Year FDA Approved [G] denotes generic availability	Relevant FDA Indication(s)	Rx Status	Available Strengths	Usual Dosage Range (starting–max)
Armodafinil [G] (Nuvigil) 2007	Excessive sleepiness (obstructive sleep apnea, narcolepsy, shift-work sleep disorder)	Schedule IV	50, 150, 200, 250 mg	150–250 mg/day
Calcium, magnesium, potassium, and sodium oxybates (Xywav) 2020	Cataplexy and excessive daytime sedation (narcolepsy) Idiopathic hypersomnia	Schedule III	0.5 g/mL	6–9 g/night
Carbidopa/levodopa [G] (Sinemet) 1975 (for Parkinson's)	Not FDA approved but used for restless legs syndrome	Rx	10/100, 25/100, 25/250 mg ODT: 10/100, 25/100, 25/250 mg ER: 25/100, 50/200 mg	12.5/50–75/300 mg/day
Gabapentin enacarbil (Horizant) 2011	Restless legs syndrome	Rx	300, 600 mg	600 mg/day
Modafinil [G] (Provigil) 1998	Excessive sleepiness (obstructive sleep apnea, narcolepsy, shift-work sleep disorder)	Schedule IV	100, 200 mg	100–400 mg/day
Pitolisant (Wakix) 2019	Cataplexy and excessive sleepiness (narcolepsy)	Rx	4.45, 17.8 mg	17.8–35.6 mg/day
Pramipexole [G] (Mirapex, Mirapex ER) 2007 (for RLS)	Restless legs syndrome	Rx	0.125, 0.25, 0.5, 0.75, 1, 1.5 mg ER: 0.375, 0.75, 1.5, 2.25, 3, 3.75, 4.5 mg	0.125–0.5 mg/day
Ropinirole [G] (Requip, Requip XL) 2005 (for RLS)	Restless legs syndrome	Rx	0.25, 0.5, 1, 2, 3, 4, 5 mg ER: 2, 4, 6, 8, 12 mg	0.25–4 mg/day
Rotigotine transdermal patch (Neupro) 2012	Restless legs syndrome	Rx	Patch: 1, 2, 3, 4, 6, 8 mg	1–3 mg/day
Sodium oxybate [G] (Xyrem) 2002	Cataplexy and excessive daytime sedation (narcolepsy)	Schedule III	0.5 g/mL	6–9 g/night
Solriamfetol (Sunosi) 2019	Excessive sleepiness (obstructive sleep apnea, narcolepsy)	Schedule IV	75, 150 mg	37.5–150 mg/day
Tasimelteon (Hetlioz) 2014	Non-24-hour sleep-wake disorder	Rx	20 mg Liquid: 4 mg/mL	20 mg/night

ARMODAFINIL (Nuvigil) Fact Sheet [G]

Bottom Line:
Armodafinil is an effective wake-promoting agent with some potential for abuse and for drug interactions. It lasts a bit longer than modafinil.

FDA Indications:
Excessive sleepiness associated with obstructive sleep apnea, narcolepsy, or shift-work sleep disorder.

Off-Label Uses:
ADHD; fatigue; treatment-resistant depression.

Dosage Forms:
Tablets (G): 50 mg, 150 mg, 200 mg, 250 mg.

Dosage Guidance:
- Obstructive sleep apnea or narcolepsy: 150–250 mg QAM.
- Shift-work sleep disorder: 150 mg QD, one hour before start of work shift.

Monitoring: No routine monitoring recommended unless clinical picture warrants.

Cost: $

Side Effects:
- Most common: Headache, nausea, dizziness, insomnia, anxiety, irritability.
- Serious but rare: Serious rash, including Stevens-Johnson syndrome, multi-organ hypersensitivity reaction, angioedema, and anaphylaxis reported rarely. Rare cases of mania, psychosis, and agitation reported.

Mechanism, Pharmacokinetics, and Drug Interactions:
- Dopamine reuptake inhibitor.
- Metabolized primarily by non-CYP450 liver pathways, but also to some degree by CYP3A4; t ½: 15 hours.
- Duration of action about eight hours.
- Potentially induces CYP1A2 and 3A4 and inhibits 2C19. Avoid concomitant use with steroidal contraceptives (hormone levels may be decreased due to 3A4 induction) and with CYP2C19 substrates (eg, omeprazole, phenytoin, diazepam); levels of these medications may be increased.

Clinical Pearls:
- Armodafinil is, as the name implies, the r-modafinil enantiomer (modafinil is a 1:1 mixture of both r- and s-enantiomers).
- Schedule IV controlled substance due to abuse potential, mostly for euphoric and stimulant-like effects.
- Increased heart rate and blood pressure may occur, particularly in patients who don't suffer from excessive sedation or fatigue and when used at higher doses.

Fun Fact:
In 2010, the FDA declined to approve use of Nuvigil to treat jet lag.

DOPAMINE AGONISTS (Mirapex, Neupro, Requip, Sinemet) Fact Sheet [G]

Bottom Line:
Dopamine agonists are effective first-line agents for restless legs syndrome (RLS), though rates of problematic impulsive or compulsive behaviors can be high. Reserve carbidopa/levodopa for intermittent use.

FDA Indications:
Parkinson's disease; RLS (except Sinemet, only approved for Parkinson's).

Off-Label Uses:
Treatment-resistant depression; cluster headache.

Dosage Forms:
- **Carbidopa/levodopa tablets (Sinemet, Sinemet CR, [G]):** IR: 10/100 mg, 25/100 mg, 25/250 mg; ER: 25/100 mg, 50/200 mg; ODT: 10/100 mg, 25/100 mg, 25/250 mg.
- **Pramipexole tablets (Mirapex, Mirapex ER, [G]):** IR: 0.125 mg, 0.25 mg, 0.5 mg, 0.75 mg, 1 mg, 1.5 mg; ER: 0.375 mg, 0.75 mg, 1.5 mg, 2.25 mg, 3 mg, 3.75 mg, 4.5 mg.
- **Ropinirole tablets (Requip, Requip XL, [G]):** IR: 0.25 mg, 0.5 mg, 1 mg, 2 mg, 3 mg, 4 mg, 5 mg; ER: 2 mg, 4 mg, 6 mg, 8 mg, 12 mg.
- **Rotigotine transdermal patches (Neupro):** 1 mg, 2 mg, 3 mg, 4 mg, 6 mg, 8 mg.

Dosage Guidance:
- Carbidopa/levodopa: Start ½ of 25/100 mg tablet QHS PRN, then increase by ½ tablet every three days as necessary to max three 25/100 mg tablets.
- Pramipexole: Start 0.125 mg taken one to three hours before HS, then double dose Q4–7 days; max 0.5 mg/day.
- Ropinirole: Start 0.25 mg taken one to three hours before HS, then increase to 0.5 mg after two to three days, 1 mg after seven days, then increase by 0.5 mg weekly until 3 mg/day, then increase by 1 mg/day to maximum 4 mg/day if necessary.
- Rotigotine transdermal patch: Start 1 mg/24 hours applied QD, can increase by 1 mg/24 hours at weekly intervals to maximum 3 mg/24 hours.

Monitoring: No routine monitoring recommended unless clinical picture warrants.

Cost: $; pramipexole ER: $$; rotigotine: $$$$$

Side Effects:
- Most common: Nausea, headache, dizziness, anxiety, insomnia. Newer data suggest nearly half of patients will develop compulsive behaviors (eg, gambling, shopping, eating, sexual activity).
- Serious but rare: Hallucinations, agitation (less common than when treating Parkinson's).

Mechanism, Pharmacokinetics, and Drug Interactions:
- Dopamine agonist.
- Metabolized primarily by: CYP450 (carbidopa/levodopa, rotigotine), renal elimination (pramipexole), CYP1A2 (ropinirole); t ½: 0.75–1.5 hours (carbidopa/levodopa), 8 hours (pramipexole), 6 hours (ropinirole), 5–7 hours (rotigotine).

Clinical Pearls:
- Avoid rotigotine in patients with sulfite allergies because it contains sodium metabisulfite, which may induce anaphylaxis or respiratory symptoms in sensitive patients. Those with history of asthma have an increased risk of sulfite sensitivity.
- Lower doses are used for RLS compared to Parkinson's.
- Onset of action: Pramipexole takes effect upon first dose. Ropinirole takes four to 10 days. Rotigotine has onset with first dose but may require up to one week for full effect.
- Caution patients about compulsive behaviors (gambling, shopping, eating). These occur commonly and can be devastating. Lower dose if such behaviors develop or discontinue if severe.
- Pramipexole showed modest efficacy for treatment-resistant depression in a controlled study. Open-label studies suggest it may work in patients who have not responded to electroconvulsive therapy.

Fun Fact:
Some Parkinson's patients have experienced an increased sex drive when taking these medications, sparking off-label use of these agents for managing low libido. Mirasex, anyone?

MODAFINIL (Provigil) Fact Sheet [G]

Bottom Line:

While modafinil can be helpful for many causes of excessive sleepiness, realize that many people end up using it off-label for lifestyle enhancement, such as working, studying, and partying.

FDA Indications:

Excessive sleepiness associated with obstructive sleep apnea, narcolepsy, or shift-work sleep disorder.

Off-Label Uses:

ADHD; fatigue; treatment-resistant depression.

Dosage Forms:

Tablets (G): 100 mg, 200 mg.

Dosage Guidance:

- Obstructive sleep apnea or narcolepsy: 100–400 mg QAM (usually 200 mg QAM).
- Shift-work sleep disorder: 100–400 mg QD (usually 200 mg QAM), one hour before start of work shift.
- ADHD (off-label): 100–400 mg QAM.
- Treatment-resistant depression, bipolar or unipolar (off-label): 100–400 mg QAM added to antidepressant.

Monitoring: No routine monitoring recommended unless clinical picture warrants.

Cost: $

Side Effects:

- Most common: Increased heart rate and blood pressure, headache, nausea, jitteriness, rhinitis, diarrhea, back pain, and insomnia.
- Serious but rare: Serious rash, including Stevens-Johnson syndrome, multi-organ hypersensitivity reaction, angioedema, and anaphylaxis reported rarely. Rare cases of mania, psychosis, and agitation reported.

Mechanism, Pharmacokinetics, and Drug Interactions:

- Dopamine reuptake inhibitor.
- Metabolized primarily by non-CYP450 liver pathways, but also to some degree by CYP3A4; t ½: 15 hours.
- Duration of action about six hours.
- Potentially induces CYP1A2 and 3A4 and inhibits 2C19. Avoid concomitant use with steroidal contraceptives (hormone levels may be decreased due to 3A4 induction) and with CYP2C9/19 substrates (eg, omeprazole, phenytoin, diazepam); levels of these medications may be increased.

Clinical Pearls:

- Schedule IV controlled substance.
- Increased heart rate and blood pressure may occur, particularly in patients who don't suffer from excessive sedation or fatigue and at higher doses.

Fun Fact:

An ADHD indication was rejected by the FDA because of modafinil's possible association with Stevens-Johnson syndrome.

OXYBATES (Xyrem, Xywav) Fact Sheet [G]

Bottom Line:

Xyrem is often used by sleep specialists as a first-line agent for narcolepsy with cataplexy. It's unlikely that many psychiatrists will prescribe it, given its side effect profile and potential for misuse. Pitolisant, which is easier to use and is not a controlled substance, may be a better option for most patients with both cataplexy and excessive daytime sedation (EDS) associated with narcolepsy.

FDA Indications:

Cataplexy and EDS in narcolepsy (ages 7 and up); idiopathic hypersomnia (Xywav).

Off-Label Uses:

Fibromyalgia; chronic pain; neuropathic pain.

Dosage Forms:

- **Sodium oxybate oral solution (Xyrem, [G]):** 0.5 g/mL.
- **Calcium, magnesium, potassium, and sodium oxybate oral solution (Xywav):** 0.5 g/mL.

Dosage Guidance:

Start 4.5 g nightly, given in two equal, divided doses (because of extremely short half-life): 2.25 g at bedtime and 2.25 g taken 2.5 to four hours later. Titrate to effect in increments of 1.5 g/night at weekly intervals (0.75 g at bedtime and 0.75 g taken 2.5 to four hours later). Usual dose 6–9 g per night. Max 9 g/night.

Monitoring: No routine monitoring recommended unless clinical picture warrants.

Cost: $$$$$

Side Effects:

- Most common: Nausea, dizziness, vomiting, somnolence, enuresis, tremor, parasomnias (sleepwalking).
- Serious but rare: Respiratory depression, depression and suicidality, impaired motor and cognitive function.

Mechanism, Pharmacokinetics, and Drug Interactions:

- CNS depressant.
- Metabolized primarily by conversion to carbon dioxide and then eliminated by expiration; t ½: 0.5–1 hour.
- Avoid concomitant use with alcohol, sedative hypnotics, and other CNS depressants. Valproic acid increases oxybate levels by 25%; adjust valproic acid dose by at least 20%.

Clinical Pearls:

- Sodium oxybate is the sodium salt of gamma hydroxybutyrate (GHB), a Schedule I controlled substance ("date rape" drug).
- Sodium oxybate is a Schedule III controlled substance and is available only through a restricted distribution program called the Xyrem REMS Program using a centralized pharmacy. Prescribers and patients must enroll in the program (www.xyremrems.com or 1-866-XYREM88).
- Patient must wait at least two hours after eating before taking a dose. Both doses should be prepared (dilute in provided vials with water) before bedtime. Dose must be taken while in bed, and patient is to lie down after dosing.
- Most patients find the taste of Xyrem to be awful.
- Xyrem alone was just as effective as modafinil alone for excessive daytime sedation, but the combination was significantly better than either medication used alone in one narcolepsy study.
- While a generic version has been approved, it's not yet available due to patent litigation.
- Xywav is the newer "mixed salts" version (patent extender?) and delivers 92% less sodium than Xyrem.
- A new indication was granted by the FDA for using Xywav to treat idiopathic hypersomnia, a rare and debilitating neurologic sleep disorder characterized by EDS, prolonged but non-restorative nighttime sleep, and severe sleep inertia (prolonged difficulty waking).

Fun Fact:

Xyrem, an orphan drug, is expensive, between $108,000 and $160,000 per year depending on the nightly dose. Jazz Pharmaceuticals is looking to expand its use by testing it in obstructive sleep apnea, Parkinson's, chronic fatigue, schizophrenia, binge eating, and cluster headache.

PITOLISANT (Wakix) Fact Sheet

Bottom Line:

Pitolisant is the only non-DEA-scheduled treatment option approved for patients with narcolepsy, but limited experience and data, plus a higher price tag, make it a second-line option after the "vigil" drugs. However, for patients with both cataplexy and excessive daytime sleepiness, it may be a better option than Xyrem or Xywav.

FDA Indications:

Cataplexy or excessive sleepiness associated with narcolepsy.

Off-Label Uses:

ADHD; fatigue; treatment-resistant depression.

Dosage Forms:

Tablets: 4.45 mg, 17.8 mg.

Dosage Guidance:

Start 8.9 mg QAM for week one. If tolerated, may increase to 17.8 mg QAM for week two. If needed, in week three or beyond, may increase to maximum dose of 35.6 mg QAM. Use lower doses in hepatic or renal impairment.

Monitoring: No routine monitoring recommended unless clinical picture warrants.

Cost: $$$$$

Side Effects:

- Most common: Insomnia, nausea, anxiety.
- Serious but rare: QT interval prolongation (4.2 msec at therapeutic doses; 16 msec at doses greater than maximum recommended).

Mechanism, Pharmacokinetics, and Drug Interactions:

- Antagonist/inverse agonist of the histamine-3 (H3) receptor.
- Metabolized primarily by CYP2D6 and, to a lesser extent, CYP3A4; t ½: 20 hours.
- Strong CYP2D6 inhibitors or in poor metabolizers: Maximum recommended dosage is 17.8 mg once daily. Strong CYP3A4 inducers may reduce pitolisant levels by 50%; adjust dose. Avoid H1 antihistaminergic agents, which may decrease effectiveness of pitolisant.

Clinical Pearls:

- Not a controlled substance.
- The H3 receptor is mainly found in the brain where it regulates wakefulness, appetite, and memory. Pitolisant blocks the H3 receptor, which has downstream effects of increased dopamine and acetylcholine in the prefrontal cortex.
- A head-to-head "non-inferiority" study with modafinil found pitolisant had nearly similar efficacy but was better tolerated.

Fun Fact:

Pitolisant is also being studied for efficacy in ADHD, dementia, obesity, and cognitive symptoms of schizophrenia.

SOLRIAMFETOL (Sunosi) Fact Sheet

Bottom Line:

Solriamfetol is a wakefulness promoter with a different mechanism of action from modafinil and armodafinil. Patients may ask you about it given all the TV ads, but time will tell how it compares with these more established (and cheaper) agents.

FDA Indications:

Excessive daytime sedation (EDS) associated with narcolepsy or obstructive sleep apnea (OSA).

Off-Label Uses:

ADHD; fatigue; treatment-resistant depression.

Dosage Forms:

Tablets: 75 mg, 150 mg (scored).

Dosage Guidance:

Start 37.5 mg QAM for sleep apnea or 75 mg QAM for narcolepsy. Increase dose at intervals of at least three days. Max dose 150 mg/day.

Monitoring: No routine monitoring recommended unless clinical picture warrants.

Cost: $$$$$

Side Effects:

• Most common: Headache, nausea, decreased appetite, and anxiety.

• Serious but rare: Increased blood pressure and pulse; psychosis or mania may occur.

Mechanism, Pharmacokinetics, and Drug Interactions:

• Dopamine and norepinephrine reuptake inhibitor (DNRI).

• Not metabolized, renally eliminated; t ½: 7 hours.

• Avoid MAOIs.

Clinical Pearls:

• This new wake-promoting drug was approved based on four studies of more than 900 adults with narcolepsy or OSA. For example, in a 12-week randomized double-blind controlled trial of 239 adults with narcolepsy, 150 mg/day of Sunosi (but not 75 mg/day) showed statistically significant improvement on tests of wakefulness.

• In a similar study of 476 adults with OSA, patients receiving 37.5 mg/day, 75 mg/day, and 150 mg/day of Sunosi showed statistically significant improvement over placebo at week 12.

• Maintenance of efficacy of up to 50 weeks was shown in two open-label extension studies of patients with EDS associated with either narcolepsy or OSA.

• Given that Sunosi is a DNRI (like bupropion) there has been interest in studying the drug for depression, though clinical trials have not yet been conducted.

• Sunosi has demonstrated abuse potential, particularly at doses higher than recommended for EDS, and has been classified as a controlled substance (Schedule IV).

Fun Fact:

Sunosi is manufactured by Jazz Pharmaceuticals, the company that sold $1.4 billion of Xyrem (sodium oxybate) in 2018. Now that generic versions of Xyrem have been approved by the FDA, Jazz will likely be looking at Sunosi as their biggest profit-maker.

TASIMELTEON (Hetlioz) Fact Sheet

Bottom Line:
Tasimelteon is a melatonin receptor agonist approved for non-24-hour sleep-wake disorder (N24SWD), which occurs primarily in blind people. Due to its high price (over $13,000 for a month's supply), you may want to consider ramelteon instead. While ramelteon hasn't been studied in patients with N24SWD, it's reasonable to try because it is so similar pharmacologically yet much more affordable.

FDA Indications:
N24SWD.

Off-Label Uses:
None recommended; potentially may be used for insomnia, jet lag, shift-work sleep disorder.

Dosage Forms:
- **Capsules:** 20 mg.
- **Oral suspension (Hetlioz LQ):** 4 mg/mL.

Dosage Guidance:
Start 20 mg QHS at the same time every night.

Monitoring: No routine monitoring recommended unless clinical picture warrants.

Cost: $$$$

Side Effects:
- Most common: Headache, increased LFTs, nightmares or unusual dreams.
- Serious but rare: None reported.

Mechanism, Pharmacokinetics, and Drug Interactions:
- Melatonin receptor agonist (at both MT1 and MT2 receptors).
- Metabolized primarily by CYP1A2 and 3A4; t ½: 1 hour.
- Smoking may reduce tasimelteon levels by 40% and lower its efficacy. Caution with 3A4 inhibitors and inducers.

Clinical Pearls:
- Like ramelteon, tasimelteon binds melatonin receptors. Tasimelteon has greater affinity for the MT2 receptor, whereas ramelteon has greater affinity for the MT1 receptor. Both are fairly non-selective, though (meaning they both bind to both MT1 and MT2), so making a clinical distinction is difficult.
- Approved as an orphan drug (a drug for rare diseases that affect fewer than 200,000 people).
- N24SWD is a circadian rhythm disorder commonly seen in blind patients with no light perception. Due to absence of environmental input, these patients experience a constant gradual shift of their sleep cycles by roughly 30 minutes per day, realigning with the 24-hour clock only once every 48 days.
- Should be used daily to maintain therapeutic effect.

Fun Fact:
The advocacy group Public Citizen accused the FDA of allowing tasimelteon's manufacturer to list N24SWD as the drug's indication without specifying that it was for use in totally blind people with N24SWD, the originally filed indication for consideration. Rather than correcting the error and adjusting the drug's label, the FDA sent out a press release officially expanding the approved indication to any patients with N24SWD (there are sighted individuals with this disorder, likely with a genetic basis).

Somatic Treatments

While devices have a long and somewhat disreputable history in psychiatry (remember Wilhelm Reich's orgonoscope?), they've undergone a resurgence, and several have been FDA approved. With the addition of this chapter in our now less accurately named "Medication" Fact Book, we created fact sheets for the four most legitimate devices in psychiatry—bright light therapy, electroconvulsive therapy, transcranial magnetic stimulation, and vagus nerve stimulation.

There are many other devices available for prescription and purchase, though none of them yet meet the Carlat standards for clinical evidence. But several are close; in particular, keep an eye out for:

- *Cranial electric stimulation (CES).* Several have been FDA cleared for depression and anxiety, but the efficacy evidence is quite weak. A couple of well-known models are the Fisher Wallace Stimulator and Alpha-Stim.

- *External trigeminal nerve stimulation (eTNS).* Recently cleared by the FDA for treatment of ADHD in kids 7–12 who are not on medication. Scant evidence; not yet available.

- *Deep brain stimulation (DBS).* A neurosurgical procedure, DBS is effective for some neurological conditions (such as Parkinson's disease and tremor), but its only approval in psychiatry thus far is a humanitarian use for treatment-resistant OCD.

Bright Light Therapy Fact Sheet

Bottom Line:

Light therapy is an effective treatment for seasonal affective disorder (SAD) and possibly for nonseasonal depression as well.

Main Uses:

SAD (not an FDA-approvable device).

Alternative Uses:

Nonseasonal depression.

Procedure:

- Establish the diagnosis of SAD, based on a clear lifelong pattern of mood worsening in the fall and winter, and improving in the spring and summer. Some clinicians use the Seasonal Pattern Assessment Questionnaire to aid with the diagnosis (free download at www.tinyurl.com/vy6ewcs2).
- Light boxes emit full-spectrum light with either fluorescent or LED bulbs (fluorescent is usually recommended). Light intensity is measured in lux, and the standard minimum intensity required is 10,000 lux (similar to light experienced if standing outside 30 minutes after sunrise).
- Light boxes should be large enough to deliver the required light intensity at a comfortable distance (usually about 24 inches away). Smaller fixtures are effective but produce more glare.
- Dawn simulator lamps are likely as effective as light boxes (Terman M and Terman JS, *Am J Psychiatry* 2006;163(12):2126–2133). These devices can be plugged into a standard lamp and cause the intensity of light to gradually increase over about an hour to mimic sunrise, with the brightness increasing to about 250 lux. Patients do not have to sit in front of these lamps after awakening.

Pre–Light Therapy Workup: No specific labs are required. No medical contraindications, but patients with ophthalmological conditions, such as glaucoma or cataracts, should be cleared by their ophthalmologist before starting the treatment.

Cost: $$; insurance coverage of light boxes is unpredictable and varies by company. Have patients contact their insurers directly; occasionally you will be asked to write a letter to support reimbursement.

Side Effects:

- Most common: Eye strain and headaches.
- Uncommon: Mania in patients with bipolar disorder, insomnia, anxiety.

Mechanism, Treatment Course, and Drug Interactions:

- Bright light apparently works by entering the eye and stimulating retinal cells, which connect to the optic nerve. The optic nerve projects to the hypothalamic suprachiasmatic nucleus, which communicates to the pineal gland, where melatonin is produced. Bright light suppresses melatonin production.
- Medications and light therapy: All psychiatric medications may be continued during light therapy.

Clinical Pearls:

- Bright light is likely most effective for patients with atypical depressive symptoms such as hypersomnia and hyperphagia.
- Meta-analyses of randomized controlled trials have reported robust response rates of bright light therapy in the range of 60% (Golden RN et al, *Am J Psychiatry* 2005;162(4):656–662). Patients who respond tend to do so in three to seven days.
- Patients should sit in front of the light box for about 30 minutes soon after awakening, preferably at the same time every morning. They can do any activity during exposure (such as reading, computer work, or running on a treadmill) as long as the light box is oriented appropriately to face them.
- While morning light is indicated for most patients, some do better with evening light. Patients can fill out the Automated Morningness-Eveningness Questionnaire to help them decide the optimal timing for their treatment. It's available free online (www.cet.org/assessments/).

Fun Fact:

According to Norman Rosenthal, the "father" of light treatment, the first person to receive the therapy was an engineer who had carefully mapped out the seasonal rhythms of his depression and suggested that NIMH devise a way of giving increased periods of light every day. Rosenthal and colleagues gave him an early version of the treatment, and he recovered from his depression (*The Carlat Psychiatry Report,* October 2006).

Electroconvulsive Therapy (ECT) Fact Sheet

Bottom Line:
ECT is one of the most effective treatments in psychiatry, but cognitive side effects understandably make patients reluctant to try it. We should recommend it to any patient with severe treatment-resistant depression or psychosis.

FDA Indications:
Treatment-resistant or severe depression (either unipolar or bipolar); catatonia.

Off-Label Uses:
Psychotic depression; severe schizophrenia; suicidality; neuroleptic malignant syndrome.

Procedure:
- Appropriate leads are placed to monitor cardiac function (via ECG), brain waves (via EEG), muscle activity (via EMG), oxygen blood saturation, and blood pressure and pulse.
- Electrodes are positioned in different areas of the scalp (bilateral, right unilateral, or bifrontal) depending on the patient and the judgment of the psychiatrist.
- Patients receive both an IV anesthetic medication (usually methohexital) to put them to sleep, and a very short-acting muscle relaxant (usually succinylcholine) to relax the muscles and thereby prevent injury during the ECT-induced seizure. Sometimes patients will also receive an anticholinergic medication to prevent bradycardia and oral secretions, as well as a beta blocker to prevent tachycardia.
- Once the patient is anesthetized, an electrical stimulus is delivered through the electrodes. The dose of the stimulus varies and is adjusted based on the patient's seizure threshold (which is determined during the first treatment). The stimulus is delivered via a brief pulse lasting anywhere from 0.5 to two milliseconds.
- Seizures usually last 30–60 seconds.

Pre-ECT Workup: No specific labs are required. There are no absolute medical contraindications. All patients should have a medical consultation prior to ECT.

Cost: $$$

Side Effects:
- Most common: Acute confusion for 30 minutes after each treatment in all patients; persistent memory loss for events occurring during the treatment period and a few weeks before and after (most patients); tension headache (30%); nausea; jaw pain.
- Longer-term memory loss occurs in about 25% of patients.
- Bilateral lead placement (electrodes on both temples) is most effective but also causes more cognitive side effects than unilateral lead placement (electrodes on right temple and scalp apex).
- Can be safely administered during pregnancy.

Mechanism, Treatment Course, and Drug Interactions:
- ECT produces a generalized seizure that has antidepressant/antipsychotic effects via unknown mechanisms—possibly by increasing monoamine neurotransmission.
- Treatments are given two or three days a week, and response usually begins after three to six treatments (one to two weeks). Patients receive seven to 10 treatments on average.
- ECT may be continued on a maintenance basis (typically, weekly ECT for two to four weeks, then tapering down to monthly or as required based on symptoms). Maintenance ECT lasts six months or more, depending on response and side effects.
- ECT can be administered on an inpatient or outpatient basis.
- All psychiatric medications may be continued during ECT. Lithium dose should be decreased to minimize cognitive side effects, and benzodiazepines and anticonvulsants should be withheld the night before ECT so as not to interfere with the seizure.

Clinical Pearls:
- ECT is the most effective treatment for depression, with a remission rate of 70%–90%.
- Elderly patients probably respond better to ECT than younger patients.
- Although ECT can be very effective, relapse rates are high in the months following treatment. Consider maintenance ECT, an antidepressant plus lithium augmentation, or psychotherapy as best approaches to maintain response.

Fun Fact:
The first ECT was conducted in 1938 by Dr. Ugo Cerletti on an Italian engineer who was hallucinating and having delusions that he was being "telepathically influenced." After 11 high-voltage treatments (without anesthesia), he made a full recovery and was discharged from the hospital.

Somatic Treatments

Transcranial Magnetic Stimulation (TMS) Fact Sheet

Bottom Line:

TMS is a reasonable option for patients who have failed several antidepressant trials and who are willing to commit to daily clinic visits for up to six weeks.

FDA Indications:

Depression that has not responded to one prior medication trial; OCD; migraine pain.

Off-Label Uses:

Post-stroke depression; Parkinson's disease; Alzheimer's disease; PTSD; chronic pain.

Procedure:

- There are several FDA-cleared TMS devices, and they all include magnetic coils, controller equipment, and a comfortable adjustable seat.
- Parameters of treatment include frequency (number of pulses per second, or hertz, typically 10–20), intensity (usually expressed as percentage of motor threshold—the threshold being the intensity of magnetic field required to elicit a motor response), train duration (how many seconds of pulsing occurs, typically four seconds), inter-train interval (time between trains, typically 26 seconds), and number of trains per session (eg, 80, assuming two trains per minute).
- During the first session, the optimal spot for stimulation is chosen by positioning the coil to elicit a motor twitch in the hand; the coil is then shifted 5 cm forward from that area.
- The standard protocol is high frequency, which is 10 hertz, or 10 pulses per second.

Pre-TMS Workup: No specific labs are required. Contraindicated in patients with increased risk for seizure or with implanted metallic hardware (such as pacemakers, cochlear implants, or aneurysm clips). All patients should have a standard history and physical prior to TMS.

Cost: $$$; insurance companies will often pay for the procedure if you can document several prior antidepressant treatment trials and failures.

Side Effects:

- Most common: Scalp discomfort, especially with high-frequency TMS, described by some patients as feeling like a woodpecker tapping on their head.
- Serious but rare: Instances of grand mal seizures and hearing loss.

Mechanism, Treatment Course, and Drug Interactions:

- TMS produces a magnetic field that modulates the activity of neurons in the cortical brain regions targeted by the coil. Theoretically, the left dorsolateral prefrontal cortex is underactive in depression, and high-frequency TMS (10 hertz) increases that activity. Low-frequency TMS (1 hertz) *inhibits* cortical activity, so it is administered over the right dorsolateral prefrontal cortex.
- Treatments are given five days a week; sessions are 30–40 minutes, and response usually begins after about 20 treatments (four weeks). Average number of treatments is about 30, or a six-week course. There is usually a three-week taper-down phase decreasing to three treatments in week one, two treatments in week two, and one treatment in week three. Some clinics do maintenance treatments of one or two treatments per month.
- TMS can be administered by trained non-MD staff. There is no requirement that the psychiatrist see patients during each appointment, and it's common for a trained operator to administer the daily treatments while the psychiatrist sees the patient once a week.
- In most naturalistic open-label studies, response rates have been in the range of 60%.
- Long-term response: About 60% of patients maintain a response at 12 months (Dunner DL et al, *J Clin Psychiatry* 2014;75(12):1394–1401).
- Medications and TMS: All psychiatric medications may be continued during TMS, but the treatment may work better for patients who can discontinue benzodiazepines or anticonvulsants.

Clinical Pearls:

- In deciding between ECT and TMS, consider that ECT works faster and is the device of choice for suicidal or psychotic depression. Patients may like the fact that TMS has fewer side effects and does not require anesthesia.
- The most commonly used form of TMS is repetitive TMS (rTMS), which stimulates the surface cortex. Deep TMS (dTMS) stimulates deeper regions. Express TMS is a rapid form of TMS for depression that reduces treatment time from 20–38 minutes to three minutes using a high-intensity magnet that produces something called intermittent theta burst stimulation (iTBS).
- The first TMS devices were approved by the FDA in October 2008.

Fun Fact:

The book *3,000 Pulses Later* describes advertising executive Martha Rhodes' positive experiences with TMS, which she credits with treating her refractory depression. "3,000 pulses" refers to the typical number of pulses delivered during a single TMS session.

Vagus Nerve Stimulation (VNS) Fact Sheet

Bottom Line:
The efficacy of VNS remains too controversial to recommend its use in all but the most desperate clinical situations. Noninvasive VNS devices may become available for depression treatment in the future.

FDA Indications:
Treatment-resistant depression (adults); refractory seizure disorder (ages 12 and up).

Off-Label Uses:
Autoimmune and chronic inflammatory disorders such as rheumatoid arthritis, Crohn's disease, irritable bowel syndrome, and fibromyalgia.

Procedure:
In a surgical procedure, a small stimulator device is implanted under the skin in the chest, and wires from the device are wound around one of the vagus nerves in the neck. After full recovery from the surgery (about two weeks), the device is programmed using a handheld transmitter. Pulses are delivered to stimulate the vagus nerve at regular intervals—usually for a 30-second period every five minutes.

Pre-VNS Evaluation: No specific labs are required. Patients will typically have a full medical workup in preparation for surgery.

Cost: $$$$$; insurance company coverage is unlikely in most cases.

Side Effects:
- Most common: Voice hoarseness or alteration (over 50%), headache, cough, neck pain, shortness of breath which may be managed by altering the stimulus parameters.
- Serious but rare: Infection, nerve damage.

Mechanism, Treatment Course, and Drug Interactions:
- VNS's mechanism is unknown. The vagus nerve (cranial nerve X) sends fibers to the median raphe nucleus and locus coeruleus, key areas of serotonergic and noradrenergic innervation relevant to depression. Stimulation of the nerve may modulate levels of both serotonin and norepinephrine.
- The device is left implanted for years, and periodic visits with neurologists and psychiatrists are necessary to monitor the device and the response.
- Medications and VNS: All psychiatric medications may be continued after implantation of VNS.

Clinical Pearls:
- The efficacy of VNS for depression is controversial. The only randomized controlled trial that randomized patients to VNS vs sham VNS found no significant difference in response rates after 10 weeks (15% for VNS vs 10% for sham). Long-term follow-up studies imply that benefits may accrue over time, with a five-year cumulative response rate of 67.6%; however, there was no comparable control group, so this could represent a nonspecific response.
- LivaNova's VNS Therapy System is a small battery-powered stimulator that requires battery removal and replacement approximately every six years.
- Noninvasive devices that stimulate the vagus nerve have been approved in Europe for depression, epilepsy, and pain. Recently, a similar device was FDA cleared in the US for cluster headache treatment (www.tinyurl.com/y6c6frv4).

Fun Fact:
Patients with seizure disorders can sometimes tell if a seizure is about to happen, and seizure patients who have VNS implanted can swipe a magnet over the stimulator area to send an extra burst of stimulation to the brain—which may prevent the seizure.

Somatic Treatments

Substance Use Disorder Medications

GENERAL PRESCRIBING TIPS

Although medications are helpful in substance use disorders, you should combine them with other approaches, such as therapy and 12-step programs. Most patients with substance use issues have co-occurring psychiatric disorders. Some clinicians prefer to get the substance use under control before treating other disorders, under the theory that substances can both obscure and aggravate the underlying psychiatric symptoms. In practice, however, it takes patients a very long time to stop use, and treatment of other conditions usually can't wait. For more detailed practical guidance on treating addiction, check out *Addiction Treatment: A Carlat Guide* by Michael Weaver, MD.

Opioid Dependence

- Methadone was first approved by the FDA for use in opioid dependence in 1947. It is a substitution therapy, and while it rarely gets patients off of opioids, it does help decrease the use of illicit forms of opioids. The problem is that patients must show up at methadone clinics to receive their dose (though they can often eventually qualify for limited take-home doses), making it hard to carve out a normal work or family life. A methadone taper can be used as part of opioid withdrawal protocols.

- Buprenorphine/naloxone (Suboxone and others) was approved in 2002, and although it is also a substitution therapy, it has advantages over methadone. You can give patients a 30-day supply, allowing them to avoid the methadone lifestyle. It's becoming easier to get a suboxone waiver. As of April 2021, as long as you are treating no more than 30 patients at a time, you don't need to do any special training and can simply apply to SAMHSA for the waiver. By the way, many clinicians don't realize that buprenorphine alone is responsible for all of buprenorphine/naloxone's beneficial effects in treating opioid use disorder, including its important ceiling effect. The naloxone is added purely to discourage users from injecting it.

- Naltrexone (ReVia, Vivitrol) blocks a specific type of opioid receptor in the brain and prevents people from feeling high when using opioids. In one study, the monthly IM formulation was found to be as effective as buprenorphine substitution for preventing opioid relapse, but only for highly motivated patients who can tolerate being opioid free for at least seven days before starting naltrexone.

- A note on terminology: Both buprenorphine/naloxone and methadone are sometimes referred to as either "substitution therapy" or "opioid agonist treatment." Sometimes you'll see the term "full agonist treatment," which refers typically to methadone, whereas "partial agonist treatment" refers to buprenorphine. On the other hand, "opioid antagonist treatment" may be used to refer to naltrexone—either in the pill version (ReVia) or the long-acting injectable version (Vivitrol).

Opioid Withdrawal

- A standard opioid withdrawal protocol relies on tapering doses of either buprenorphine (with or without naloxone) or methadone. Buprenorphine is more commonly used because it is safer than methadone and more available.

- Comfort meds:
  - Acetaminophen or ibuprofen for flu-like aches and pains
  - Clonidine for anxiety
  - Baclofen for muscular spasms
  - Benzodiazepines for anxiety/agitation
  - Hypnotics for insomnia (such as trazodone, low-dose quetiapine, diphenhydramine)
  - Antinausea medications (such as ondansetron, trimethobenzamide)
  - Antidiarrhea medications (such as loperamide)

Alcohol Dependence

- Disulfiram (Antabuse) is an aversive treatment, causing patients to become ill if they drink while taking the medication. For a long time it was the only approved medication for treating alcohol dependence, and it still has a place in treatment for patients who are very highly motivated to not drink at all (for example, those who are on probation after a DUI, or those who are about to lose jobs or partners if they go on just one more bender).

- Naltrexone (ReVia, Vivitrol) blocks a specific type of opioid receptor in the brain and is thought to act by reducing cravings and the rewarding effects of alcohol. Most substance use specialists consider it the treatment of choice for alcohol use disorder.

- Acamprosate (Campral) is effective in maintaining abstinence after detox. It is thought to "normalize" the brain glutamate system, which becomes unstable after many years of heavy alcohol use. It may work best in patients who are not using other substances, who are alcohol free before starting it, and who have a strong commitment to abstinence.

- Combining medications is another strategy. For example, the combination of acamprosate and disulfiram seems to be more effective than acamprosate alone; however, the combination of naltrexone and acamprosate has not been shown to be more effective than naltrexone alone.

Alcohol Withdrawal

- The most common medications used for alcohol withdrawal are benzodiazepines, which, like ethanol, act by enhancing the effects of the neurotransmitter GABA. It is thought that chronic alcohol causes overstimulation of GABA receptors, and those receptors compensate by becoming less sensitive to GABA. When there's no alcohol around, those less sensitive receptors cannot get enough GABA endogenously and get "thirsty" for more GABA—leading to typical alcohol withdrawal symptoms such as anxiety, tremor, sweating, etc. When benzos are given, they act as substitute GABA juice and stop withdrawal symptoms.

- Among benzodiazepines, the most common drugs used are chlordiazepoxide (Librium) and diazepam (Valium). Both have long half-lives and active metabolites, factors that help ensure benzo serum levels stay consistent between doses, preventing breakthrough symptoms. For patients with significant liver disease (eg, cirrhosis) or elderly patients, however, levels of chlordiazepoxide and diazepam (plus their metabolites) can build up, causing excess sedation. In these patients, we tend to choose either oxazepam (Serax) or more often lorazepam (Ativan), both of which have shorter half-lives and no active metabolites.

- Other medications to consider:
  - Anticonvulsants are sometimes used, both for core withdrawal symptoms and to prevent seizures—most commonly carbamazepine, valproic acid, or gabapentin.
  - For elevated vital signs and anxiety, consider adrenergic agents (eg, clonidine, propranolol).
  - Baclofen, a muscle relaxant, can be helpful in addition to benzodiazepines for core symptoms, dosed at 5–10 mg TID.
  - Miscellaneous comfort meds, eg, acetaminophen or ibuprofen for headache, bismuth (Pepto-Bismol) or trimethobenzamide (Tigan) for nausea, trazodone for insomnia.

Smoking Cessation

See our special smoking cessation fact sheet in this chapter for more information.

Alcohol Use Disorder Treatment Algorithm

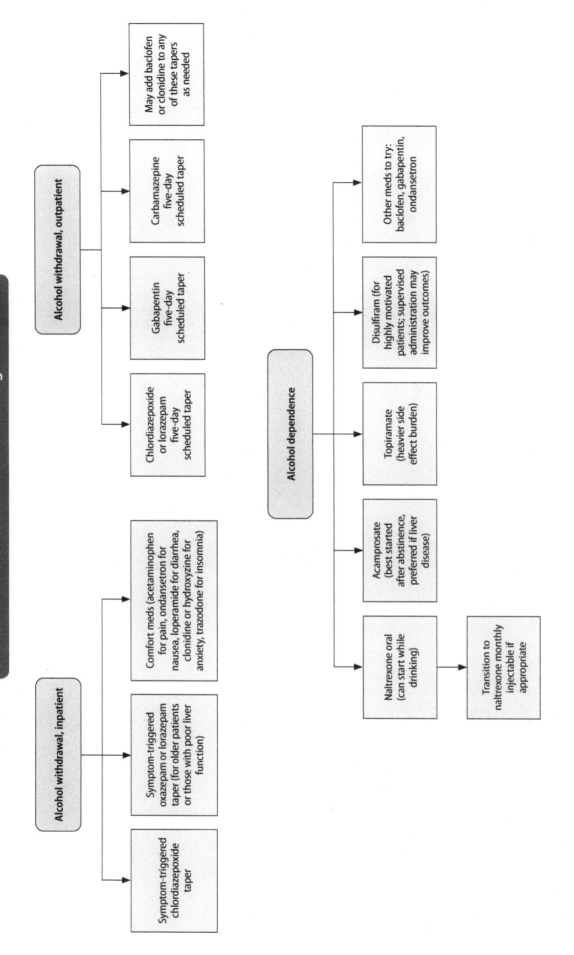

Alcohol withdrawal, outpatient
- Chlordiazepoxide or lorazepam five-day scheduled taper
- Gabapentin five-day scheduled taper
- Carbamazepine five-day scheduled taper
- May add baclofen or clonidine to any of these tapers as needed

Alcohol withdrawal, inpatient
- Symptom-triggered chlordiazepoxide taper
- Symptom-triggered oxazepam or lorazepam taper (for older patients or those with poor liver function)
- Comfort meds (acetaminophen for pain, ondansetron for nausea, loperamide for diarrhea, clonidine or hydroxyzine for anxiety, trazodone for insomnia)

Alcohol dependence
- Naltrexone oral (can start while drinking)
  - Transition to naltrexone monthly injectable if appropriate
- Acamprosate (best started after abstinence, preferred if liver disease)
- Topiramate (heavier side effect burden)
- Disulfiram (for highly motivated patients; supervised administration may improve outcomes)
- Other meds to try: baclofen, gabapentin, ondansetron

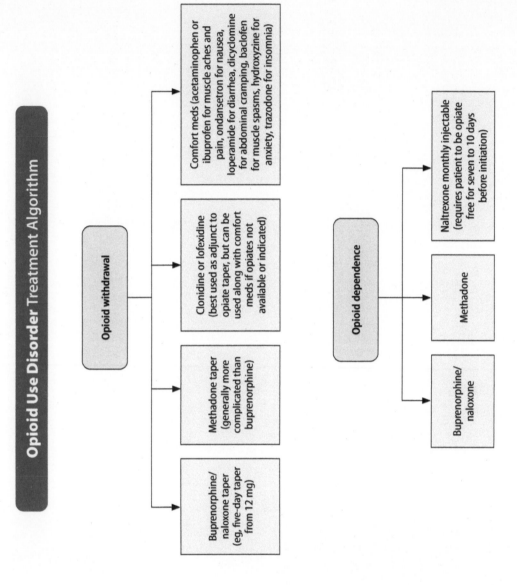

Opioid Use Disorder Treatment Algorithm

Opioid withdrawal

- Buprenorphine/naloxone taper (eg, five-day taper from 12 mg)
- Methadone taper (generally more complicated than buprenorphine)
- Clonidine or lofexidine (best used as adjunct to opiate taper, but can be used along with comfort meds if opiates not available or indicated)
- Comfort meds (acetaminophen or ibuprofen for muscle aches and pain, ondansetron for nausea, loperamide for diarrhea, dicyclomine for abdominal cramping, baclofen for muscle spasms, hydroxyzine for anxiety, trazodone for insomnia)

Opioid dependence

- Buprenorphine/naloxone
- Methadone
- Naltrexone monthly injectable (requires patient to be opiate free for seven to 10 days before initiation)

Table 20: Substance Use Disorder Medications

Generic Name (Brand Name) Year FDA Approved (Rx status) [G] denotes generic availability	Relevant FDA Indication(s)	Available Strengths (mg)	Usual Dosage Range (mg)
Acamprosate [G] (Campral) 2004 (Rx)	Alcohol use. Best when started after a period of abstinence.	333	666 TID
Buprenorphine [G] (Belbuca, Buprenex, Butrans) 2002 (Schedule III)	Opioid use. Substitution therapy.	2, 8 SL (Subutex [G]) 0.075, 0.15, 0.3, 0.45, 0.6, 0.75, 0.9 buccal film (Belbuca, [G]) (used for pain) 0.3 mg/mL injection (Buprenex, [G]) (used for pain) 5, 7.5, 10, 15, 20 mcg/hr patch (Butrans) (used for pain)	8–16 QD SL
Buprenorphine extended-release injection (Sublocade) 2017 (Schedule III)	Opioid use. Substitution therapy.	100, 300	300 mg monthly ×2 doses, then 100 mg monthly
Buprenorphine and naloxone [G] (Bunavail, Suboxone, Zubsolv) 2002 (Schedule III) Generic available for 2/0.5, 8/2 mg SL tablets and SL film strips only	Opioid use. Substitution therapy formulated to prevent misuse and diversion.	2.1/0.3, 4.2/0.7, 6.3/1 buccal film (Bunavail) 2/0.5, 4/1, 8/2, 12/3 SL film strip (Suboxone, [G]) 2/0.5, 8/2 SL tablet (generic only) 0.7/0.18, 1.4/0.36, 2.9/0.71, 5.7/1.4, 8.6/2.1, 11.4/2.9 SL tablet (Zubsolv)	4–24 QD
Bupropion SR [G] (Zyban) 1997 (Rx)	Tobacco use. Decreases craving.	150	150 QAM–150 BID
Clonidine [G] (Catapres, Kapvay) 1974 (Rx)	Opioid use. Decreases withdrawal symptoms.	0.1, 0.2, 0.3 IR tablet 0.1, 0.2 ER tablet 0.1, 0.2, 0.3 mg/day patch	0.1–0.2 Q4–Q6 hours PRN (IR tablet)
Disulfiram [G] (Antabuse) 1951 (Rx)	Alcohol use. Aversive treatment.	250, 500	125–500 QPM
Lofexidine (Lucemyra) 2018 (Rx)	Opioid use. Decreases withdrawal symptoms.	0.18	3–4 tablets QID, then taper
Methadone [G] (Dolophine, Methadose) 1947 (Schedule II)	Opioid use. Substitution therapy.	5, 10, 40 10 mg/mL, 10 mg/5 mL, 5 mg/5 mL oral liquid	20–120 QD
Naloxone [G] (Narcan Nasal Spray, Kloxxado, Zimhi) 2015 (intranasal) (Rx)	Opioid use. Emergency opioid overdose rescue.	4 mg/0.1 mL intranasal (Narcan) 8 mg/0.1 mL intranasal (Kloxxado) 5 mg/0.5 mL intramuscular or subcutaneous (Zimhi)	×1; may repeat every 2–3 minutes

Generic Name (Brand Name) Year FDA Approved (Rx status) [G] denotes generic availability	Relevant FDA Indication(s)	Available Strengths (mg)	Usual Dosage Range (mg)
Naltrexone [G] (ReVia) 1984 (Rx)	Alcohol use. Decreases alcohol euphoria. Opioid use. Blocks opioid effects.	50	25–50 QD
Naltrexone ER (Vivitrol) 2006 (Rx)		380	380 Q4week
Nicotine inhaled (Nicotrol Inhaler) 1997 (Rx)	Tobacco use. Substitution therapy.	4 mg delivered/cartridge	6–16 cartridges per day
Nicotine nasal spray (Nicotrol NS) 1996 (Rx)		0.5 mg delivered/spray	1–2 sprays/hour PRN
Nicotine polacrilex [G] (Nicorette Gum, others) 1992 (OTC)		2, 4	1 piece PRN up to 24/day
Nicotine polacrilex [G] (Nicorette Lozenge, others) 2009 (OTC)		2, 4	1 piece PRN up to 20/day
Nicotine transdermal [G] (Habitrol, Nicoderm CQ, others) 1991 (OTC)		7, 14, 21/24 hr	14–21 QD
Varenicline [G] (Chantix) 2006 (Rx)	Tobacco use. Decreases craving.	0.5, 1	0.5 QD–1 BID

Smoking Cessation

(The following is adapted from a Carlat One-Pager that was originally created for the June 2015 issue of the *Carlat Addiction Treatment Report*. See that issue for the full article.)

Assessment

DSM-5: "Problematic pattern" of tobacco use leading to "significant distress" that lasts at least 12 months.

1. *Determine daily nicotine use.* How many packs per day (20 mg nicotine is typically absorbed per 20-cigarette pack)? E-cigarettes (nicotine varies)? Chewing tobacco (one pouch = ¼ pack)? Hookah?
2. *Determine the usage pattern.* When does the patient have their first cigarette of the day? Does the patient smoke when sick?
3. *Determine past quitting techniques.* Have any worked—or *not* worked?

Pharmacological Treatment: Which to Choose?

- **Nicotine replacement therapy (NRT).** Start most patients on NRT. Prescribe patch based on nicotine load: One cigarette delivers about 1 mg of nicotine; so one pack per day = 21 mg patch. Place it at the same time each day, usually in the morning. Start above the heart and rotate left around the body to prevent skin irritation. Use 0.5% cortisone cream for irritation/rash. Initial dose for four to eight weeks, then taper monthly or every two months. Advise no smoking—patients may note nausea or racing heart if they do.

- **Combination NRT.** As effective as varenicline. If there are cravings throughout the day even with a patch, add a short-acting agent (gum, lozenge, spray, inhaler). Discuss chewing technique for gum: Chew a few times to activate the release (the sign is bad peppery taste), then park between cheek and gum, switching sides every few minutes. Each piece is 2 mg or 4 mg and lasts about 30 minutes. Spray and inhaler are available by prescription only.

- **Varenicline (Chantix).** Most effective single medication for smoking. Start 0.5 mg per day for three days, increase to twice daily for seven to 10 days, then quit smoking, then increase gradually to 1 mg twice daily for three months. Discuss possible insomnia and vivid dreams (common). Psychiatric side effects, such as depression, suicidal ideation, and aggression, are unusual and likely caused by nicotine withdrawal rather than varenicline.

- **Bupropion (Wellbutrin SR, Zyban).** Effective, but less effective than varenicline. 150 mg/day is just as effective as the manufacturer's recommended dose of 150 mg BID and carries fewer side effects. Possible side effects of insomnia, nervousness, weight loss (potentially good, especially since many people gain weight after quitting).

Tips to Improve Success of Treatment

- Normalize failure. Most people need multiple quit attempts before success; if patients know this in advance, they might be more willing to come back and try again.
- The first week after quitting is the hardest in terms of craving. Craving spells last 10–20 minutes; distraction techniques can work to deal with them. Patients can try drinking a large glass of cold water, playing a video game, etc.
- Warn patients that they might cough temporarily after they quit—this is a normal lung response to healing.
- Give phone number 1-800-QUIT-NOW for free support.

ACAMPROSATE (Campral) Fact Sheet [G]

Bottom Line:

Acamprosate is best for maintaining abstinence in patients who have already quit, but it can be helpful even after patients relapse. Naltrexone is the better choice for patients who are still drinking, since it is better at helping patients quit. Acamprosate is also preferred over naltrexone in patients with hepatic impairment.

FDA Indications:

Alcohol dependence.

Dosage Forms:

Delayed-release tablets (G): 333 mg.

Dosage Guidance:

- Start 666 mg TID. Give 333 mg TID in patients with renal impairment.
- Can give 999 mg twice a day if patients can't remember to take it three times daily.

Monitoring: No routine monitoring recommended unless clinical picture warrants.

Cost: $$

Side Effects:

- Most common: Diarrhea (dose related, transient), weakness, peripheral edema, insomnia, anxiety.
- Serious but rare: Acute renal failure reported in a few cases; suicidal ideation, attempts, and completions rare but greater than with placebo in studies.

Mechanism, Pharmacokinetics, and Drug Interactions:

- Mechanism of action is not fully defined; it appears to work by promoting a balance between the excitatory and inhibitory neurotransmitters, glutamate and GABA, respectively (GABA and glutamate activities appear to be disrupted in alcohol dependence).
- Not metabolized, cleared unchanged by kidneys; t ½: 20–33 hours.
- No significant drug interactions.

Clinical Pearls:

- Approved by the FDA in 2004, but it has been used in France and other countries since 1989.
- Does not eliminate or treat symptoms of alcohol withdrawal. Usually prescribed for maintenance of abstinence; may continue even if patient relapses with alcohol.
- Clinically, acamprosate has demonstrated efficacy in more than 25 placebo-controlled trials and has generally been found to be more effective than placebo in reducing risk of returning to any drinking and increasing the cumulative duration of abstinence. However, in reducing heavy drinking, acamprosate appears to be no better than placebo.
- Acamprosate can be used with naltrexone or disulfiram (different mechanism of action), although the combination with naltrexone may not increase efficacy per available studies.
- Taking with food is not necessary, but it may help compliance to do so.
- Compared to naltrexone and disulfiram, acamprosate is not metabolized by the liver and is not impacted by alcohol use, so it can be administered to patients with hepatitis or liver disease and to patients who continue drinking alcohol.

Fun Fact:

Each 333 mg tablet contains 33 mg of elemental calcium (because it is available as acamprosate calcium salt).

BUPRENORPHINE (Sublocade) Fact Sheet [G]

Bottom Line:

Buprenorphine (Subutex, available now only as generic) is the active ingredient in Suboxone (buprenorphine/naloxone) and is responsible for the effectiveness of the combination medication in opioid use disorder. In the past, buprenorphine alone was preferred for the initial (induction) phase of treatment, while Suboxone was preferred for maintenance treatment (unsupervised administration). Currently, the combination is favored for both induction and maintenance as it decreases abuse or diversion potential.

FDA Indications:

Opioid dependence: induction, maintenance (Sublocade); moderate-severe pain (Belbuca, Buprenex, Butrans).

Dosage Forms:

- **SL tablets (G):** 2 mg, 8 mg (scored).
- **Extended-release injection (Sublocade):** 100 mg/0.5 mL, 300 mg/1.5 mL prefilled syringes.
- **Buccal film (Belbuca, [G]):** 0.075 mg, 0.15 mg, 0.3 mg, 0.45 mg, 0.6 mg, 0.75 mg, 0.9 mg (used for pain).
- **Injection (Buprenex, [G]):** 0.3 mg/mL (used for pain).
- **Transdermal patch (Butrans):** 5 mcg/hr, 7.5 mcg/hr, 10 mcg/hr, 15 mcg/hr, 20 mcg/hr (used for pain).

Dosage Guidance:

- Induction procedure:
  - Begin at least four hours after last use of heroin or other short-acting opioids and when first signs of withdrawal appear; otherwise, you may trigger withdrawal symptoms.
  - Start 2–8 mg SL day one; then 8–16 mg SL QD (usual initial dose range is 12–16 mg/day and accomplished over three to four days).
  - Other than extended-release injection, not for maintenance treatment; patients should be switched to the buprenorphine/naloxone combination product for maintenance and unsupervised therapy.
- Patients with moderate to severe opioid use disorder who have been stabilized with SL or buccal buprenorphine for greater than seven days may convert to monthly subcutaneous injections. Start 300 mg monthly for two months, then give 100 mg monthly maintenance doses. Some patients may require higher doses.

Monitoring: No routine monitoring recommended unless clinical picture warrants.

Cost: SL: $$; monthly injection: $$$$$

Side Effects:

- Most common: Headache, pain, insomnia, nausea, anxiety.
- Serious but rare: Hepatitis reported rarely, ranging from transient, asymptomatic transaminase elevations to hepatic failure; in many cases, patients had preexisting hepatic dysfunction. QT prolongation with higher doses of transdermal patch.

Mechanism, Pharmacokinetics, and Drug Interactions:

- Opioid agonist (delta and mu receptors) and antagonist (kappa receptors).
- Metabolized primarily through CYP3A4; t ½: 24–48 hours.
- Avoid concomitant use with opioid analgesics (diminished pain control). Additive effects with CNS depressants. CYP3A4 inhibitors and inducers may affect levels of buprenorphine.

Clinical Pearls:

- Schedule III controlled substance. Prescribing of SL tablets for opioid dependence is limited to providers who have met qualification criteria and have received a DEA number specific to buprenorphine (see www.buprenorphine.samhsa.gov).
- Monthly injection offers alternative that may be convenient for some patients.

Fun Fact:

The subcutaneous implant formulation of buprenorphine (Probuphine) was discontinued. Its use was severely limited as it was invasive, expensive, and an option only for patients stable on ≤8 mg/day. Other implants currently in development include medications for schizophrenia, breast cancer, photosensitivity, and Parkinson's disease.

BUPRENORPHINE/NALOXONE (Bunavail, Suboxone, Zubsolv) Fact Sheet [G]

Bottom Line:

Buprenorphine/naloxone is the definitive partial agonist treatment for opioid use disorder. The combination product is preferred over buprenorphine alone for maintenance because the addition of naloxone lowers its potential for injection abuse. The SL film formulation is priced a little higher than the SL tablets yet provides very little (if any) meaningful benefit; generic SL tablets should be used as a cost-saving measure.

FDA Indications:

Opioid dependence (induction and maintenance).

Dosage Forms:

- **SL tablets (G):** 2/0.5 mg, 8/2 mg (scored).
- **SL film strips (Suboxone, [G]):** 2/0.5 mg, 4/1 mg, 8/2 mg, 12/3 mg.
- **SL tablets (Zubsolv):** 0.7/0.18 mg, 1.4/0.36 mg, 2.9/0.71 mg, 5.7/1.4 mg, 8.6/2.1 mg, 11.4/2.9 mg.
- **Buccal film (Bunavail):** 2.1/0.3 mg, 4.2/0.7 mg, 6.3/1 mg.

Dosage Guidance:

- Induction procedure:
  - Begin at least four hours after last use of heroin or other short-acting opioids and when first signs of withdrawal appear; otherwise, you may trigger withdrawal symptoms.
  - Start 2–8 mg SL day one; then 8–16 mg SL QD (usual initial dose range is 12–16 mg/day and accomplished over three to four days).
- Maintenance treatment: give combination product (Suboxone or [G]) daily in the equivalent buprenorphine dose on last day of induction; adjust dose in increments of 2 mg or 4 mg to a level that maintains treatment and suppresses opioid withdrawal symptoms (usually 4–24 mg/day); max 32 mg/day.
- Zubsolv 5.7/1.4 mg SL tablet provides equivalent buprenorphine to a Suboxone 8/2 mg SL tablet.
- Bunavail 4.2/0.7 mg buccal film provides equivalent buprenorphine to a Suboxone 8/2 mg SL tablet.

Monitoring: No routine monitoring recommended unless clinical picture warrants.

Cost: SL tablet, film, Bunavail: $–$$ depending on dose; Zubsolv: $$$$

Side Effects:

- Most common: Headache, pain, vomiting, sweating.
- Serious but rare: Hepatitis reported rarely, ranging from transient, asymptomatic transaminase elevations to hepatic failure; in many cases, patients had preexisting hepatic dysfunction.

Mechanism, Pharmacokinetics, and Drug Interactions:

- Buprenorphine: Opioid agonist (delta and mu receptors) and antagonist (kappa receptors); naloxone: Opioid antagonist.
- Metabolized primarily through CYP3A4; t ½: 24–48 hours (naloxone: 2–12 hours).
- Avoid concomitant use with opioid analgesics (diminished pain control). Additive effects with CNS depressants. CYP3A4 inhibitors and inducers may affect levels of buprenorphine.

Clinical Pearls:

- Schedule III controlled substance. Prescribing is limited to physicians who have met qualification criteria and have received a DEA number specific to buprenorphine (see www.buprenorphine.samhsa.gov).
- Naloxone is an opioid antagonist that is active only when injected; it is added to buprenorphine in order to reduce misuse via intravenous injection of a dissolved tablet.
- The SL film formulation's manufacturer claims it dissolves faster and tastes better than SL tablets. Actually, it is more likely a way for the manufacturer to switch users to a "new" product (with patent protection until 2025) rather than lose patients to generics.
- SL film should be placed at base of tongue to the side of midline; this allows patient to use two films at the same time if dose dictates.
- Zubsolv and Bunavail formulations have better bioavailability, hence the dose equivalencies noted above.
- Prescribers should be aware of the risk for diversion and sale of buprenorphine films and tablets. Some regular opioid users periodically buy buprenorphine "off the street" and use it to combat cravings and withdrawal symptoms if their drug of choice is not readily available.

Fun Fact:

The manufacturer of Suboxone, Reckitt Benckiser, generates most of its revenue from selling home and personal care products like Lysol cleaners and Durex condoms.

BUPROPION SR (Zyban) Fact Sheet [G]

Bottom Line:
Bupropion SR is somewhat less effective in smoking cessation than varenicline, but given the high rate of comorbidity between smoking and depression, it is an attractive option for many patients. It is also a particularly good choice for patients who are not able to set a quit date prior to initiating treatment.

FDA Indications:
Smoking cessation.

Off-Label Uses:
ADHD; sexual dysfunction; bipolar depression.

Dosage Forms:
SR tablets (G): 150 mg ER.

Dosage Guidance:
Start 150 mg QAM for three days, then 150 mg BID; separate doses by at least eight hours and administer last dose no later than 6 p.m. to minimize insomnia. Target smoking quit dates are generally in the second week of treatment.

Monitoring: No routine monitoring recommended unless clinical picture warrants.

Cost: $

Side Effects:
- Most common: Agitation, insomnia, headache, nausea, vomiting, tremor, tachycardia, dry mouth, weight loss.
- Serious but rare: Seizures; risk higher with rapid and large dose increases and in patients at risk for seizures. Anaphylactoid reactions (eg, pruritus, urticaria, angioedema, dyspnea) reported rarely; reports include Stevens-Johnson syndrome and anaphylactic shock. Class warning regarding suicide risk (see Antidepressants chapter).

Mechanism, Pharmacokinetics, and Drug Interactions:
- Norepinephrine and dopamine reuptake inhibitor.
- Metabolized primarily through CYP2B6; may inhibit CYP2D6; t ½: 21 hours.
- Avoid use with MAOIs. Levels of drugs metabolized by CYP2D6 (eg, paroxetine, fluoxetine, aripiprazole, iloperidone, atomoxetine, beta blockers) may be increased. Successful cessation of smoking may alter pharmacokinetic properties of other medications (eg, clozapine, olanzapine, theophylline, warfarin, insulin).

Clinical Pearls:
- If patient successfully quits smoking after seven to 12 weeks, may consider maintenance therapy based on individual patient risk-benefit. Efficacy of maintenance therapy (150 mg BID) has been shown for up to six months. However, if patient has not made significant progress by the seventh week of therapy, success is unlikely and discontinuation should be considered.
- Bupropion slows the weight gain that often occurs in the initial weeks after smoking cessation, but with time, this effect becomes negligible.
- Bupropion and nicotine replacement therapy show similar quit rates: About 25% of patients, or double that seen with placebo, are abstinent at six months.
- Equally effective in smokers with or without history of depression.

Fun Fact:
Much of the initial direct-to-consumer advertising that was done for Zyban was via print ads in smoke-free places such as airports.

DISULFIRAM (Antabuse) Fact Sheet [G]

Bottom Line:

Disulfiram is an aversive treatment, causing a buildup of ethanol's metabolite acetaldehyde in the serum, which in turn causes symptoms such as flushing, dizziness, nausea, and vomiting. Since disulfiram does not reduce cravings and any alcohol ingestion could result in a reaction, noncompliance can be common. Its use should be reserved for selective, highly motivated patients in conjunction with supportive and psychotherapeutic treatment.

FDA Indications:

Alcohol dependence.

Dosage Forms:

Tablets (G): 250 mg, 500 mg.

Dosage Guidance:

Start 125 mg QPM (must be abstinent from alcohol >12 hours); increase to 250 mg QPM after several days. Maintenance is usually 250–500 mg QPM, but some patients can drink alcohol without a reaction at the 250 mg/day dose.

Monitoring: LFTs if liver disease is suspected.

Cost: $

Side Effects:

- Most common: Skin eruptions (eg, acne, allergic dermatitis), drowsiness, fatigue, impotence, headache, metallic taste.
- Serious but rare: Severe (very rarely fatal) hepatitis or hepatic failure reported and may occur in patients with or without prior history of abnormal hepatic function. Rare psychotic episodes have been reported. Rarely may cause peripheral neuropathy or optic neuritis.

Mechanism, Pharmacokinetics, and Drug Interactions:

- Aldehyde dehydrogenase inhibitor.
- Metabolized primarily through CYP450; t ½ is not defined, but elimination from body is slow, and effects may persist for one or two weeks after last dose.
- While taking disulfiram, and for one to two weeks after stopping, avoid concomitant use of any medications containing alcohol (including topicals), metronidazole, or "disguised" forms of ethanol (cough syrup, some mouthwashes, oral solutions or liquid concentrates containing alcohol such as sertraline). Avoid vinegars, cider, extracts, and foods containing ethanol.

Clinical Pearls:

- Disulfiram inhibits the enzyme aldehyde dehydrogenase; when taken with alcohol, acetaldehyde levels are increased by five- to 10-fold, causing unpleasant symptoms that include flushing, nausea, vomiting, palpitations, chest pain, vertigo, hypotension, and (in rare instances) cardiovascular collapse and death. This is the basis for its use as aversion therapy. Common advice to patients: "You'll wish you were dead, but it likely won't kill you."
- Reaction may last from 30–60 minutes to several hours or as long as alcohol remains in the bloodstream.
- Advise patients to carry an identification card or a medical alert bracelet that states they are taking the medication and lists the symptoms of the reaction and clinician contact information.
- Therapy lasts until the patient is fully recovered and a basis for permanent self-control has been established; maintenance therapy may be required for months or even years.

Fun Fact:

Disulfiram's anti-protozoal activity may be effective in *Giardia* and *Trichomonas* infections.

LOFEXIDINE (Lucemyra) Fact Sheet

Bottom Line:

Lofexidine is an alpha-2 agonist (similar to clonidine and guanfacine) that is used to reduce the intensity of opioid withdrawal symptoms. It effectively blunts some of the most disturbing symptoms of detox such as anxiety and tachycardia, but is generally not effective for withdrawal pain symptoms such as myalgias and headache, so it should be used with an analgesic like ibuprofen or acetaminophen. Some data indicate that lofexidine is more effective than clonidine for management of opioid withdrawal; however, given its much higher price tag, we recommend you stick to clonidine.

FDA Indications:

Opioid withdrawal.

Dosage Forms:

Tablets: 0.18 mg.

Dosage Guidance:

- Start three 0.18 mg tablets QID at five- to six-hour intervals during peak withdrawal symptoms (typically the first five to seven days after last use of opioid). Withdrawal symptoms should be used clinically to guide gradual dose reduction.
- Maximum daily dose is 2.88 mg (16 tablets), and no single dose should exceed 0.72 mg (four tablets).
- Discontinue over a two- to four-day period by gradually reducing in increments of one tablet per dose every one to two days. Treatment course should be no more than 14 days.

Monitoring: Monitor blood pressure and pulse. Monitor ECG in patients with congestive heart failure, bradyarrhythmia, or risk for QT prolongation.

Cost: $$$$$

Side Effects:

- Most common: Orthostatic hypotension, bradycardia, dizziness, somnolence, sedation, dry mouth.
- Serious but rare: Syncope, QT interval prolongation.

Mechanism, Pharmacokinetics, and Drug Interactions:

- Alpha-2 receptor agonist.
- Metabolized primarily by CYP450 2D6; t ½: 11–12 hours.
- Caution when used with CYP450 2D6 inhibitors (such as paroxetine) or in poor 2D6 metabolizers as there may be an increased risk for hypotension. Caution with other agents that may increase QT interval (eg, methadone). Caution when used with CNS depressants (additive CNS depression).

Clinical Pearls:

- Analog of clonidine, another alpha-2 agonist, available since 1992 in the UK (you can find the clonidine fact sheet in the ADHD Medications chapter).
- Has been approved for use in Europe since the 1990s, but was not approved by the FDA until 2018. Approval was based on two randomized, double-blind, placebo-controlled clinical trials of 866 adults with opioid dependence; lofexidine lessened severity of withdrawal symptoms more than placebo.
- Decide on how rapidly to taper the dose by using a symptom-triggered assessment such as the Clinical Opiate Withdrawal Scale (COWS), an 11-item scale measuring opioid withdrawal symptoms including stomach cramps, muscle spasms/twitching, feeling of coldness, heart pounding, muscle tension, aches, pains, yawning, runny eyes, and insomnia or sleep problems.
- Lower the dose if symptomatic hypotension or bradycardia occurs, and in patients with impaired hepatic or renal function.
- Some patients may experience markedly increased blood pressure when lofexidine is discontinued.
- Has been studied for alcohol withdrawal but was not found to be effective.

Fun Fact:

Case reports support its use for hot flashes associated with menopause.

METHADONE (Methadose) Fact Sheet [G]

Bottom Line:

Methadone is a long-acting opioid and is one of the mainstays of opioid substitution therapy, along with buprenorphine. Although it is tantamount to replacing one addiction for another, it has the harm reduction benefits of avoiding the infectious diseases that accompany sharing needles and preventing dangerous behaviors used to obtain illicit opioids (such as theft or prostitution). Disadvantages include the need to go to a methadone clinic daily, the potential for diversion, and the potential for accumulation with repeated doses.

FDA Indications:

Opioid dependence; severe pain.

Dosage Forms:

- **Tablets (G):** 5 mg, 10 mg, 40 mg (scored).
- **Oral solution (G):** 10 mg/5 mL, 5 mg/5 mL.
- **Oral concentrate (G):** 10 mg/mL.

Dosage Guidance:

Start 15–30 mg single dose; then 5–10 mg every two to four hours. Adjust dose to prevent withdrawal symptoms; max 40 mg on day one. 80–120 mg per day is a common maintenance dose for opioid dependence.

Monitoring: ECG if cardiac disease.

Cost: $

Side Effects:

- Most common: Constipation, dizziness, sedation, nausea, sweating.
- Serious but rare: May prolong the QTc interval and increase risk for torsades de pointes; caution in patients at risk for QTc prolongation; usually with doses >100 mg/day. Severe respiratory depression may occur; use extreme caution during initiation, titration, and conversion from other opioids to methadone. Respiratory depressant effects occur later and persist longer than analgesic effects, possibly contributing to cases of overdose.

Mechanism, Pharmacokinetics, and Drug Interactions:

- Opioid agonist.
- Metabolized primarily through CYP2B6, 2C19, and 3A4 (major); inhibits CYP2D6; t ½: 8–59 hours.
- High potential for interactions. Avoid concomitant use with other potent sedatives or respiratory depressants. Use with caution in patients on medications that are metabolized by CYP2D6, inhibit CYP3A4, prolong the QTc interval, or promote electrolyte depletion.

Clinical Pearls:

- Schedule II controlled substance; distribution of 40 mg tablets restricted to authorized opioid addiction treatment facilities.
- May only be dispensed according to the SAMHSA Center for Substance Abuse Treatment guidelines. Regulations vary by area; consult regulatory agencies and/or methadone treatment facilities.
- Methadone accumulates with repeated doses; dose may need reduction after three to five days to prevent CNS depressant effects.

Fun Fact:

A persistent but untrue urban legend claims the name "Dolophine" was coined in tribute to Adolf Hitler by its German creators. The name was in fact created after the war by the American branch of Eli Lilly, and the pejorative term "adolphine" (never an actual name of the drug) didn't appear in the US until the early 1970s.

NALOXONE (Kloxxado, Narcan Nasal Spray, Zimhi) Fact Sheet [G]

Bottom Line:

Naloxone is an opioid antagonist that is used to rapidly reverse opioid overdose. It's important to prescribe this life-saving treatment to all your opioid-dependent patients.

FDA Indications:

Emergency treatment of known or suspected opioid overdose.

Dosage Forms:

- **Intranasal (Narcan Nasal Spray):** 4 mg/0.1 mL.
- **Intranasal (Kloxxado):** 8 mg/0.1 mL.
- **Injectable prefilled syringe (Zimhi):** 5 mg/0.5 mL.
- Generic intranasal kit may be assembled using 2 mg/2 mL prefilled needleless syringe and a mucosal atomization device nasal adapter (requires assembly at time of administration).

Dosage Guidance:

Intranasal: Bystander to spray in one nostril; may repeat into other nostril with additional doses every two to three minutes if no or minimal response and until emergency response arrives. The drug is absorbed automatically into the nasal mucosa, which is why it is effective in patients who are unconscious and cannot sniff it.

Monitoring: No routine monitoring recommended unless clinical picture warrants.

Cost: Intranasal: $$$; generic kit: $

Side Effects:

Most common: Symptoms of opioid withdrawal, including body aches, fever, sweating, runny nose, sneezing, piloerection, yawning, weakness, shivering or trembling, nervousness, restlessness or irritability, diarrhea, nausea or vomiting, abdominal cramps, increased blood pressure, and tachycardia.

Mechanism, Pharmacokinetics, and Drug Interactions:

- Opioid antagonist.
- Metabolized primarily by conjugation (non-P450) in the liver; t ½: 1.36 hours.

Clinical Pearls:

- Because treatment of overdose with this opioid antagonist must be performed by someone other than the patient, instruct prescription recipients to inform those around them that they have naloxone rescue and ensure that those people have been instructed in recognizing overdose symptoms and administering the medication.
- Evzio 2 mg auto-injector offered a novel device with voice instructions but was very expensive; it has been discontinued by the manufacturer and is no longer available. Zimhi is a new injectable (intramuscular or subcutaneous) prefilled syringe for layperson use but comes in a much higher 5 mg dose and delivers nearly five-fold higher peak serum concentrations, which could result in very severe precipitated withdrawal symptoms.
- Most opioids have a longer duration of action than naloxone, so it's likely that overdose symptoms (CNS depression and respiratory depression) will return after initial improvement. Therefore, patients should continue to be monitored and should receive medical attention after emergency dose(s) provided.
- Intranasal forms of naloxone rescue administration, if broadly distributed to those at risk, could make overdose rescue a more acceptable and widespread practice.
- Like Zimhi, Kloxxado is a higher-dose formulation that was developed to combat the presumed need for repeated doses of naloxone after overdose with higher-potency opioids such as fentanyl. Whether multiple doses are required has been controversial, and use of this ultra-potent antagonist could result in severe precipitated withdrawal. Kloxxado is likely overkill for most patients—stick to the 4 mg nasal formulation.
- Check out the Prescribe to Prevent website (www.prescribetoprevent.org) for prescriber resources such as webinars, toolkits, patient education materials, and medical-legal resources. This website also provides guidance to physicians on writing a prescription for naloxone.

Fun Fact:

Naloxone was first approved for opioid overdose treatment in 1971 and is available as a very inexpensive injectable generic. Newer formulations come at a much higher price because of the way they are formulated, making them easier to use by non-emergency provider bystanders.

NALTREXONE (ReVia, Vivitrol) Fact Sheet [G]

Bottom Line:

Naltrexone, an opioid antagonist, is the first-line medication for alcohol use disorder—though it is also approved for opioid use disorder. By reducing the endorphin-mediated euphoria of drinking, it helps people moderate, preventing that first drink from leading to several more. Avoid naltrexone in patients with hepatic impairment or those taking opioid-based pain medications. For opioid dependence, methadone and buprenorphine are more effective for most, although naltrexone may be appropriate for highly motivated opioid-dependent patients, with injectable preferred over oral.

FDA Indications:

Alcohol dependence; opioid addiction (relapse prevention following detox).

Off-Label Uses:

Self-injurious behavior.

Dosage Forms:

- **Tablets (ReVia, [G]):** 50 mg (scored).
- **Long-acting injection (Vivitrol):** 380 mg.

Dosage Guidance:

- Opioid dependence: Start 25 mg for one day; if no withdrawal signs, increase to and maintain 50 mg/day (with food); doses >50 mg may increase risk of hepatotoxicity.
- Alcohol dependence: Start at 50 mg QD; can increase to 100 mg QD after 12 weeks if no response.
- Injection: 380 mg IM (gluteal) Q4 weeks (for opioid or alcohol dependence). Do not initiate therapy until patient is opioid free for at least seven to 10 days (by urinalysis).

Monitoring: LFTs if liver disease is suspected.

Cost: Tablet: $; injection: $$$$$

Side Effects:

- Most common: Headache, nausea, somnolence, vomiting.
- Serious but rare: Black box warning regarding dose-related hepatocellular injury; the difference between apparent safe and hepatotoxic doses appears to be five-fold or less (narrow therapeutic window). Discontinue if signs/symptoms of acute hepatitis develop.

Mechanism, Pharmacokinetics, and Drug Interactions:

- Opioid antagonist.
- Metabolized primarily through non-CYP450 pathway; t ½: 4 hours (5–10 days for IM).
- No significant interactions other than avoiding use with opioids (see below).

Clinical Pearls:

- May precipitate acute withdrawal (pain, hypertension, sweating, agitation, and irritability) in opioid-using patients; ensure patient is opioid free for at least seven to 10 days prior to initiating.
- In naltrexone-treated patients requiring emergency pain management, consider alternatives to opioids (eg, regional analgesia, non-opioid analgesics, general anesthesia). If opioid therapy is required, patients should be under the direct care of a trained anesthesia provider.
- Efficacy of oral naltrexone in alcohol dependence (craving and relapse) is more convincing than in opioid dependence. In opioid dependence, craving is not decreased but euphoric effects are blocked. Monthly IM naltrexone may be more effective than oral at maintaining abstinence in opioid dependence, without concern for daily medication adherence.

Fun Fact:

Methylnaltrexone, a closely related drug, is marketed as Relistor for the treatment of opioid-induced constipation.

NICOTINE GUM/LOZENGE (Nicorette, others) Fact Sheet [G]

Bottom Line:
First-line intervention for those patients who can stop smoking at initiation of therapy; nicotine in the form of gum or lozenge may act as a substitute oral activity, which may aid in behavior modification.

FDA Indications:
Smoking cessation.

Dosage Forms:
- **Gum (G):** 2 mg, 4 mg (over the counter).
- **Lozenge (G):** 2 mg, 4 mg (over the counter).

Dosage Guidance:
- For gum: Chew one piece of gum PRN urge to smoke, up to 24 pieces/day. Patients who smoke <25 cigarettes/day should start with the 2 mg strength; patients smoking ≥25 cigarettes/day should start with the 4 mg strength. Use the following 12-week dosing schedule: For weeks one through six, chew a piece of gum every one to two hours; to increase chances of quitting, chew at least nine pieces/day. For weeks seven through nine, chew a piece of gum every two to four hours. For weeks 10–12, chew a piece of gum every four to eight hours. Patients should not chew more than one piece of gum at a time.
- For lozenges: Patients who smoke their first cigarette within 30 minutes of waking should use the 4 mg strength; otherwise the 2 mg strength is recommended. Use the following 12-week dosing schedule: For weeks one through six, use a lozenge every one to two hours; to increase chances of quitting, use at least nine lozenges/day. For weeks seven through nine, use a lozenge every two to four hours. For weeks 10–12, use a lozenge every four to eight hours. Maximum dose is five lozenges every six hours or 20 lozenges/day. Patients should not use more than one lozenge at a time.
- Patients should be advised to completely stop smoking upon initiation of therapy.

Monitoring: No routine monitoring recommended unless clinical picture warrants.

Cost: $

Side Effects:
Most common: Headache; indigestion; nausea; hiccups; tongue, mouth, and throat irritation or tingling; jaw ache (gum).

Mechanism, Pharmacokinetics, and Drug Interactions:
- Nicotinic-cholinergic receptor agonist.
- Metabolized primarily through liver as well as kidneys and lungs; t ½: 1–2 hours.
- Minimal risk for drug interactions. Successful cessation of smoking may increase serum levels of medications metabolized by CYP1A2 (eg, clozapine, olanzapine, theophylline), which is induced by hydrocarbons in smoke; nicotine itself has no effect.

Clinical Pearls:
- Chew gum slowly until it tingles (about 15 chews), then park gum between cheek and gum until tingle is gone (about one minute); repeat until most of tingle is gone (~30 minutes).
- Lozenges should not be chewed or swallowed; allow them to dissolve slowly (~20–30 minutes).
- Heavy smokers should use higher-dose gum or lozenge and at least nine pieces/day to maximize chances of success. Do not use more than one piece at a time.
- Each 4 mg lozenge or gum results in 2 mg of absorbed nicotine, equivalent to two cigarettes.

Fun Fact:
Nicotine gum is available in a variety of flavors (fruit, mint, cinnamon, orange, cherry, and "original").

NICOTINE INHALED (Nicotrol Inhaler) Fact Sheet

Bottom Line:
Inhaled nicotine is expensive and can cause unpleasant side effects, both of which make this form of nicotine replacement therapy difficult to recommend as a first-line option since no single therapy has been shown to be more effective than another.

FDA Indications:
Smoking cessation.

Dosage Forms:
Cartridge: 4 mg delivered per 10 mg cartridge (prescription required).

Dosage Guidance:
- Use frequent continuous puffing for 20 minutes with each cartridge; 80 deep inhalations over 20 minutes releases 4 mg nicotine, of which 2 mg is absorbed. Use six to 16 cartridges per day. Taper after six to 12 weeks of use by gradual dose reduction over six to 12 additional weeks.
- Patients should be advised to completely stop smoking upon initiation of therapy.

Monitoring: No routine monitoring recommended unless clinical picture warrants.

Cost: $$$$

Side Effects:
Most common: Headache, mouth/throat irritation, dyspepsia, cough, unpleasant taste, rhinitis, tearing, sneezing.

Mechanism, Pharmacokinetics, and Drug Interactions:
- Nicotinic-cholinergic receptor agonist.
- Metabolized primarily through liver as well as kidneys and lungs; t ½: 1–2 hours.
- Minimal risk for drug interactions. Successful cessation of smoking may increase serum levels of medications metabolized by CYP1A2 (eg, clozapine, olanzapine, theophylline), which is induced by hydrocarbons in smoke; nicotine itself has no effect.

Clinical Pearls:
- Insert cartridge into inhaler and push hard until it pops into place. Replace mouthpiece and twist the top and bottom so that markings do not line up. Inhale deeply into the back of the throat or puff in short breaths. Nicotine in cartridge is used up after about 20 minutes of active puffing.
- Do not eat or drink 15 minutes before or during use. To minimize coughing, puff lightly rather than inhaling into lungs.
- Local irritation in the mouth and throat may occur in as many as 40% of patients; coughing (32%) and rhinitis (23%) are also common. These effects are generally mild and occur less frequently with continued use. Use with caution in patients with bronchospastic disease due to potential airway irritation (other forms of nicotine replacement may be preferred).
- Higher ambient temperatures deliver more nicotine; lower temperatures deliver less.
- One cartridge delivers 80 puffs or about 2 mg of absorbed nicotine. Roughly 10 cartridges per day is equivalent to the nicotine of smoking one pack per day.

Fun Fact:
A nicotine inhaler is not really a true inhaler; puffing deposits the nicotine into the mouth, and it is then absorbed in the same manner as the nicotine gum or lozenge preparations.

NICOTINE NASAL SPRAY (Nicotrol NS) Fact Sheet

Bottom Line:

The idea of nasal administration of nicotine is appealing in that it more closely approximates the time course of plasma nicotine levels observed after cigarette smoking than other dosage forms; however, the high cost and unpleasant side effects make this difficult to recommend as a first-line treatment, especially since no one form of nicotine replacement therapy has been shown to be more effective than another.

FDA Indications:

Smoking cessation.

Dosage Forms:

10 mL bottle: 10 mg/mL delivering 0.5 mg/spray in 200 sprays (prescription required).

Dosage Guidance:

- Use one or two sprays/hour as needed; do not exceed more than five doses (10 sprays) per hour. Max dose is 40 doses/day (80 sprays). Each dose (two sprays) contains 1 mg of nicotine.
- After initial eight weeks of treatment, taper dose gradually over four to six weeks.
- Patients should be advised to completely stop smoking upon initiation of therapy.

Monitoring: No routine monitoring recommended unless clinical picture warrants.

Cost: $$$$

Side Effects:

Most common: Headache, dyspepsia, rhinitis, nasal irritation, sneezing, coughing.

Mechanism, Pharmacokinetics, and Drug Interactions:

- Nicotinic-cholinergic receptor agonist.
- Metabolized primarily through liver as well as kidneys and lungs; t ½: 1–2 hours.
- Minimal risk for drug interactions. Successful cessation of smoking may increase serum levels of medications metabolized by CYP1A2 (eg, clozapine, olanzapine, theophylline), which is induced by hydrocarbons in smoke; nicotine itself has no effect.

Clinical Pearls:

- Prime pump prior to first use. Blow nose gently prior to use. Tilt head back slightly, breathe through mouth, and spray once in each nostril. Do not sniff, swallow, or inhale through nose.
- Moderate to severe nasal irritation in 94% of patients in the first two days of use; severity decreases over time. Nasal congestion and transient changes in sense of smell and taste also reported. Avoid in patients with chronic nasal disorders (eg, allergy, rhinitis, nasal polyps, and sinusitis). Exacerbations of bronchospasm reported in patients with asthma.
- Heavy smokers may well use the maximum amount of 80 sprays/day, meaning they would need a new bottle every two to three days. This can be tremendously and prohibitively expensive.
- Potential for abuse and dependence appears to be greater than with other nicotine replacement therapies.

Fun Fact:

In a published case report (Myrick H et al, *Am J Psychiatry* 2001;158(3):498), a 54-year-old man who could no longer afford his Nicotrol NS prescription found a commercial source for nicotine on the internet (sold as an insecticide). He purchased 25 g in a 1 g/mL solution for $30, diluted the nicotine solution with distilled water to 10 mg/mL, and then placed the solution into empty spray bottles.

NICOTINE PATCH (Nicoderm CQ, others) Fact Sheet [G]

Bottom Line:
Nicotine patches are a first-line intervention in patients who are able to quit smoking at initiation of treatment and who are regular and constant smokers.

FDA Indications:
Smoking cessation.

Dosage Forms:
Transdermal patch (G): 7 mg, 14 mg, 21 mg/24 hour (over the counter).

Dosage Guidance:
- Patients smoking >10 cigarettes/day: Start with 21 mg/day for six weeks, then 14 mg/day for two weeks, then 7 mg/day for two weeks. Patients smoking ≤10 cigarettes/day: Start with 14 mg/day for six weeks, then 7 mg/day for two weeks.
- Apply new patch every 24 hours (same time each day, usually after awakening) to non-hairy, clean, dry skin on the upper body or upper outer arm; each patch should be applied to a different site. Adjustment may be required during initial treatment (move to higher dose if experiencing withdrawal symptoms, or lower dose if side effects are experienced).
- Patients should be advised to completely stop smoking upon initiation of therapy.

Monitoring: No routine monitoring recommended unless clinical picture warrants.

Cost: $

Side Effects:
Most common: Application site reactions (itching, burning, or redness), diarrhea, dyspepsia, abdominal pain.

Mechanism, Pharmacokinetics, and Drug Interactions:
- Nicotinic-cholinergic receptor agonist.
- Metabolized primarily through liver as well as kidneys and lungs; t ½: 3–6 hours.
- Minimal risk for drug interactions. Successful cessation of smoking may increase serum levels of medications metabolized by CYP1A2 (eg, clozapine, olanzapine, theophylline), which is induced by hydrocarbons in smoke; nicotine itself has no effect.

Clinical Pearls:
- Patch may be worn for 16 or 24 hours. If craving upon awakening, wear patch for 24 hours; if vivid dreams or sleep disruptions occur, wear patch for 16 hours, removing at bedtime.
- Do not cut patch; this causes rapid evaporation, making the patch useless.
- Up to 50% of patients will experience a local skin reaction, which is usually mild and self-limiting but may worsen with continued treatment. Local treatment with hydrocortisone cream 1% or triamcinolone cream 0.5% and rotating patch sites may help. In fewer than 5% of patients, such reactions require discontinuation.

Fun Facts:
Studies have found that smoking seems to provide short-term relief from symptoms of ulcerative colitis; recent data have suggested the use of nicotine patches in some patients with flare-ups of ulcerative colitis (not maintenance treatment).

VARENICLINE (Chantix) Fact Sheet [G]

Bottom Line:
Varenicline is the most effective tobacco cessation medication. Psychiatric side effects are usually limited to insomnia or abnormal dreams, but more dramatic reactions are possible, though rare.

FDA Indications:
Smoking cessation.

Dosage Forms:
Tablets (G): 0.5 mg, 1 mg.

Dosage Guidance:
Start 0.5 mg QD for three days; ↑ to 0.5 mg BID for four days then ↑ to 1 mg BID for 11 weeks. Titrate slowly and take with food and a full glass of water to decrease GI upset. Start one week before target quit date; consider setting a quit date up to 35 days after starting varenicline (may improve likelihood of abstinence).

Monitoring: No routine monitoring recommended unless clinical picture warrants.

Cost: $$$$

Side Effects:
- Most common: Nausea, insomnia, headache, abnormal dreams, constipation, flatulence.
- Serious but rare: Warning for serious neuropsychiatric events (including depression, suicidal thoughts, suicide, psychosis, hostility), even in those without preexisting psychiatric disease, guidance was recently revised to indicate that risk is lower than previously suspected.

Mechanism, Pharmacokinetics, and Drug Interactions:
- Nicotine receptor partial agonist.
- Excreted mostly unchanged with minimal hepatic (non-CYP450) metabolism; t ½: 24 hours.
- Potential lowered tolerance to alcohol, with psychiatric reactions. H2 blockers, quinolones, and trimethoprim may increase varenicline levels. Successful cessation of smoking may alter pharmacokinetic properties of other medications (eg, clozapine, olanzapine, theophylline, warfarin, insulin).

Clinical Pearls:
- Dual mechanism of action: Partial agonist at nicotinic receptors, mimicking nicotine effects on the brain and reducing withdrawal symptoms; blocks nicotine from binding to these receptors, thereby decreasing the reinforcing effect of smoking.
- If patient successfully quits smoking after 12 weeks, may continue for another 12 weeks. If not successful in first 12 weeks, then discontinue and reassess factors contributing to failure.
- Similar quit rates as bupropion at six months (25%), but higher quit rates compared to bupropion at one year if a second 12-week course of varenicline is used.
- Can be combined with bupropion; use with nicotine replacement therapies likely to lead to increased side effects, particularly nausea, headache, vomiting, and dizziness.
- Generic varenicline has been newly approved; look for a significant price drop in the months to come.

Fun Fact:
The show *Saturday Night Live* aired a parody of a Chantix commercial suggesting that side effects of *quitting* smoking could be dangerous (it's on YouTube).

Appendices

APPENDIX A: DRUG INTERACTIONS IN PSYCHIATRY

In this appendix you'll find three tables related to drug interactions. For an in-depth discussion of the complexities of drug interactions, please read our new Carlat Guide, *Prescribing Psychotropics: From Drug Interactions to Pharmacogenetics*. See www.thecarlatreport.com/prescribing for more information.

Generally, when pressed for time, most clinicians will use one of the following online drug interaction checkers:

Free
- Medscape (https://reference.medscape.com/drug-interactionchecker)
- www.epocrates.com (you'll need to register first)
- www.drugs.com/drug_interactions.html

Paid
- Lexi-Interact (https://www.wolterskluwer.com/en/solutions/lexicomp), $119 for one-year subscription

However, it's helpful to review drug interaction tables occasionally because they will give you context and allow you to begin to memorize which medications are most likely to cause troublesome interactions. The majority of interactions in psychiatry will **not** result in a serious outcome. Many interactions, however, may result in decreased efficacy or increased adverse effects, and these can be easily avoided.

To understand drug-drug interactions, you'll need to refamiliarize yourself with some basic terms. Drugs are **substrates** of specific enzymes (the medication relies on specific enzymatic pathway(s) for metabolism). An **inhibitor** is a drug that binds more tightly to an enzyme than the usual substrate and prevents the enzyme from doing its job; as a result, the substrate for that enzyme gets stuck in a game of musical chairs as it scurries around looking for a free enzyme system to break it down. Since this drug is not getting metabolized as quickly as it otherwise would (the inhibitor is preventing it from doing so), its serum levels become higher than expected. On the other hand, **inducers** stimulate the production of extra enzymes. With more enzymes around, the substrate for that enzyme is broken down more rapidly, leading to lower serum drug levels.

Another important concern with drug interactions is timing. **Inhibition** happens quickly. It can occur with the first dose of a medication and can subside quickly when an inhibitor is discontinued. How long it takes to subside depends on the inhibitor's half-life. Generally, the inhibition will stop after five half-lives of the inhibitor drug. On the other hand, for **induction** to occur, the body has to synthesize more CYP450 enzymes, and this can take up to four weeks. This accounts for the delayed "auto-induction" of carbamazepine. Likewise, for induction to subside, these extra enzymes need to be broken down, a process that could also take several weeks. As a general rule of thumb, any drug prescribed with its inhibitor should be started at half the usual dose and titrated more slowly. Conversely, a drug prescribed with its inducer may need to be dosed higher after the few weeks it takes for induction to occur. One exception to the rule of inhibitors increasing substrate levels is when the substrate is a prodrug. Tamoxifen, hydrocodone, and tramadol are prodrugs that rely on CYP450 2D6 to be converted into an active metabolite. In the presence of a potent inhibitor like fluoxetine or paroxetine, patients may see a drop in therapeutic effects rather than increased effects.

Practical Tips for Quickly Identifying Significant Drug Interactions
- Identify the 10 drugs that you most commonly prescribe and memorize the major drug interactions for each one.
- Antidepressants, antipsychotics, antibiotics, antiretrovirals, and older anticonvulsants have a high likelihood of significant drug interactions—so be particularly vigilant if your patient is taking any of these.
- Recognize the drugs with a narrow therapeutic window, ie, drugs for which the toxic dose is not much higher than the therapeutic dose. Commonly used drugs with narrow therapeutic windows include lithium, carbamazepine (Tegretol), warfarin (Coumadin), digoxin (Lanoxin), phenytoin (Dilantin), and phenobarbital.
- Recognize drugs that cause serious side effects and outcomes if blood levels are significantly increased or decreased (eg, oral contraceptives, lamotrigine, clozapine, tricyclic antidepressants, warfarin).
- Drugs with long half-lives, such as diazepam (Valium) or aripiprazole (Abilify), can be particularly troublesome when involved in drug interactions, because metabolic inhibitors—or hepatic dysfunction—can make them ultra-long lasting. Be cautious with any new or rarely prescribed drugs: Neither you nor anybody else has had much experience with them, and unreported drug interactions can appear.
- The risk of drug interactions can increase exponentially as the number of drugs increases. Setting a threshold to check for interactions is helpful (eg, any patient on three or more drugs).

Appendix Table A1: CYP450 Drug Interactions for Some Common Psychiatric Medications

CYP450 Family	Inducers	Inhibitors	Substrates ("Victim" Drugs)	Symptoms When Induced	Symptoms When Inhibited
1A2	Armodafinil Carbamazepine Cigarette smoke Modafinil St. John's wort	Fluvoxamine Melatonin	Asenapine	Loss of efficacy (psychosis)	Insomnia/EPS
			Caffeine	Withdrawal headaches	Jitteriness
			Clozapine	Loss of efficacy (psychosis)	Seizures/sedation/anticholinergic effects
			Duloxetine	Loss of efficacy (depression)	Increased blood pressure
			Fluvoxamine	Loss of efficacy (depression/OCD)	GI/sedation
			Melatonin	Loss of efficacy (insomnia)	Sedation
			Mirtazapine	Loss of efficacy (depression)	Sedation
			Olanzapine	Loss of efficacy (psychosis)	Sedation
			Ramelteon	Loss of efficacy (insomnia)	Sedation
			Ropinirole	Loss of efficacy (RLS, Parkinson's)	Insomnia/anxiety/compulsive behavior
			Thiothixene	Loss of efficacy (psychosis)	Sedation/EPS
			Trifluoperazine	Loss of efficacy (psychosis)	Sedation/EPS
2B6	Carbamazepine Phenobarbital		Bupropion	Loss of efficacy (depression)	N/A
			Methadone	Opioid withdrawal	N/A
			Selegiline	Loss of efficacy (depression)	N/A
2C9	Carbamazepine St. John's wort	Fluoxetine Fluvoxamine	Methadone	Opioid withdrawal	CNS and respiratory depression
2C19	Carbamazepine Phenytoin	Armodafinil Fluoxetine Fluvoxamine Modafinil Oxcarbazepine	Barbiturates	Loss of efficacy (insomnia/anxiety/seizures)	Sedation/barb intoxication
			Citalopram	Loss of efficacy (depression/anxiety)	GI effects
			Diazepam	Loss of efficacy (insomnia/anxiety/seizures)	Sedation/BZD intoxication
			Doxepin	Loss of efficacy (depression/anxiety/insomnia)	Seizures/arrhythmia/anticholinergic effects
			Escitalopram	Loss of efficacy (depression/anxiety)	GI effects
			Methadone	Opioid withdrawal	CNS and respiratory depression
			Sertraline	Loss of efficacy (depression/anxiety)	GI effects

( ) indicates less potent inhibitory effect, therefore generally less of a risk except at higher doses

CYP450 Family	Inducers	Inhibitors	Substrates ("Victim" Drugs)	Symptoms When Induced	Symptoms When Inhibited
2D6	Not inducible	Asenapine Bupropion Duloxetine Fluoxetine Haloperidol Methadone Paroxetine Thioridazine Venlafaxine	Amphetamine	N/A	Insomnia/decreased appetite
			Aripiprazole	N/A	Akathisia/sedation
			Atomoxetine	N/A	GI/constipation
			Brexpiprazole	N/A	Akathisia/sedation
			Chlorpromazine	N/A	Seizures/sedation/anticholinergic effects
			Clonidine	N/A	Hypotension/dizziness/sedation
			Clozapine	N/A	Seizures/sedation/anticholinergic effects
			Codeine/hydrocodone	N/A	Less/no analgesia (not converted to morphine)
			Deutetrabenazine	N/A	Sedation/QT prolongation
			Dextroamphetamine	N/A	Insomnia/decreased appetite
			Dextromethorphan	N/A	Difficulty breathing, dizziness, drowsiness, anxiety, or confusion
			Diphenhydramine	N/A	Sedation/anticholinergic
			Donepezil	N/A	GI effects
			Doxepin	N/A	Sedation/anticholinergic
			Doxylamine	N/A	Sedation/anticholinergic
			Duloxetine	N/A	Increased BP
			Fluoxetine	N/A	GI effects
			Fluphenazine	N/A	EPS
			Fluvoxamine	N/A	GI effects/sedation
			Galantamine	N/A	GI effects
			Haloperidol	N/A	EPS
			Iloperidone	N/A	Tachycardia/hypotension/stiffness
			Lisdexamfetamine (prodrug of dextroamphetamine)	N/A	Insomnia/decreased appetite
			Lofexidine	N/A	Hypotension/dizziness/sedation
			Loxapine	N/A	EPS/sedation
			Methamphetamine	N/A	Insomnia/decreased appetite
			Mirtazapine	N/A	Somnolence
			Mixed amphetamine salts	N/A	Insomnia/decreased appetite
			Paroxetine	N/A	GI effects/anticholinergic/sedation
			Perphenazine	N/A	EPS/sedation
			Pitolisant	N/A	Insomnia/anxiety
			Propranolol	N/A	Decreased BP/pulse

( ) indicates less potent inhibitory effect, therefore generally less of a risk except at higher doses

CYP450 Family	Inducers	Inhibitors	Substrates ("Victim" Drugs)	Symptoms When Induced	Symptoms When Inhibited
2D6	Not inducible	Asenapine Bupropion Duloxetine Fluoxetine Haloperidol Methadone Paroxetine Thioridazine Venlafaxine	Risperidone	N/A	EPS/orthostasis
			Thioridazine	N/A	Seizures/sedation/anticholinergic effects/QT prolongation
			Trazodone	N/A	Sedation
			Tricyclics	N/A	Seizures/arrhythmia/anticholinergic
			Valbenazine	N/A	Sedation/QT prolongation
			Venlafaxine	N/A	GI effects
			Vortioxetine	N/A	GI effects
3A4	Armodafinil Carbamazepine Modafinil Oxcarbazepine St. John's wort	Fluvoxamine Grapefruit juice Nefazodone	Alprazolam	Loss of efficacy (insomnia/anxiety/seizures)	Sedation/BZD intoxication
			Aripiprazole	Loss of efficacy (psychosis)	Akathisia/sedation
			Armodafinil	Loss of efficacy (narcolepsy)	Insomnia/increased pulse
			Avanafil	Loss of efficacy (sexual dysfunction)	Headache/flushing/prolonged erection
			Brexpiprazole	Loss of efficacy (psychosis)	Akathisia/sedation
			Buprenorphine	Opioid withdrawal	CNS and respiratory depression
			Buspirone	Loss of efficacy (anxiety)	GI effects/jitteriness
			Carbamazepine	Loss of efficacy/seizures	Sedation/arrhythmia
			Cariprazine	Loss of efficacy (psychosis)	Akathisia/sedation
			Citalopram	Loss of efficacy (depression/anxiety)	GI effects
			Clonazepam	Loss of efficacy (insomnia/anxiety/seizures)	Sedation/BZD intoxication
			Clozapine	Loss of efficacy (psychosis)	Seizures/sedation/anticholinergic effects
			Diazepam	Loss of efficacy (insomnia/anxiety/seizures)	Sedation/BZD intoxication
			Escitalopram	Loss of efficacy (depression/anxiety)	GI effects
			Eszopiclone	Loss of efficacy (insomnia)	Sedation/confusion
			Flibanserin	Loss of efficacy (sexual desire)	Nausea/dizziness/sedation
			Flurazepam	Loss of efficacy (insomnia)	Sedation/BZD intoxication
			Galantamine	Loss of efficacy (dementia)	GI effects
			Guanfacine	Loss of efficacy (ADHD)	Sedation/dry mouth/dizziness
			Iloperidone	Loss of efficacy (psychosis)	Sedation/dizziness
			Lemborexant	Loss of efficacy (insomnia)	Sedation/confusion
			Levomilnacipran	Loss of efficacy (depression)	GI effects
			Loxapine	Loss of efficacy (psychosis)	EPS/sedation
			Lurasidone	Loss of efficacy (psychosis)	Sedation/akathisia
			Methadone	Opioid withdrawal	CNS and respiratory depression
			Mirtazapine	Loss of efficacy (depression/insomnia)	Somnolence

( ) indicates less potent inhibitory effect, therefore generally less of a risk except at higher doses

CYP450 Family	Inducers	Inhibitors	Substrates ("Victim" Drugs)	Symptoms When Induced	Symptoms When Inhibited
3A4	Armodafinil Carbamazepine Modafinil Oxcarbazepine St. John's wort	Fluvoxamine Grapefruit juice Nefazodone	Modafinil	Loss of efficacy (narcolepsy)	Insomnia/increased pulse
			Nefazodone	Loss of efficacy (depression)	Sedation/orthostasis
			Oral contraceptives	Loss of efficacy (pregnancy)	GI effects
			Pimavanserin	Loss of efficacy (psychosis)	Nausea/confusion
			Pitolisant	Loss of efficacy (EDS)	Insomnia/anxiety
			Quetiapine	Loss of efficacy (psychosis)	Sedation/orthostasis
			Sildenafil	Loss of efficacy (sexual dysfunction)	Headache/flushing/prolonged erection
			Suvorexant	Loss of efficacy (insomnia)	Sedation/confusion
			Tadalafil	Loss of efficacy (sexual dysfunction)	Headache/flushing/prolonged erection
			Trazodone	Loss of efficacy (insomnia)	Sedation/orthostasis
			Triazolam	Loss of efficacy (insomnia)	Sedation/BZD intoxication
			Tricyclics	Loss of efficacy (depression/anxiety)	Seizures/arrhythmia/anticholinergic
			Valbenazine	N/A	Sedation/QT prolongation
			Vardenafil	Loss of efficacy (sexual dysfunction)	Headache/flushing/prolonged erection
			Vilazodone	Loss of efficacy (depression/anxiety)	GI effects
			Zaleplon	Loss of efficacy (insomnia)	Sedation/confusion
			Ziprasidone	Loss of efficacy (psychosis)	Sedation/akathisia
			Zolpidem	Loss of efficacy (insomnia)	Sedation/confusion

( ) indicates less potent inhibitory effect, therefore generally less of a risk except at higher doses

Clinical Consequence	Medications Most Commonly Contributing	Comments
Decreased efficacy of psychiatric medications	Carbamazepine, St. John's wort, cigarette smoking strongly induce metabolism and decrease serum levels of many psychotropics (see Table A1 for details)	Smoking may reduce olanzapine, clozapine levels; carbamazepine can reduce levels of many medications
Decreased efficacy of opioids	Potent 2D6 inhibitors (paroxetine, fluoxetine, duloxetine, bupropion) prevent conversion of certain opioids (codeine, hydrocodone, oxycodone) to active metabolites, thereby decreasing pain relief	Use alternative antidepressants (eg, sertraline, citalopram, escitalopram)
Decreased efficacy of oral contraceptive pills (OCPs)	Carbamazepine, St. John's wort, cigarette smoking strongly induce metabolism and decrease serum levels of OCPs	Avoid these meds in women taking OCPs
Increased side effects or toxicity of psychiatric medications	The most common and potent CYP450 inhibitors are paroxetine, fluoxetine, duloxetine, bupropion, valproic acid, asenapine, and grapefruit juice—all may lead to increased substrate levels and increased side effects or toxicity (see Table A1 for interaction details)	Adjust dose of substrate or use alternative medications
Serotonin syndrome	High doses or combinations of the following: SSRIs, SNRIs, TCAs, MAOIs, buspirone, dextromethorphan, lithium, tramadol, trazodone	Caution patients to report new sudden onset of fever, agitation, tremor, sweating, diarrhea; discontinue offending agents and provide supportive care
QT prolongation	Monotherapy or combined therapy with the following: ziprasidone, thioridazine, TCAs, methadone, and certain cardiac meds and antibiotics (amiodarone, ciprofloxacin, clarithromycin, erythromycin, ketoconazole, quinidine)	May lead to potentially fatal arrhythmias; monitor ECG and electrolytes and use alternative medications in patients with borderline or increased QT interval
Increased risk for bleeding	Serotonergic antidepressants (SSRIs, SNRIs) especially when combined with anticoagulants (warfarin), antiplatelets (aspirin), or NSAIDs	May lead to bruising or minor bleeding (nosebleed, gum bleed); GI bleeds and more severe bleeding also rarely reported; use alternative in patients at highest risk, such as the elderly
Lowered seizure threshold	Bupropion, clozapine	Use with caution in patients with a history of seizures, electrolyte disturbances, or head trauma; consider concomitant antiepileptic for seizure prophylaxis
Lithium toxicity	Lithium used in combination with NSAIDs, ACE inhibitors, angiotensin II receptor blockers, diuretics (especially thiazides)	Use alternative agents or monitor lithium levels closely and adjust dosing
Anticholinergic delirium	Anticholinergics (benztropine, trihexyphenidyl), antihistamines (diphenhydramine, doxylamine), low-potency first-generation antipsychotics (chlorpromazine), olanzapine, clozapine, TCAs, others (oxybutynin)	High anticholinergic burden may lead to confusion and delirium, particularly in older patients; minimize use or use alternative medications

What Causes the MAOI-Food Interaction?

Tyramine is an amino acid naturally found in our bodies and in some foods. It's responsible for norepinephrine release, which can lead to elevated blood pressure. Normally, the monoamine oxidase (MAO) enzyme breaks down norepinephrine, keeping blood pressure in check. Blocking MAO-A in the GI tract with an MAOI, combined with eating foods high in tyramine, can lead to a "cheese reaction" or hypertensive crisis. Patients taking any MAOI (with the exception of the lowest dose of the selegiline patch) should adhere to this diet while they are taking the MAOI and for two weeks after stopping the MAOI (that's the time it takes to regenerate new MAO enzymes after irreversible inhibition by the MAOI).

Appendix Table A3: MAOI Dietary and Medication Restrictions

Food or Drink Category	Avoid	Minimize Intake[1]	Allowed[2]
Meat, poultry, fish	• Aged, air dried, fermented, smoked, pickled, or cured meats, poultry, fish (cacciatore), bacon, aged or dried sausage, salami, mortadella, corned beef, pastrami, pickled herring, lox, smoked salmon, smoked trout, shrimp paste, liverwurst, meat extracts (flavor cubes, bouillon) • Spoiled or improperly stored meat, poultry, fish, or animal livers (discolored, malodorous, or moldy)	• Processed meats, cooked ham, hot dogs, pepperoni, bologna • Properly stored smoked fish	• Fresh, fresh frozen, or fresh processed (not aged or smoked) meat, poultry, fish • Fresh breakfast sausage • Fresh gravy
Dairy, eggs, cheese	Aged cheeses: blue/bleu, camembert, cheddar, gorgonzola, gouda, gruyere, provolone, Roquefort, Stilton, Swiss (fermentation holes, strong smells, salty or biting taste)	• Cheeses: Parmesan, Romano • Soy milk • (limit these to 1 half-cup serving) • 1–2 slices of pizza from large chain commercial outlets (generally made with low-tyramine cheese); avoid larger quantities, extra cheese, or pizzas containing aged cheese	• Cheeses: mozzarella, American, ricotta, cottage, cream, farmer, or pot • Fresh pasteurized milk • Pasteurized cream • Yogurt • Sour cream • Ice cream • Pudding • Butter • Eggs
Fruit	• Overly ripened banana, banana peel • Overly ripened avocado • Dried fruit	• Avocado (not over-ripened) • Canned figs • Raspberries	Fresh, frozen, or canned and properly stored fruits and fruit juices
Vegetables	• Broad bean pods (fava beans, Italian green beans) • Soy beans • Bean pastes • Edamame beans • Kimchee (kimchi) • Snow peas	Chili peppers	• Fresh, frozen, canned, or dried and properly stored vegetables, leafy salad greens, lentils, beans (except fava and soy) • Veggie burgers containing no soy product
Soy	Soy products (soy sauce, tofu, tempeh)	Soy milk (1 half-cup serving)	
Beverages	• Tap (draft) beer, non-pasteurized beer, Korean beer (including non-alcoholic) • Vermouth	• Caffeine-containing drinks • Clear alcoholic spirits (gin, vodka, rum) • Red or white wine (no more than two 4-oz servings per day) • Bottled or canned beer, including non-alcoholic (no more than two 12-oz servings per day)	Decaffeinated beverages (coffee, tea)
Breads, cereal, crackers	• Sourdough bread • Crackers and breads that contain aged cheese		Commercial yeast breads, hot and cold cereals, most crackers (containing no aged cheese)
Condiments and miscellaneous	• Concentrated yeast extract (marmite, vegemite) • Soy products (soy sauce, tofu, teriyaki, soy paste, Thai or Vietnamese fish sauce) • Sauerkraut	Chocolate (limit to 2 oz, or 4 oz of chocolate-containing dessert)	• Brewer's yeast or baker's yeast • Monosodium glutamate (MSG) • Ketchup, mustard, mayonnaise, salt, spices, herbs • Non-cheese salad dressings • Worcestershire sauce

[1] "Minimize Intake" items should be eaten only occasionally; no more than one serving (½ cup) of one to three of these per day.

[2] "Allowed" items become "Avoid" items if spoiled or improperly stored. No leftover, improperly stored, handled, or spoiled foods of any type should be consumed. Purchase and consume only fresh meats, poultry, and fish that are properly wrapped and stored under refrigeration and eaten the same day or frozen right away. Fresh produce should be consumed within 48 hours of purchase and not eaten if overripe.

Food or Drink Category	Avoid	Minimize Intake[1]	Allowed[2]
Medications			
Pain medications	Opioids including meperidine (Demerol), propoxyphene (Darvon), tramadol (Ultram), fentanyl, methadone		Acetaminophen Ibuprofen
Cold/allergy medications	Any combination product with a "-D" for decongestant (eg, Zyrtec-D) Dextromethorphan (Delsym) Pseudoephedrine (Sudafed) Decongestant nasal sprays		Menthol lozenges Plain nasal saline spray Robitussin alone (guaifenesin) Cetirizine (Zyrtec), fexofenadine (Allegra), loratadine (Claritin) without the "-D" for decongestant
Antidepressants	Avoid all unless prescribed by doctor who has experience prescribing MAOIs; includes buspirone, OTC antidepressants (St. John's wort, SAMe)		
Stimulants	Avoid all use including prescription, illicit stimulants (methamphetamine, cocaine, ecstasy), or OTC diet pills (may contain stimulants)		

[1] "Minimize Intake" items should be eaten only occasionally; no more than one serving (½ cup) of one to three of these per day.

[2] "Allowed" items become "Avoid" items if spoiled or improperly stored. No leftover, improperly stored, handled, or spoiled foods of any type should be consumed. Purchase and consume only fresh meats, poultry, and fish that are properly wrapped and stored under refrigeration and eaten the same day or frozen right away. Fresh produce should be consumed within 48 hours of purchase and not eaten if overripe.

References

- Flockhart DA. Dietary restrictions and drug interactions with monoamine oxidase inhibitors: an update. *J Clin Psychiatry* 2012;73 Suppl 1:17–24. doi:10.4088/JCP.11096su1c.03.
- Gardner DM et al. The making of a user friendly MAOI diet. *J Clin Psychiatry* 1996;57(3):99–104.
- Hirsch M & Birnbaum RJ. Monoamine oxidase inhibitors (MAOIs) for treating depressed adults. *UpToDate* 2018.

APPENDIX B: PSYCHIATRIC MEDICATIONS IN PREGNANCY AND LACTATION

Determining the risk of medications in pregnancy used to be a simple matter of looking up a drug's pregnancy categorization in the *PDR*. This went from category "A," the lowest risk, to "X," contraindicated in pregnancy. But this ABCDX system provided very little practical or clinically useful information. In 2014, the FDA came up with a new system of labeling, which requires descriptive subsections on different aspects of pregnancy and lactation, and omits the letter categories—though you'll still see the old system in use for drugs approved before 2015.

Pregnancy presents a unique problem to the psychiatrist. Contrary to what many may think or assume, pregnancy does not protect a woman from an acute episode, a recurrence, or an exacerbation of psychiatric illness. Withholding medications during pregnancy can *sometimes* be an appropriate option, but this is generally not recommended. And since all psychotropic medications cross the placenta to at least *some* degree, their potential effects on the fetus, on labor and delivery, and on the neonate must be considered and balanced with the risk of *not* treating the mother with medication (see our July/August 2016 double issue of *TCPR* for an overview). A similar risk-benefit assessment must be considered in the case of a mother who wishes to breastfeed her child, as psychotropic medications are excreted into breast milk to varying degrees.

One of us (TP) is a pharmacist specializing in psychopharmacology who is commonly consulted by psychiatrists to provide updated information on the safety of medications in pregnancy and breastfeeding. It is a difficult task, because the quantity and quality of data vary greatly. The accompanying table was developed by pulling together a variety of sources, including isolated case reports, case series, birth registries, retrospective surveys, prospective comparative cohort studies, case control studies, and meta-analyses. Making judgments about which medication to use—or not use—in a pregnant or lactating woman is a delicate balancing act, involving an assessment of the severity of the underlying illness versus the uncertainties inherent in prescribing medications when the available data are limited.

In reading the table, keep the following in mind: In the general US population, the baseline rate of major malformations is between 1% and 4%, depending on the population studied and the definitions of "malformations" used. If treatment is necessary, monotherapy with the lowest *effective* dose and for the shortest duration is prudent. Safety data are generally more robust with older agents, and for that reason older agents—with a few key exceptions—are more preferable than newer drugs with less established safety profiles.

Almost all drugs enter breast milk. The exposure to the infant is described as a percentage of the maternal dose—that is, how much of the weight-adjusted maternal dose is actually excreted into the breast milk. When less than 10% of a mother's dose of medication is excreted into the breast milk, it is generally considered compatible with breastfeeding (with some exceptions) since these low serum levels are unlikely to lead to adverse effects in the infant.

While the table summarizes the current knowledge about psychotropic medication in pregnancy and lactation, information in this area is constantly evolving. If you regularly treat women of childbearing age, we suggest that you keep up with new data, consult with experts, and use resources such as:

- Organization of Teratology Information Specialists at www.mothertobaby.org or 866-626-6847
- LactMed peer-reviewed database of the National Library of Medicine, updated monthly at https://www.ncbi.nlm.nih.gov/books/NBK501922
- MGH Center for Women's Mental Health at www.womensmentalhealth.org
- The CDC's wide range of offerings at https://www.cdc.gov/pregnancy/meds

And, if you don't mind paying a fee (or if you are a trainee and have free access), you can check out www.reprotox.org, an online database of summaries. Another source of information can be the drug labeling, which, as of 2015, is more detailed than in the past. These resources, along with our table, provide information based upon the available evidence (or lack thereof), but the ultimate clinical decision comes down to careful and individualized consideration between the physician and the patient and her family.

Additional References

- Besag FM. ADHD treatment and pregnancy. *Drug Saf* 2014;37(6):397–408.
- Chisolm MS et al. Management of psychotropic drugs during pregnancy. *BMJ* 2016;352:h5918.
- Khan SJ et al. Bipolar disorder in pregnancy and postpartum: Principles of management. *Curr Psychiatry Rep* 2016;18(2):13.
- McLafferty LP et al. Guidelines for the management of pregnant women with substance use disorders. *Psychosomatics* 2016;57(2):115–130.
- Muzik M et al. Use of antidepressants during pregnancy?: What to consider when weighing treatment with antidepressants against untreated depression. *Matern Child Health J* 2016;20(11):2268–2279.
- Ornoy A et al. Antidepressant, antipsychotics, and mood stabilizers in pregnancy: What do we know and how should we treat pregnant women with depression? *Birth Defects Res* 2017:109(12):933–956.

- Oyebode F et al. Psychotropics in pregnancy: Safety and other considerations. *Pharmacol Ther* 2012;135(1):71–77.
- Payne JL. Psychopharmacology in pregnancy and breastfeeding. *Med Clin North Am* 2019;103(4):629–650.
- Rowe H et al. Maternal medication, drug use, and breastfeeding. *Child Adolesc Psychiatr Clin N Am* 2015;24(1):1–20.
- Sachs HC et al. The transfer of drugs and therapeutics into human breast milk: An update on selected topics. *Pediatrics* 2013;132(3):e796–e809.
- Vigod S et al. Depression in pregnancy. *BMJ* 2016;352:i547.

Appendix Table B: Psychiatric Medications in Pregnancy and Lactation

Medication	Pregnancy	Breastfeeding	Recommendations
Anxiolytics/Hypnotics			
Benzodiazepines (various agents)	Possible increased incidence of cleft lip or palate (with first trimester exposure); floppy infant syndrome (with exposure just before delivery); neonatal withdrawal syndrome; lower Apgar scores	Excretion less than 10%. Excessive sedation in infant, lethargy with consequent feeding difficulty and weight loss reported.	• Try to avoid in first trimester and late in pregnancy (although intermittent use less likely to induce withdrawal symptoms in neonate) • Lorazepam (Ativan) may be best in class to use due to lack of active metabolites and relatively shorter half-life • Monitor sedation in breastfed infants; use of shorter-acting agents preferred
Buspirone (BuSpar)	Minimal data; difficult to determine risks	Low to undetectable infant levels reported	• Avoid in pregnancy due to limited data • Likely safe in breastfeeding
Diphenhydramine (Benadryl)	Fairly consistent data show lack of associated malformations	Larger doses or more prolonged use may cause adverse effects in the infant	• Considered to be the safest hypnotic in pregnancy and breastfeeding
Non-benzodiazepines: Eszopiclone (Lunesta) Zaleplon (Sonata) Zolpidem (Ambien)	No increased risk of malformations, but data fairly sparse	Relatively low levels in breast milk. Most data are with zolpidem. Zolpidem is relatively hydrophilic and excreted rapidly; therefore, may be favored.	• Reserve for second-line use due to paucity of data • Zolpidem at low dose is the best option when non-benzos are needed
Suvorexant (Belsomra), lemborexant (Dayvigo)	No data	No data	• Use other agents with more data and longer record of experience
Trazodone	Fewer data show no increased risk of malformations	<1% excretion; not expected to cause adverse effects in breastfed infants	• Probably safe in pregnancy and breastfeeding
Mood Stabilizers			
Carbamazepine (Tegretol)	Rate of major malformation 2.2%–7.9%. Neural tube defects (0.5%–1%), craniofacial defects, cardiovascular malformations, and hypospadias reported.	Relatively high levels in breast milk but with few adverse effects reported. Sedation, poor sucking, withdrawal reactions, and three cases of hepatic dysfunction have been reported.	• Avoid if possible • If use unavoidable, add high-dose (4 mg) folic acid supplementation
Lamotrigine (Lamictal)	Rate of major malformations 1%–5.6%. Increased risk of oral clefts (0.4%).	Based on limited data, thought to be safe; however, infant exposure can be high and can vary widely (reports of 18%–60% of maternal concentrations); monitor infant. Relatively high infant exposure (22.7%); avoid or exercise caution.	• Safest of the anticonvulsants in pregnancy, though good safety data are sparse. Serum levels should be monitored; levels usually decrease over course of pregnancy.
Lithium (Eskalith, Lithobid)	Rate of major malformations 4%–12%. Risk of Ebstein's anomaly (cardiac problem) is lower than previously thought (0.05%–0.1%). Increased maternal risk of diabetes, polyhydramnios, thyroid dysfunction during pregnancy.	30%–50% excretion; not recommended due to high risk of toxicity	• Try to avoid, particularly in first trimester • If first trimester use required, fetal echocardiogram recommended • Check serum levels and thyroid function frequently during pregnancy, since changes in metabolism and total body water require dose adjustments, particularly in third trimester • Avoid in breastfeeding if possible
Oxcarbazepine (Trileptal)	Danish study showed no increased risk of major malformation. However, data are limited.	Possible adverse effects in breastfed infants; monitor infant for drowsiness, adequate weight gain, and developmental milestones	• Relatively safe, though more data are needed

Medication	Pregnancy	Breastfeeding	Recommendations
Valproate (Depakote)	Most teratogenic of all mood stabilizers, with a 6.2%–20.3% rate of congenital malformations, with neural tube defects most prominent. Teratogenic effects are dose-related with greatest risk at doses >1000 mg per day. Recently, exposure linked to autism.	Relatively low excretion (0.68%); considered compatible with breastfeeding	• Avoid in pregnancy unless absolutely required • If use unavoidable, add high-dose (4 mg) folic acid supplementation • Safe in breastfeeding
Antipsychotics			
First-generation	No increased risk of malformations seen with high-potency agents. Small increased risk with low-potency agents such as chlorpromazine (Thorazine). Transient extrapyramidal side effects; sedation; withdrawal symptoms in neonates.	Relatively low excretion reported although little data available. Sedation and Parkinsonism effects possible in breastfed infants.	• Haloperidol (Haldol), fluphenazine (Prolixin) favored during pregnancy because of long history of safe use • Relatively safe in breastfeeding
Second-generation	Fewer data available, most showing no increased risk of malformations. Maternal hyperglycemia, impaired glucose tolerance, and weight gain may lead to maternal complications. Large-for-gestational-age infants reported. Floppy infant syndrome reported in clozapine exposure; monitor neutrophils in neonate for six months.	Excretion low, usually <3%, with exception of clozapine (Clozaril), which is seen in relatively high concentrations in breast milk	• Overall, relatively safe in pregnancy; not treating serious mental illness in pregnancy poses greater risk. Most data with risperidone, olanzapine, quetiapine. • Avoid clozapine in breastfeeding if possible.
Antidepressants			
Bupropion (Wellbutrin)	No increased risk of malformation	<1% excretion with no adverse outcomes reported	• Safe for use in pregnancy and breastfeeding
Duloxetine (Cymbalta)	Little data	No published data, though exposure is low	• Not enough data to recommend
Levomilnacipran (Fetzima)	No data	No published data	• Not enough data to recommend
Mirtazapine (Remeron)	Sparse data, but one small study suggests no increased rate of major malformation	Low excretion; compatible with breastfeeding	• Likely safe in pregnancy and breastfeeding
SSRIs	Controversial data regarding cardiovascular malformation with first trimester paroxetine (Paxil) exposure. Larger and more recent studies show no overall increased risk for malformations with SSRIs. Conflicting reports, with some showing decreased gestational age, low birth weight, poor neonatal adaptation, low Apgar scores (some of which could be due to underlying depression or anxiety). Conflicting reports regarding SSRI use in later pregnancy and persistent pulmonary hypertension (PPHN). Neonatal toxicity reported as transient jitteriness, tremulousness, and tachypnea. No problems detected in behavioral or cognitive development—greatest data with fluoxetine (Prozac).	Relatively low excretion, varies by agent: Citalopram (Celexa): 5%–10% Fluoxetine: 3%–9% Fluvoxamine (Luvox): <2% Paroxetine: <4% Sertraline (Zoloft): <2%	• SSRIs are relatively safe in pregnancy; avoid paroxetine if possible • Sertraline is safest in breastfeeding • Avoid fluoxetine in breastfeeding due to long half-life and active metabolite

Medication	Pregnancy	Breastfeeding	Recommendations
Tricyclics	Relatively large database; recent meta-analysis of 300,000 live births revealed no increased risk of malformations. Neonatal anticholinergic effects. Transient neonatal withdrawal symptoms reported.	<1%–5% excretion; appear relatively safe during breastfeeding, with possible exception of doxepin	• Safe in pregnancy; desipramine and nortriptyline preferred due to lower anticholinergic and orthostatic hypotension risks • Relatively safe in breastfeeding; monitor infant for sedation
Venlafaxine (Effexor)/ desvenlafaxine (Pristiq)	Earlier data regarding major malformations reassuring, but one more recent study suggested a possible association with birth defects; additional studies needed. Increased maternal blood pressure may be a concern during pregnancy, particularly at higher doses.	2%–9.2% excretion; no adverse outcomes reported	• Less recommended than other antidepressants
Vilazodone (Viibryd)	No data	No published data	• Not enough data to recommend
Vortioxetine (Trintellix)	No data	No published data	• Not enough data to recommend
Stimulants			
Amphetamines and methylphenidates	No apparent congenital malformations; may constrict blood flow to placenta, which reduces oxygen flow to developing fetus. May cause premature delivery, small for gestational age and low-birth-weight babies; however, data inconclusive. Neonatal withdrawal possible.	0.2% excreted into breast milk; adverse effects usually not observed	• Not recommended in pregnancy due to possibility of vasoconstriction and ability to disrupt blood flow to the fetus • Likely safe in breastfeeding

APPENDIX C: CLASSIFICATIONS OF CONTROLLED SUBSTANCES

In 1970, under the Controlled Substances Act, the FDA created classification schedules that organize drugs into groups based on their risk of abuse or harm. There are five classifications of controlled substances (Schedule I, II, III, IV, and V), and drugs with the highest risk-to-benefit ratio are considered Schedule I drugs. Most drugs used in psychiatry are not scheduled at all (antidepressants, antipsychotics, etc). Some of us get confused about whether the most restricted drugs are Schedule I or V. Here's a mnemonic: The number 1 looks like a needle, and a needle is used to inject heroin—which is the prototypical Schedule I drug. The DEA's more comprehensive and regularly updated listing can be found here: http://goo.gl/Mo6KEQ

Prescription drug monitoring programs (PDMPs) are searchable databases that can help prescribers identify potential abuse or diversion of controlled substances in individual patients. If you prescribe controlled substances like benzodiazepines and stimulants, it's a good idea to learn about your state's PDMP laws, consider your search results in the context of all available information, and watch for regulatory changes over the next few years. To find your state's program, check with the PDMP Training and Technical Assistance Center (www.pdmpassist.org/content/state-pdmp-websites).

Appendix Table C: **Classifications of Controlled Substances**

Schedule	Description	Prescribing Implications	Some Examples
I	No accepted medical use, high potential for abuse, illegal to possess or use	Can't be prescribed at all (with the exception of medical marijuana in some states)	• Heroin, LSD, ecstasy, and others • Marijuana (though legalized in some states, it is still illegal at the federal level)
II	High potential for abuse, but legal for medical use	Can be prescribed only 1 month at a time, cannot be refilled, cannot be called in, and patient must give pharmacy a paper script (unless you use an e-prescribing program that is certified by DEA to allow prescribing of controlled substances)	• All psychostimulants, such as amphetamine and methylphenidate • Opiates that are especially potent, such as oxycodone, fentanyl, and others • Vicodin (hydrocodone and acetaminophen) was recently reclassified from Schedule III to Schedule II
III	Lower potential for abuse than Schedule I or II, but still pretty abusable	Can be refilled up to 5 times (no more than 6 months), can be called in	• Anabolic steroids • Barbiturates • Dronabinol (Marinol) • Esketamine (Spravato) • Ketamine • Suboxone (buprenorphine/naloxone) • Xyrem (sodium oxybate) • Xywav (mixed-salts oxybate)
IV	Lower potential for abuse than Schedule III	Can be refilled up to 5 times (no more than 6 months), can be called in	• All benzodiazepines (eg, clonazepam, lorazepam, etc) • Carisoprodol (Soma) • Lorcaserin (Belviq), an anti-obesity drug • Tramadol (Ultram) • Various hypnotics, like lemborexant (Dayvigo), suvorexant (Belsomra), zaleplon, zolpidem • Wake-promoting agents, like modafinil and armodafinil and solriamfetol (Sunosi)
V	Lowest potential for abuse	Can be refilled as many times as prescriber chooses (eg, for 1 year or more), can be called in	• Antidiarrheal Lomotil (diphenoxylate/atropine) • Cough preparations with small amounts of codeine, such as Robitussin AC • Pregabalin (Lyrica)

An updated and more complete list of the schedules is published annually in Title 21 *Code of Federal Regulations* and can be found here: www.deadiversion.usdoj.gov/schedules/orangebook/c_cs_alpha.pdf

APPENDIX D: LAB MONITORING FOR PSYCHIATRIC MEDICATIONS

This is a short and sweet table listing the medications that most psychiatrists would agree require lab monitoring. Our recommendations are quite abbreviated, and we haven't spelled out whether you should order labs before or after starting the medications, nor how you should do follow-up monitoring. There's just too much variation in practice for us to give authoritative detailed guidelines. These medications are mainly here to jog your memory so you don't forget to at least consider what type of monitoring to do.

Appendix Table D: **Recommended Laboratory Tests for Psychiatric Medications**

Medications	Recommended Laboratory Tests
Acamprosate	BUN/creatinine if renal impairment is suspected
Amantadine	BUN/creatinine if renal impairment is suspected
Antipsychotics—second-generation, primarily clozapine, olanzapine, quetiapine, paliperidone, risperidone[1, 2]	Fasting glucose and lipids
Atomoxetine	LFTs
Carbamazepine	Complete blood count (CBC), sodium, LFTs, pregnancy test, HLA-B*1502 in Asians[3] Carbamazepine level (at least 3 days on stable dose, trough level, 12 hours after last dose); target: 4–12 mcg/mL
Chlorpromazine	ECG if cardiac disease
Citalopram	ECG if cardiac disease, dose ≥40 mg/day
Clomipramine	Clomipramine/norclomipramine levels (at least 5 days on stable dose, trough level, 12 hours after last dose); target: 220–500 ng/mL
Clozapine	Fasting glucose and lipids, CBC Clozapine/norclozapine level (at least 3 days on stable dose, trough level, 12 hours after last dose); target: >350 ng/mL; toxicity >700 ng/mL
Desvenlafaxine	Periodic BP
Deutetrabenazine	ECG if cardiac disease
Disulfiram	LFTs if liver disease is suspected
Duloxetine	LFTs if liver disease is suspected[4]
Gabapentin	BUN/creatinine if renal impairment is suspected
Levomilnacipran	Periodic BP/pulse rate
Lithium	TSH, BUN/creatinine[5], pregnancy test, ECG if cardiac disease Lithium level (at least 5 days on stable dose, trough level, 12 hours after last dose); target: 0.8–1.2 mEq/L (acute mania) and 0.6–1.0 mEq/L (maintenance)
Methadone	ECG if cardiac disease
Mirtazapine	Lipids
Naltrexone	LFTs if liver disease is suspected
Nortriptyline	Nortriptyline level (at least 5 days on stable dose, trough level, 12 hours after last dose); target: 50–150 ng/mL
Oxcarbazepine	Sodium, HLA-B*1502 in Asians[3]
Paliperidone	Prolactin if symptoms, fasting glucose and lipids
Pregabalin	BUN/creatinine if renal impairment is suspected
Risperidone	Prolactin if symptoms, fasting glucose and lipids
SSRIs	Sodium in elderly if fatigue, dizziness, confusion
Stimulants	ECG if cardiac disease
Thioridazine	ECG if cardiac disease
Topiramate	Bicarbonate
Tricyclic antidepressants	ECG if cardiac disease
Valbenazine	ECG if cardiac disease
Valproic acid	LFTs, CBC for platelets, pregnancy test, ammonia if confusion Valproic acid level (at least 3 days on stable dose, trough level, 12 hours after last dose with IR or 21–24 hours with ER); target: 50–125 mcg/mL
Venlafaxine	Periodic BP
Ziprasidone	ECG if cardiac disease

[1] Some guidelines recommend monitoring glucose and lipids with all second-generation antipsychotics.

[2] Utility of routine therapeutic monitoring is unclear for antipsychotic medications other than clozapine; reference ranges are available for many agents, and blood levels may help in establishing whether a patient is taking the medication.

[3] HLA-B*1502 is a gene that increases the risk of developing toxic epidermal necrolysis (TEN) and Stevens-Johnson syndrome (SJS) in response to taking carbamazepine. Asians, especially Han Chinese, are much more likely to have the gene than other populations.

[4] Duloxetine should not be prescribed in patients with significant alcohol use or evidence of chronic liver disease as it can lead to hepatic failure in rare cases (Cymbalta prescribing information). While the manufacturer does not recommend baseline LFTs for all patients, some clinicians do so anyway to be extra cautious.

[5] The serum creatinine is used to compute the estimated glomerular filtration rate (eGFR), a more precise measure of kidney functioning. Increasingly, laboratory test results include the eGFR. You can calculate it yourself using an online calculator at www.niddk.nih.gov/health-information/communication-programs/nkdep/laboratory-evaluation/glomerular-filtration-rate-calculators. See also Appendix H for dosing in renal disease.

APPENDIX E: URINE TOXICOLOGY SCREENING

Drug screening is a routine part of psychiatric practice. It can help assessment and diagnosis, monitoring of therapeutic goals in patients with substance use disorders, and identifying diversion of controlled substances. Specimens of urine, blood, hair, saliva, sweat, and even nails can be used to do lab drug testing, and some tests are more specific, sensitive, and accurate than others. Urine drug screening is most commonly used because it's noninvasive, available in large volume, and generally has high concentrations of drug and metabolites, which allows for longer detection than in blood.

Remember that a drug screen, while quick and inexpensive, should be considered preliminary as it may be subject to false results or unable to detect all substances. A more accurate, sensitive, and reliable test, such as gas chromatography-mass spectrometry or high-performance liquid chromatography, may be ordered for confirmation.

Appendices

Appendix Table E: Urine Drug Testing

Drug	Detection Period	Agents Potentially Causing Positive Result
Alcohol	7–12 hours (80 hours for alcohol metabolites EtG and EtS)	Short-chain alcohols (eg, isopropyl alcohol)
Amphetamine/methamphetamine	1–2 days	ADHD medications (atomoxetine, stimulants) Amantadine (Symmetrel) Antipsychotics (aripiprazole, chlorpromazine, thioridazine) Bupropion (Wellbutrin) Ephedrine (Primatene, Bronkaid) Isometheptene (Midrin) MDMA (ecstasy) Phentermine (Adipex-P, Qsymia) Phenylephrine (Sudafed PE) Promethazine (Phenergan) Pseudoephedrine (Sudafed) Ranitidine (Zantac) Selegiline (Eldepryl, Emsam) TCAs (desipramine, trimipramine) Trazodone (Desyrel) Trimethobenzamide (Tigan)
Barbiturates	2–4 days (2–3 weeks for long-acting phenobarbital)	Ibuprofen (Advil, Motrin) Naproxen (Naprosyn)
Benzodiazepines (alprazolam, clonazepam, lorazepam, triazolam may not be detected on some assays)	24 hours (short-acting); 2–4 days (long-acting); >7 days for chlordiazepoxide, diazepam	Oxaprozin (Daypro) Sertraline (Zoloft)
Cocaine	6–8 hours (2–4 days for benzoylecgonine metabolite)	Coca leaf tea Topical anesthetics containing cocaine
LSD	2–4 days	Trazodone (Desyrel)
Marijuana	3 days for single use; 5–7 days for moderate use (4x/week); 10–15 days for daily use; >30 days for long-term heavy use	Dronabinol (Marinol) Efavirenz (Sustiva) Hemp-containing foods NSAIDs Proton pump inhibitors
MDMA	1–2 days	
Nicotine	12 hours	
Opioids: Buprenorphine Codeine Heroin, hydromorphone, morphine, oxycodone Methadone	2–3 days (5–7 days for metabolites) 1–2 days 2–4 days 2–3 days; 7–9 days for chronic use	Dextromethorphan (Robitussin DM) Diphenhydramine (Benadryl) Doxylamine (Unisom) Poppy seeds Quinolones Rifampin (Rifadin) Verapamil (Calan)
PCP	2–8 days; up to 30 days for chronic use	Dextromethorphan (Robitussin DM) Diphenhydramine (Benadryl) Doxylamine (Unisom) Ibuprofen (Motrin) Imipramine (Tofranil) Ketamine (Ketalar, Spravato) Lamotrigine (Lamictal) MDPV (bath salts) Meperidine (Demerol) Tramadol (Ultram) Venlafaxine (Effexor), desvenlafaxine (Pristiq)

Adapted from: Moeller KE et al, *Mayo Clin Proc* 2008;83(1):66–76; Moeller KE et al, *Mayo Clin Proc* 2017;92:774–796; Verebey KG, Meenan G. Diagnostic laboratory: Screening for drug abuse. In: Ruiz P, Strain E, eds. *Lowinson and Ruiz's Substance Abuse: A Comprehensive Textbook.* 5th ed. Philadelphia: Wolters Kluwer, Lippincott Williams & Wilkins, 2011:123–137; Warner EA, Sharma N. Laboratory diagnosis. In: Ries RK, Miller SC, Fiellen DA, Saitz R, eds. *Principles of Addiction Medicine.* 4th ed. Philadelphia: Lippincott Williams & Wilkins; 2009:295–304

APPENDIX F: PHARMACOGENETIC TESTING

The Basics

Variations in patients' genetic profiles can affect how they respond to medications. While the actual clinical importance of this phenomenon is not yet clear, it's likely that genetic variations in pharmacokinetic genes have some effect on serum levels of medications in many patients. Based on these CYP450 polymorphisms, individuals are categorized in different ways with respect to specific enzymes:

- *Extensive metabolizers.* Otherwise known as "normal" metabolizers, these people have normally active CYP450 genes on both chromosomes, meaning that they see an average level of drug in the body.

- *Intermediate metabolizers.* These people metabolize drugs a bit more slowly than extensive metabolizers, but not dramatically so.

- *Poor metabolizers.* These people carry inactive or partially active CYP450 genes, and therefore metabolize drugs significantly more slowly than extensive metabolizers. This may result in more side effects since serum drug levels are higher.

- *Ultrarapid metabolizers.* With extra copies of certain genes, these people metabolize drugs more quickly than extensive metabolizers, sometimes requiring unusually high doses of medications to achieve a therapeutic level.

There are also genetic variations in pharmacodynamic genes that might increase or decrease the efficacy of drugs, but the evidence for this effect is less robust than for pharmacokinetic effects.

Pharmacogenetic Testing in Clinical Practice

The science of pharmacogenetic testing is complex, which makes it hard for us mere mortals to evaluate the claims of the many commercial test kits flooding the market.

In March 2017, *TCPR* explored this topic and focused on three tests: Genesight, Genecept, and CNSDose. We concluded that the evidence was not yet robust enough to recommend any of these tests. However, we did review information from FDA drug labels and created a table listing FDA recommendations for pharmacogenetic testing relevant to specific psychotropic drugs.

Many of the recommendations are to lower starting doses in patients who are poor metabolizers. For example, in aripiprazole's label, you'll read: "Dosing recommendation in patients who are classified as CYP450 2D6 poor metabolizers (PM): The aripiprazole dose in PM patients should initially be reduced to one-half (50%) of the usual dose and then adjusted to achieve a favorable clinical response."

While the FDA does not specifically ask you to order genetic testing, you will not know whether your patient is a poor metabolizer unless someone has ordered it. Therefore, a case could be made for selectively ordering CYP450 testing to ensure you dose drugs in accordance with FDA labeling. Whether you do this is a judgment call; most of us are content to skip the genetic testing, and instead choose to start most medications at a low dose and titrate up gradually in order to prevent side effects.

Appendix Table F: FDA Label Information Relevant to Pharmacogenetic Testing for Psychiatric Drugs

Medication	FDA Recommendations	Clinical Rationale
Amphetamines Aripiprazole Atomoxetine Brexpiprazole Deutetrabenazine Iloperidone Lofexidine Perphenazine Pimozide Pitolisant Tetrabenazine Thioridazine Valbenazine Venlafaxine Vortioxetine	Reduce dose in CYP2D6 PMs[1]	Usual starting dose is too high in PMs, so start lower and increase gradually
Amitriptyline Clomipramine Clozapine Desipramine Doxepin Imipramine Nortriptyline Protriptyline Trimipramine	Monitor levels in CYP2D6 PMs	These medications, most of which are tricyclic antidepressants, can cause life-threatening side effects if levels are too high; consider monitoring serum levels in PMs
Carbamazepine Oxcarbazepine	Avoid or use cautiously in individuals with the HLA-B*1502 allele (applicable to Asians)	Risk of serious rashes such as Stevens-Johnson syndrome
Citalopram	Maximum recommended daily dose of 20 mg (rather than 40 mg) for CYP2C19 PMs	Risk of QT prolongation and cardiac arrhythmia
Flibanserin	Monitor for adverse reactions in CYP2C9 PMs	Risk of hypotension and dizziness
Pimozide	In CYP2D6 PMs, dose should not exceed 4 mg/day in adults	Risk of QT prolongation and cardiac arrhythmia
Thioridazine	Contraindicated in CYP2D6 PMs, due to risk of QT prolongation	Risk of QT prolongation and cardiac arrhythmia

[1] PM = poor metabolizer

Source: www.fda.gov/medical-devices/precision-medicine/table-pharmacogenetic-associations

Medications with a high anticholinergic "load" can negatively affect memory and cognition, particularly in the elderly. This is often a dose-related effect, with a potential for high doses to cause confusion and delirium. Use alternatives to these medications when possible, especially in older patients or those with dementia.

Appendix Table G: Some Commonly Used Highly Anticholinergic Medications

Therapeutic Class	Medication
Antidepressants	Amitriptyline (Elavil) Amoxapine (Asendin) Clomipramine (Anafranil) Desipramine (Norpramin) Doxepin >6 mg (Sinequan) Imipramine (Tofranil) Nortriptyline (Pamelor) Paroxetine (Paxil) Protriptyline (Vivactil) Trimipramine (Surmontil)
Antiemetics	Prochlorperazine (Compazine) Promethazine (Phenergan)
Antihistamines (first generation)	Brompheniramine (Dimetapp) Chlorpheniramine (Chlor-Trimeton) Cyproheptadine (Periactin) Dicyclomine (Bentyl) Dimenhydrinate (Dramamine) Diphenhydramine (Benadryl) Doxylamine (Unisom) Hydroxyzine (Vistaril, Atarax) Meclizine (Antivert)
Antimuscarinics (urinary incontinence)	Fesoterodine (Toviaz) Oxybutynin (Ditropan) Tolterodine (Detrol)
Antiparkinsonian agents	Benztropine (Cogentin) Trihexyphenidyl (Artane)
Antipsychotics	Chlorpromazine (Thorazine) Clozapine (Clozaril) Loxapine (Loxitane) Olanzapine (Zyprexa) Perphenazine (Trilafon) Thioridazine (Mellaril) Trifluoperazine (Stelazine)
Skeletal muscle relaxants	Cyclobenzaprine (Flexeril) Methocarbamol (Robaxin) Orphenadrine (Norflex)

Appendices

APPENDIX H: DOSING OF PSYCHOTROPIC MEDICATIONS IN PATIENTS WITH HEPATIC OR RENAL IMPAIRMENT

Hepatic and renal disease (whether hepatitis, alcohol related, or cirrhosis) can significantly affect the pharmacokinetics of medications by altering metabolism, protein binding, and elimination. When prescribing psychiatric medications for these patients, sound clinical judgment would dictate to use lower doses and titrate more slowly. Some medications require extra consideration, and we've included those here. For patients with severe hepatic or renal impairment, consider consultation with specialists.

Medication	Hepatic Impairment	Renal Impairment
ADHD Medications		
Atomoxetine	Mod: Decrease dose by 50% Sev: Decrease dose by 75%	No change
Lisdexamfetamine	Consider dose reduction	CrCl 15–30 mL/min: Max 50 mg/day CrCl <15 mL/min: Max 30 mg/day
Viloxazine	Avoid use	Sev: Reduce dose by 50%
Antidepressants		
Bupropion	Mod-sev: Max 75 mg/day or 150 SR/XL mg QOD	Consider dose reduction
Citalopram	Sev: Max 20 mg/day	Sev: Use with caution
Desvenlafaxine	Mod: Max 100 mg/day Sev: Max 50 mg/day	Mod: Max 50 mg/day Sev: Max 50 mg QOD
Duloxetine	Avoid use	Mild-mod: Consider dose reduction Sev: Avoid use
Escitalopram	Sev: Max 10 mg/day	Sev: Use with caution
Esketamine	Mod: Use caution Sev: Avoid use	Use caution
Isocarboxazid	Avoid use	Mild-mod: Use with caution Sev: Avoid use
Ketamine	Use caution	Use caution
Levomilnacipran	No change	Mod: Max 80 mg/day Sev: Max 40 mg/day ESRD: Avoid use
Mirtazapine	Consider dose reduction	Use with caution Mod-sev: Consider dose reduction
Nefazodone	Avoid use	No change
Paroxetine	Sev: Max 40 mg/day	Sev: Max 40 mg/day
Phenelzine	Avoid use	Mild-mod: Use with caution Sev: Avoid use
Venlafaxine	Mild-mod: Reduce dose by 50% Sev: Use with caution	Mild-mod: Reduce dose by 25% Sev: Reduce dose by 50% or more
Antipsychotics		
Brexpiprazole	Mod-sev: Max 3 mg/day	Mod-sev: Max 3 mg/day
Lumateperone	Mod-sev: Avoid use	Use with caution
Lurasidone	Mod: Max 80 mg/day Sev: Max 40 mg/day	Mod-sev: Max 80 mg/day
Paliperidone	Sev: Use with caution	CrCl 50–70 mL/min: Max 6 mg/day CrCl 10–49 mL/min: Max 3 mg/day ESRD: Avoid use LAI: Adjust dose in CrCl 50–79 mL/min; avoid use CrCl <50 mL/min
Risperidone	Mild-mod: Consider dose reduction Sev: Max 4 mg/day	Mild-mod (CrCl ≥30 mL/min): Consider dose reduction Sev (CrCl <30 mL/min): Max 4 mg/day
Ziprasidone	No change	PO: No change Use IM with caution (cyclodextrin excipient renally eliminated)
Anxiolytics		
Buspirone	Sev: Avoid use	Mild-mod: Consider dose reduction Sev: Avoid use
Clonazepam	Sev: Avoid use	Use with caution
Diazepam	Mild-mod: Use with caution Sev: Avoid use	Use with caution

CrCl = creatinine clearance; Mild (Child-Pugh Class A or CrCl 51–80 mL/min); Mod = moderate (Child-Pugh Class B or CrCl 31–50 mL/min); Sev = severe (Child-Pugh Class C or CrCl ≤30 mL/min); ESRD = end-stage renal disease (CrCl <10 mL/min): LAI = long-acting injectable

Appendices

Medication	Hepatic Impairment	Renal Impairment
Lorazepam	Sev: Consider dose reduction, avoid IM/IV	Use with caution Sev: Avoid IM/IV
Dementia Medications		
Aducanumab	Use with caution	Use with caution
Galantamine	Mod: Max 16 mg/day Sev: Avoid use	CrCl 9–59 mL/min: Max 16 mg/day CrCl <9 mL/min: Avoid use
Memantine	Sev: Use caution	CrCl 5–29 mL/min: Max 10 mg/day CrCl <5 mL/min: Avoid use
Rivastigmine	Mild-mod: Max 4.6 mg/day patch Sev: Use caution	No change
Hypnotics		
Eszopiclone	Sev: Max 2 mg/day	No change
Flurazepam	Mild-mod: Use with caution Sev: Avoid use	Use with caution
Lemborexant	Mod: Max 5 mg/day Sev: Avoid use	No change
Zaleplon	Mild-mod: Max 5 mg/day Sev: Avoid use	Sev: Use with caution
Zolpidem	Mild-mod: Max 5 mg/day Sev: Avoid use	Sev: Use with caution
Mood Stabilizers and Anticonvulsants		
Gabapentin	No change	CrCl 30–59 mL/min: Max 1400 mg/day divided BID CrCl 16–29 mL/min: Max 700 mg/day CrCl ≤15 mL/min: 100–300 mg/day
Lamotrigine	Mod-sev: Reduce dose by 25% Sev with ascites: Reduce dose by 50%	Use with caution Mod-sev: Reduce dose by 25% ESRD: Max 100 mg QOD
Lithium	No change	Mild-mod: Consider dose reduction Sev: Avoid use
Oxcarbazepine	Sev: Use with caution	Sev: Reduce dose by 25%–50%
Pregabalin	No change	CrCl 30–59 mL/min: Max 300 mg/day divided BID–TID CrCl 16–29 mL/min: Max 150 mg/day given QD–BID CrCl ≤15 mL/min: 25–75 mg/day QD
Topiramate	Use with caution	Mod-sev: Reduce dose by 50%
Valproic acid	Mild-mod: Use with caution Sev: Avoid use	Consider dose reduction (reduced protein binding may result in higher active free fraction not reflected in total serum level)
Side Effect Medications		
Amantadine	Use with caution	CrCl 30–50 mL/min: Max 100 mg/day CrCl 15–29 mL/min: Max 100 mg QOD CrCl <15 mL/min: 200 mg Qweek
Metformin	Avoid use	Mild-mod: Use with caution Sev: Avoid use
Valbenazine	Mod-sev: Max 40 mg/day	No change
Sleep Disorder Medications		
Armodafinil	Sev: Reduce dose by 50%	Use with caution
Carbidopa/levodopa	Use with caution	CrCl <50 mL/min: Reduce dose by up to 50%
Modafinil	Sev: Reduce dose by 50%	Use with caution
Oxybates	Reduce dose by 50%	Use with caution
Pitolisant	Mod: Max 17.8 mg/day Sev: Avoid use	Mild: Use with caution Mod: Max 17.8 mg/day Sev: Avoid use
Pramipexole	No change	CrCl 20–60 mL/min: Max 0.5 mg/day CrCl <20 mL/min: Avoid use

CrCl = creatinine clearance; Mild (Child-Pugh Class A or CrCl 51–80 mL/min); Mod = moderate (Child-Pugh Class B or CrCl 31–50 mL/min); Sev = severe (Child-Pugh Class C or CrCl ≤30 mL/min); ESRD = end-stage renal disease (CrCl <10 mL/min): LAI = long-acting injectable

Medication	Hepatic Impairment	Renal Impairment
Solriamfetol	Use with caution	Mild-mod: Max 75 mg/day Sev: Max 37.5 mg/day
Substance Use Disorder Medications		
Acamprosate	Sev: Use with caution	CrCl 30–50 mL/min: 333 mg TID CrCl <30 mL/min: Avoid use
Buprenorphine	Mod-sev: Use with caution	No change
Bupropion SR	Mod-sev: Max 150 SR mg QOD	Consider dose reduction
Disulfiram	Use with caution	Use with caution
Lofexidine	Mild: Max 3 tabs Q5–6H Mod: Max 2 tabs Q5–6H Sev: Max 1 tab Q5–6H	CrCl 30–89 mL/min: Max 2 tabs Q5–6H CrCl <30 mL/min: Max 1 tab Q5–6H
Methadone	Consider reduced dose	ESRD: Reduce dose by 25%–50%
Naltrexone	Sev: Use with caution	Sev: Use with caution
Varenicline	No change	CrCl <30 mL/min: Max 0.5 mg BID

CrCl = creatinine clearance; Mild (Child-Pugh Class A or CrCl 51–80 mL/min); Mod = moderate (Child-Pugh Class B or CrCl 31–50 mL/min); Sev = severe (Child-Pugh Class C or CrCl ≤30 mL/min); ESRD = end-stage renal disease (CrCl <10 mL/min): LAI = long-acting injectable

Appendices

Index

Note: Trade names are capitalized, bolded page numbers are for fact sheets, italic page numbers are for treatment algorithms, and non-bolded page numbers are for quick-scan tables and other miscellaneous entries.

propranolol, 111, **124,** 245
ProSom, 111
Provigil, 17, 206, **209**
Prozac, 38, 40, 41, **51**
Prozac Weekly, 38, 40, **51**

Q

Qelbree, 17, **31**
QT interval prolongation, **196,** 248
quazepam, 111
Qudexy XR, 144, **151**
quetiapine, 73, 74, **94,** 247, 258
Quillichew ER, 15, 18, **28**
Quillivant XR, 15, 18, **28**
quinidine, 248

R

ramelteon, 111, **125,** 244
Razadyne, 134, **137**
Razadyne ER, 134, **137**
Remeron, 39, 42, **55,** 254
Remeron SolTab, 39, **55**
renal impairment, 264–267
Requip, 206, **208**
Requip XL, 206, **208**
Restoril, 110, 111, **127**
ReVia, 226, **236**
Rexulti, 72, **77**
Riomet, **178**
Risperdal, 73, **95**
Risperdal Consta, **95,** 104
Risperdal M-Tab, 73, **95**
risperidone, 73, 74, **95,** 104, 246, 258, 265
Ritalin, 14, **27**
Ritalin LA, 15, **28**
Ritalin SR, 14, **28**
rivastigmine, 134, **140,** 266
ropinirole, 206, **208,** 244
rotigotine transdermal patch, 206, **208**
Rozerem, 111, **125**

S

S-adenosyl-L-methionine (SAMe), 153, **160**
Saphris, 72, **76**
Secuado, 72, **76**
selective serotonin reuptake inhibitors (SSRIs), 38, 40, 41, 248, 254, 258
selegiline transdermal, 39, 42, **59,** 244
Serax, 111

serdexmethylphenidate/ dexmethylphenidate, 14, **22**
Seroquel, 73, **94**
Seroquel XR, 73, **94**
serotonin norepinephrine reuptake inhibitors (SNRIs), 38, 41, 248
serotonin syndrome, **197,** 248
sertraline, 38, 40, 41, **60,** 244
Serzone, 39, 42, **57**
sexual dysfunction, **198**
sexual dysfunction medications, 163–164
sialorrhea (hypersalivation), **199**
side effect management, 173, 266
sildenafil, 164, **169,** 247
Silenor, 110, **117**
Silexan, 153, **154**
Sinemet, 206, **208**
Sinemet CR, **208**
skeletal muscle relaxants, 263
sleep disorder medications, 205–206, 266–267
smoking cessation, **227**
sodium oxybate, 206, **210**
solriamfetol, 206, **212,** 267
somatic treatments, 215
Sonata, 110, **129,** 253
Spravato, 39, **50**
Staxyn, 164, **172**
Stelazine, 71, **98**
Stendra, 164, **165**
stimulants, 255, 258
St. John's wort, 153, **161,** 244, 246, 247, 248
Strattera, 17, **20**
Striant, 164, **171**
Sublocade, 225, **229**
Suboxone, 225, **230**
substance use disorder medications, 221–222, *223–224,* 225–226, 267
substrates, 244–247
Subvenite, 144, **147**
Sunosi, 206, **212**
suvorexant, 110, **126,** 247, 253
Symbyax, **90**
Symmetrel, **175**
Synthroid, **61**

T

tadalafil, 164, **170,** 247
tardive dyskinesia, **200**
tasimelteon, 206, **213**
Tegretol, 144, **145,** 253
Tegretol XR, 144, **145**
temazepam, 110, 111, **127**
Tenex, 17, **24**

Teril, 144, **145**
testosterone, 164, **171**
tetrabenazine, **179**
thiazides, 248
thioridazine, 71, 74, **96,** 245, 246, 248, 258
thiothixene, 71, 74, **97,** 244
Thorazine, 71, **79**
thyroid augmentation, **61**
Tofranil, 39, 41
Topamax, 144, **151**
topiramate, 144, **151,** 258, 266
tramadol, 248
transcranial magnetic stimulation (TMS), **218**
Tranxene, 111
tranylcypromine, 39, 42, **56**
trazodone, 39, 42, **62,** 111, 246, 247, 248, 253
tremor, **202**
triazolam, 110, 111, **128,** 247
tricyclic antidepressants, 38–39, 41, **63,** 246, 247, 248, 255, 258
trifluoperazine, 71, 74, **98,** 244
trihexyphenidyl, **180,** 248
Trilafon, 71, **92**
Trileptal, 144, **149,** 253
Trintellix, 39, 42, **66,** 255
Trokendl XR, 144, **151**

U

Unisom, 110
urine toxicology screening, 259–260

V

vagus nerve stimulation (VNS), **219**
valbenazine, **181,** 246, 247, 258, 266
Valium, 110, 111, **116**
valproate, 254
valproic acid, 144, **152,** 248, 258, 266
vardenafil, 164, **172,** 247
vardenafil ODT, 164, **172**
varenicline, 226, **241,** 267
venlafaxine, 38, 41, **64,** 245, 246, 255, 258, 265
venlafaxine ER, 38, **64**
Versacloz, 72, **80**
Viagra, 164, **169**
Viibryd, 39, 42, **65,** 255
vilazodone, 39, 42, **65,** 247, 255
viloxazine, 265
viloxazine XR, 17, **31**
Vistaril, 110, **120**
vitamin D, 153, **162**
Vivitrol, 226, **236**
vortioxetine, 39, 42, **66,** 246, 255

Vraylar, 72, **78**
Vyleesi, 164, **166**
Vyvanse, 16, 18, **25**

W
Wakix, 206, **211**
warfarin, 248
weight gain, **203**
Wellbutrin, 17, 39, **44,** 254
Wellbutrin SR, 39, 42, **44**
Wellbutrin XL, 39, 42, **44**

X
Xanax, 110, 111, **112**
Xanax XR, 110, **112**
Xenazine, **179**
xerostomia (dry mouth), **187**
Xyrem, 206, **210**
Xywav, 206, **210**

Z
zaleplon, 110, **129,** 247, 253, 266
Zenzedi, 16, **23**
Z-hypnotics, 110–111

Zimhi, 225, **235**
ziprasidone, 73, 74, **99,** 247, 248, 258, 265
Zoloft, 38, 40, 41, **60**
zolpidem, 111, **130,** 247, 253, 266
zolpidem low dose, 111
Zolpimist, 111, **130**
Zubsolv, 225, **230**
Zulresso, 39, **43**
Zyban, 225, **231**
Zyprexa, 72, **90**
Zyprexa Relprevv, **90,** 104
Zyprexa Zydis, 72, **90**

CPSIA information can be obtained
at www.ICGtesting.com
Printed in the USA
LVHW070806130622
721006LV00031BA/2229